MW00475731

A Comprehensive Guide to Music Therapy

of related interest

Clinical Applications of Music Therapy in Psychiatry
Edited by Tony Wigram and Jos De Backer
ISBN 978 1 85302 733 8

**Clinical Applications of Music Therapy in Developmental
Disability, Paediatrics and Neurology**
Edited by Tony Wigram and Jos De Backer
ISBN 978 1 85302 734 5

Music Therapy in Health and Education
Edited by Margaret Heal and Tony Wigram
ISBN 978 1 85302 175 6

Analytical Music Therapy
Edited by Johannes Th. Eschen
ISBN 978 1 84310 058 4

Music Therapy – Intimate Notes
Mercédèss Pavlicevic
ISBN 978 1 85302 692 8

Music for Life
Aspects of Creative Music Therapy with Adult Clients
Gary Ansdell
ISBN 978 1 85302 299 9 pb
ISBN 978 1 85302 300 2 CD

A Comprehensive Guide to Music Therapy

Theory, Clinical Practice, Research and Training

*Tony Wigram, Inge Nygaard Pedersen
and Lars Ole Bonde*

Jessica Kingsley Publishers
London and Philadelphia

First published in Danish in 2001 under the title of *Musikterapi: Når Ord Ikke Slår Til – En håndbog I musikterapiens teori og praksis I Danmark* by Klim, Århus.

First published in the United Kingdom in 2002
by Jessica Kingsley Publishers
116 Pentonville Road
London N1 9JB, UK
and
400 Market Street, Suite 400
Philadelphia, PA 19106, USA
www.jkp.com

Copyright © Tony Wigram, Inge Nygaard Pedersen
and Lars Ole Bonde 2002

The right of Tony Wigram, Inge Nygaard Pedersen and Lars Ole Bonde, to be identified
as authors of this work has been asserted by them in accordance with the Copyright,
Designs and Patents Act 1988

All rights reserved. No part of this publication may be reproduced in any material form
(including photocopying or storing it in any medium by electronic means and whether or
not transiently or incidentally to some other use of this publication) without the written
permission of the copyright owner except in accordance with the provisions of the
Copyright, Designs and Patents Act 1988 or under the terms of a licence issued by the
Copyright Licensing Agency Ltd, Saffron House, 6-10 Kirby Street, London EC1N 8TS.
Applications for the copyright owner's written permission to reproduce any part of this
publication should be addressed to the publisher.

Warning: The doing of an unauthorised act in relation to a copyright work may result in
both a civil claim for damages and criminal prosecution.

Library of Congress Cataloging in Publication Data
A CIP catalog record for this book is available from the Library of Congress

British Library Cataloguing in Publication Data
A CIP catalogue record for this book is available from the British Library

ISBN 978 1 84310 083 6

Printed and Bound in Great Britain by
Athenaeum Press, Gateshead, Tyne and Wear

Table of Contents

List of Figures

List of Tables

Foreword

Many books have been written about music therapy, mostly catering for the specialized market of music therapists and music therapy students. Frequently these texts are specific and focus on a defined area of clinical practice or research. There is, therefore, a need for a more general overview and guide to the complex field of music therapy that can give a comprehensive understanding of the many different theories and clinical methods that have developed internationally.

This book was originally published in Danish (*Musikterapi, Når Ord Ikke Slår Til: En håndbog i musikterapiens teori og praksis i Danmark*: Klim, Aarhus), and was directed towards the Nordic countries where there are still only a limited number of books written in Scandinavian languages. The high standards in university-based music therapy education, research and clinical practice in Denmark ensure that the content of this book is very inclusive in order to present a broad perspective of the field. The project – to write a short primer on music therapy that gave information to medical, clinical, academic and social milieus and professionals – was originally planned as a 120-page book, but during the writing it rapidly expanded to a 320-page book with a CD of musical and clinical examples.

The decision to translate the book into English, and modify the text with additional material, was taken in order to present this unique overview of the field of music therapy to an English-speaking audience. The book will still retain some characteristics that identify its origins from a Danish perspective. However, this enhances, rather than limits, the quality and content of the book, using a model of theory, clinical practice and research that is not only international in style, but is also recognized and referenced internationally as a fine model at a high level and standard. The university requirement for a comprehensive academic and clinical training program in music therapy in Denmark at Master's level, full-time over five years, has ensured that the music therapy profession is recognized at the same professional level as medical doctors and psychologists in Denmark. The established international PhD program and Research Training School in Music Therapy at Aalborg University has also attracted students and researchers from all over Europe, the USA and Australia, and nurtures and promotes both qualitative and quantitative research in a wide range of clinical and theoretical areas.

This book is intended as a wide-ranging foundation text for students and professionals, academics and clinicians. It is particularly intended for the lay public and related professionals who may be interested to find out about the theoretical foundations, clinical practice, research and training in music therapy. It is, by nature, a 'primer' for the field, giving an overview of the multifaceted and fascinating world that is music therapy. However, it is not in any way superficial, and while we have attempted to keep the material presented very readable and user friendly, some of the chapters go into considerable detail and depth. In this way, the book will act as a resource, and as a guide, with information that can answer questions and supply knowledge to a wide range of different readers.

Wherever this book does not include sufficient detail, due to limitations of space, it more than compensates in providing information on how to access other resources, websites, databases and a wide range of literature. This is provided in Chapter 7 and the bibliography. In this way, the book can act as a point of reference, *guiding the way* to further sources.

The world is becoming smaller, day by day, thanks to the Internet, e-mail and a significant increase in international travel. In a relatively small field like music therapy this allows for, but also demands, a fast and free-flowing exchange of ideas, research results and clinical outcomes. This book is intended as a *general guide* to understanding the field, and accessing that information, but also as a reference book. Although the predominant model of music therapy in Europe is improvisational, insight-based therapy, all forms of music therapy theory and practice used within a wider international field are referred to and briefly explained. As in medical and paramedical professions, the profession of music therapy contains a rich diversity of approaches and methods, often developed with specific relevance to meet the needs of certain client populations. This book attempts to reflect the many facets of that diversity in order to enable the reader to see the panorama of music therapy.

Tony Wigram PhD, Aalborg University, 2002

Introduction

Music has been a medium of therapy for centuries, and there are numerous examples of the curative or healing powers of music in the historical records of different cultures (Campbell 1991; Gouk 2000; Horden 2000; Pratt and Jones 1988; Wigram *et al.* 1995 – see the overview in Chapter 1.1).

Over the last fifty years, music therapy has developed as a clinically applied treatment administered by trained professionals in countries where the development of graduate and post-graduate level training and *clinical* practice has resulted in qualified and recognized practitioners. Music therapy is now accepted as a discipline alongside other paramedical professions such as physiotherapy, occupational therapy, speech therapy and psychology in paramedical services and special educational services provided by health and education authorities.

In some countries, music therapy is officially recognized by political, clinical and academic institutions or organizations, and also by employment agencies. In other countries music therapy still has not found recognition as a science and as a profession. Styles of work vary considerably, and are influenced by the clinical field within which the music therapists are working, and the training and cultural background from which they come. Recent publications have highlighted the wide application and enormous diversity of music therapy (Aigen 1998; D. Aldridge 1996a; D. Aldridge 1998a; D. Aldridge 2000; Aldridge *et al.* 2001; Benenzon 1997; Bruscia 1987, 1991, 1998a, 1998b; Bunt 1994; Decker-Voigt and Knill 1996; Dileo 1999; Heal and Wigram 1993; Kenny 1995; Pratt and Grocke 1999; Tomaino 1998; Wigram and De Backer 1999a, 1999b; Wigram, Saperston and West 1995).

In Europe, music therapy traditions have developed on the foundations of more psychodynamic and psychotherapeutically orientated approaches. Frequently one finds here a model where the therapist is actively using music-making through the medium of *clinical improvisation* in order to establish a *musical relationship* with the patients through which he or she will be able to help them understand the nature of their problem. This active form of music therapy has involved the development of music therapy training programs which require, at entry level, highly trained musicians in order to develop their skills in the therapeutic field. Therapists require a knowledge of the potential in therapy of the various elements of music for helping the patient, together with a theoretical framework of therapeutic intervention (Alvin 1975, 1976, 1978; Austin 1991; Bang 1980; Bean 1995; Bunt 1987; De Backer 1993; Flower 1993; Nordoff and Robbins 1971, 1977; Odell-Miller 1995; Oldfield 1995; Priestley 1975, 1995; Wigram 1995b; Wigram, Saperston and West 1995).

With certain clinical populations (patients), music therapy has been found to be effective and beneficial. For example, there is much documented material on the efficacy of music therapy intervention to improve and develop communication and relationship-building with patients with autistic disability, and in assessing communication disorder (Edgerton 1994; Howat 1995; Muller and Warwick 1993; Warwick 1995; Wigram 1991c, 1995a, 1999c). Neurological disorders, including Alzheimer's disease, Huntington's chorea and Parkinson's disease have apparently responded positively to music therapy, in terms of movement activities, singing and music listening (Bonny 1989; Bright 1981; Erdonmez 1993; Selman 1988).

Behavioural approaches in music therapy have emerged mainly in the United States of America and they have frequently developed the use of music as a stimulant, a relaxant or a reward. In addition, the structure and properties of music have been applied and manipulated to achieve development, growth and improvement in patients. In this sense, the therapeutic process does not involve a dynamic and responsive *interaction* with the patient, but the music is structured in order to help the patient overcome emotional, physical or psychological problems from which they are suffering. This is a more prescriptive and applied use of music (Clair 1991a; Darrow and Cohen 1991; Davis *et al.* 1999; Grant 1995; Hanser 1987, 1995; Unkefer 1990).

In Europe, there has been a strong tradition for using live, improvised music in music therapy. Participation in active music-making has traditionally been the method by which music therapists are trained to engage and treat patients. An understanding of the nature of a patient's *musical behaviour*, the way they play, and the non-verbal and musically communicative interaction which they have developed is the method by which the process of therapy is undertaken, and through which a patient will achieve progress.

This book is structured to follow a path starting in history and leading the reader through to current research and clinical practice. The authors have tried to present the information, for example in Chapter 3, using a specific format so that each section and subject area has a similar design and content style to make it easier for readers to find the information they need.

Chapter 1 gives an historic introduction to music therapy as a method of treatment. A general historical overview goes back to the concept of music developed by Pythagoras, and then explores the connection between music and medicine. The chapter continues with a review of the way music therapy as a discipline is defined, and the variability and differences inherent when considering different models, approaches and methods of music therapy. The chapter finishes with a consideration of different theories regarding our understanding of music and introduces a music therapy theoretical perspective on music and music experiences.

Chapter 2 addresses the theoretical foundations of music therapy. To begin, the wide-ranging and diverse field of the psychology of music is described, drawing on the main areas of study that have relevance for music therapy. The chapter continues with a comprehensive overview of the many different theories and approaches in therapy and psychotherapy that have influenced and underpinned the philosophies and theories of music therapy. How the theory of music therapy is connected to psychoanalytic, psychodynamic and transpersonal theories from psychology is addressed, including a section by Dr Niels Hannibal on the relationship between music therapy and the theories of child development advanced by Daniel Stern. A final section focuses on the concepts of how music and music experience is presented as analogy and metaphor – how music and musical interaction ('musicking', Small 1998) reflects psychological processes, qualities and problems. Finally it exemplifies how music itself (selected baroque movements) can be understood as a metaphor for psychological processes in three specific levels.

Chapter 3 is a presentation of some of the most important traditions, models and methods in music therapy – taking an international perspective. The models coming from pioneers in music therapy are reviewed, and the essential elements of their historical development, characteristic methods used in sessions, clinical application, documentation and level of intervention are systematically reported. Later in the chapter, methods and traditions including the physiological, medical and healing applications of music are reported.

Chapter 4 presents a broad picture of the area of clinical practice. The most prominent and typical areas within which music therapy is practised are reviewed, and different styles and methods of clinical work are discussed. The needs of various client populations are reflected in the approaches that are described in this chapter. Two PhD students at Aalborg University have contributed here with material from their own specialized areas – Hanne Mette Ochsner Ridder in the field of older adults, and Dr Ulla Holck writing about communication-disordered children. As no single chapter could begin to comprehensively cover the wide range of clinical practices, the chapter finishes with an overview of the clinical literature where case studies have documented the broad field.

Chapter 5 focuses on music therapy research and *clinical assessment*. It goes through different methods of research and gives examples from research projects in the literature. A focus is then placed on the development of a research milieu, research school and PhD program, using the International Research School in Music Therapy at Aalborg University as an example. This chapter continues by looking at assessment and evaluation in music therapy, considering different methods and tools. The authors attempt to bring into focus the importance of professional and scientific documentation of the goals and expectations of therapy, giving, at the end, the reference frame of evidence-based practice.

Chapter 6 is a short, concentrated look at the elements of a music therapist's education, using the five-year, full-time course in music therapy (Bachelor's/Master's) at Aalborg University as an example of a comprehensive education. Starting with the process of the entrance tests, the chapter works through the four main areas of study and skill development in music therapy training – musical skills, theoretical knowledge, clinical practice and self-experience.

Chapter 7 is informative in character and considers practical tools and resources. Here one can see some of the organizations, publications (journals and books), websites and Internet-based resources that will guide the reader to many fruitful areas of exploration beyond this book.

Chapter 8 is a glossary or lexicon compiled to offer definitions of some of the terms that are frequently used in the book as an attempt to clarify some of the 'jargon' of music therapy, psychology of music and 'musicmedicine'. In many cases they are formulated by the authors, therefore they are not taken from dictionary sources.

The bibliography at the end is comprehensive, and includes not only direct resources from the field of music therapy, but also references from many associated disciplines.

The book is accompanied by a CD that gives the clinical and musical examples referred to in many of the chapters.

The book is an exciting and productive collaboration between the three authors, who have worked together for the last ten years at the University of Aalborg in Denmark. We have discussed each chapter so much, and so often, feeding off and gaining from each other's ideas and critique that it seems irrelevant to specify who has written what in the book. However, we would like to offer our thanks to the many colleagues who have contributed material and information for us to include in this book, and who have reviewed the text in order to offer feedback so that we can improve our work. In addition to the PhD students previously mentioned, we would like to record our gratitude to many music therapists in Denmark – Ole Agger,

Bolette Daniels Beck, Morten HjØgaard, Ingrid Irgens-MØller, Helle Nystrup Lund, Hilde Skrudland and Ellen ThØmasen.

The work of translating the original Danish book, undertaken by the three authors, has been aided very significantly by Ingrid Iregens-MØller, who assisted with extremely well-formulated English versions of the original Danish text.

Note

Words that are defined in the Glossary are italicised the first time they appear in the text.

CHAPTER I

Introduction to Music Therapy

1.1 Music Therapy – A Historical Perspective

Music for a while shall all your cares beguile

(Shakespeare)

Since antiquity, music has been used as a therapeutic tool, and ancient healing rituals including sound and music have survived in many cultures (Gouk 2000). Shamanism has been studied in depth within social anthropology, and modified shamanism is often an integrated part of modern self-developmental work. Myths and narratives on the healing power of music are numerous in most cultures. The tale of Saul and David (1 Samuel, Chapter 16) is one of the best known in the Western hemisphere. Orpheus is another mythological figure with appeal to many music therapists – as mentioned by Alvin (1975) and Bunt (1994).

However, the question is whether there exists a continuous, unbroken tradition connecting modern, scientific music therapy with the practice and philosophy of music and medicine handed down from antiquity. This is what Kümmel (1977) claimed in his doctoral thesis, but this notion has met serious criticism in a recent book on the history of music therapy (Horden 2000). It can hardly be questioned that the healing power of music is a common theme in literature on philosophy and music theory since Plato, but Horden has demonstrated that the medical literature from its very early days (the time of Hippocrates) had a sceptical attitude towards the speculative and metaphysical doctrine on the nature of music, and that treatises taking music seriously are few and far between in the history of medicine. 'It is philosophy and religion that make conceptual room for music therapy' (p.44). Horden has also noticed that music is not included as a subject in two standard British works on the history of medicine and psychiatry.

The tradition of including a chapter on the healing power of music in a treatise on music goes back probably to Boethius (circa AD 600). His famous treatise *De Institutione Musica* was spread all over Europe in the Middle Ages; it was part of the reading requirement in the university 'Quadrivium' (see Figure 1.1) and thus also included in the syllabus of medical students. Anecdotes, phrases and statements from Boethius are repeated over and over in the medieval music literature, as the connection between music and medicine (or health) was based on a few, but concise, theoretical assumptions (Gouk 2000; Horden 2000):

1. In (Neo)Platonic theory the harmonic vibrations system of music as sound was interpreted as a microcosmic reflection of the vibrations and number proportions found in macrocosmos, e.g. in the periods of revolution of planets and celestial bodies – or in 'the World Soul'.

2. The medical theory of the four bodily fluids (the so-called humoral medicine, or *pathology*) maintained that health is a matter of balance between the fluids/humours, i.e. that disturbances of the human mind (mental illness) have a somatic origin, and that the balance of humours can be influenced by the vibrations of music.

3. The ethos doctrine maintained that music in different modes has specific properties and potentials of influencing the human mind.

4. Consciousness (the mind) can promote or impair health, and music can – through the susceptible mind – influence the individual following certain principles.

These four assumptions are discussed in the following pages. We agree with Horden that the antique and classic theories of the healing power of music are above all speculative thoughts on the relationship between music, body, mind and spirit. Even if a psychosomatic element often plays a prominent part in a treatise, we are not dealing with historical or empirical documentations of the healing effects of music – rather with anecdotes and hypotheses tenacious of life, and repeatedly stated through the centuries in treatises on music and, rarely, medicine. As Horden formulates it, music therapy was a 'fringe discipline' of medicine.

The speculative, metaphysical element is also common in the 'New Age' literature on music and healing (see Chapter 3.8). Contemporary music therapy is based on scientific thinking and empirical documentation; however, the theories mentioned constitute an important part of the history of ideas within the profession. The ancient speculative theories can still provide useful, relevant and inspiring analogies, metaphors or images (Horden 2001).

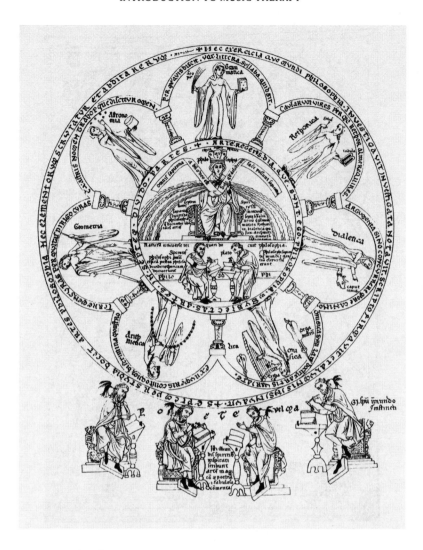

Figure 1.1: Artes Liberales

Allegorical representation of the seven free arts ('Artes Liberales') from the medieval manuscript *Hortus Deliciarum* by the Abbess Herrad of Landsberg (middle of the twelfth century).

In the centre, above Socrates and Plato, we see Philosophia (divine wisdom) on her throne. 'I, philosophy, divide my subjects in seven areas.' They pour out of her breasts, four to the left, three to the right. Trivium to the right: Grammatica (on top) is depicted with a handbook, Retorica with a table, Dialectica with a dog's head. Quadrivium follows: Musica with three string instruments (a harp and two lyres), Arithmetica with a counting device, Geometria with measure and compass, and finally Astronomia with a round measure for the zodiac. Musica says: 'I am Musica, and my science is comprehensive and diverse.' Below, and outside the circle inspired by the Holy Ghost, we find four poets. They are inspired by the unholy ghost when writing about Fate, Mythology and Magic.

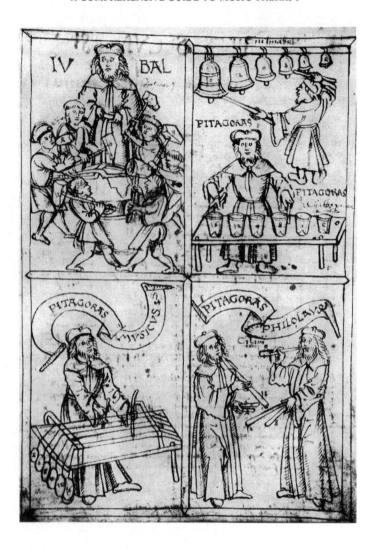

Figure 1.2: Pythagoras – the four fields

The music theorists of the Middle Ages disagreed on the question: who 'invented' music? Some said Pythagoras, others the biblical figure Jubal, of whom Genesis 4:21 tells that 'he was the progenitor of harpists and flutists'. The theorist and poet Johannes Hollandrinus suggests a typical compromise, also including two medieval theorists. He writes: 'Pythagoras invented music, and Boethius passed it on. Guido examined the notes, and Jubal recorded the melody.'

The picture is from Franchinus Gaffurius' *Theorica Musica*. The upper left scanning field shows Jubal and represents the interval proportions between two pairs of blacksmiths' hammers: 4:8:16 to the left, and 6:9:12 to the right, producing the following intervals: fifth (4:6), fourth (6:8), major second (8:9) and fourth (9:12 and 12:16), and the tone row: A-E-a-h-e-a'. The same row appears in the other three scanning fields, where we see Pythagoras conducting various experiments: playing bells, glasses, a monochord with six strings, and two times three flutes (assisted by his pupil Philolaos).

The theory of vibrations in micro- and macrocosmos

In our post-modern era most people of the Western hemisphere consider music a commodity, i.e. a consumer good. A person is free to choose between (commercially distributed) music experiences, be it concerts, CDs, MP3 files or music videos – and free to use them anywhere and anytime.

But in the not-so-distant past it was still a tradition in Western cultures to maintain that music and health (physiological as well as psychological) were closely related.

This tradition goes back to the legendary Greek philosopher Pythagoras (circa 500 BC) and early Greek medical science of his time. It was not broken (maybe just marginalized) until the eighteenth and nineteenth century witnessed the development of modern natural and medical science, based on empirical and statistical principles.

Recently – after nearly 250 years of separation – medicine, health psychology and music therapy are approaching each other again, realizing that man is *not* a (ever so fantastic) 'machine', but a complex, bio-psycho-social being. Or, as we prefer to see it, man is a unity of body, mind and spirit placed into a social order, and music has comprehensive effects and meaning on all levels.

Pythagoras realized this 2500 years ago, and even if his philosophy (communicated to us by his disciples) may be hard to grasp, his basic discoveries are simple. Pythagoras was (as far as we know) both a mystic and a serious scientist, who also worked empirically. He studied the surrounding world with his senses and thought deeply about the implications of his discoveries for man and culture. One of his working tools was a so-called *monochord* – a measure and music 'instrument' with only one string. On this instrument he could experiment with notes and intervals, with the proportions of two or more notes – and their relationship to human consciousness. The discoveries of Pythagoras are still relevant.

Music exists on a *physical level*. A string produces a tone by vibrating at a specific speed, and today we say that the concert pitch of A equals 440 vibrations per minute (measured in hertz, Hz), and that it becomes audible by making the molecules of the surrounding air vibrate at the same speed. When these vibrations meet a human listener's ear, complicated perceptual and cognitive operations in the brain lead him/her to the conclusion that the tone is the A played by the oboe to initiate the orchestra's tuning. 'Concert pitch' is in fact a historical compromise. At the end of the seventeenth century an A was equal to 415 Hz. In modern orchestras like the Berlin Philharmonic the pitch is 445 Hz, which gives the orchestral sound some extra brilliance. Today the vibration speed of a note can be measured exactly. Of course, this was not possible for Pythagoras. What he measured – exactly – were the mathematical proportions between tones and intervals, as produced by a string. Using the monochord he discovered a series of laws of the relationship between length of a string and pitch.

An example: If the string of the monochord vibrates freely the fundamental note corresponds to the string length of '1' (e.g. 440 Hz). If the string is divided into halves, they vibrate at double speed (2:1 – 880 Hz). If it is divided into thirds, the vibration will be three times faster (3:1 – 1320 Hz). There is a regular, mathematical (proportional) relationship between string length and vibration speed. However, this is all physics, numbers, 'body'.

How does the human mind experience music at the *psychological level*? We experience vibrations as notes, and (maybe) the interplay of notes as music. String lengths and vibration speeds are measurable, exact proportions in the physical world – quantities. Notes (and music) are qualities – the vibrational phenomena, as they are interpreted by the human mind. When studying the vibrations from a qualitative point of view it is revealed that the string divided into halves produces the same note as before, but an octave higher. The octave is a fundamental principle of acoustics and psychoacoustics, and everyone has experienced it. Without the octave it would not be possible for men and women (and children) to sing in unison. The octave is a universal phenomenon, and music (defined as humanly produced sound ordered in time) would also be impossible without it. But the octave can be distributed and ordered in modes and scales in many ways, and these are culturally specific.

The string length of two-thirds (of the full string) produces a fifth. A string length of one fourth will produce a note two octaves higher than the fundamental; a string length of one fifth will produce a note two octaves plus a major third higher. And so forth. It is possible for anyone to perform experiments with this on a guitar, for example, using a single string, and thus experience that we are dealing with a law of nature – and a relationship between a quantitative/physical phenomenon and a qualitative/psychological experience.

The relationship between intervals can be expressed as proportional numbers or ratios:

- octave = 2:1
- fifth = 3:2
- fourth = 4:3
- major third = 5:4.

Then it begins to be more complicated. For instance, a minor third, a major third and a major second can be defined as different proportions, due to the nature of the overtone or nature row. We will not go into this here.

Pythagoras knew that tones are also produced in nature, e.g. in 'wind harps' where the wind makes the air in a stone cylinder vibrate (as heard in certain rock formations). However, he did not know the physical principles for the production of nature tones, and they were theoretically irrelevant for him. Such a natural 'cylinder' can not only produce a fundamental but also natural overtones (partial tones) depending on how strong the wind is. Overtones are also called partial tones, counting from the fundamental as No.1. The relative power of the partial tones is different from instrument to instrument, thus contributing to the specific timbre of an instrument. These overtones are produced in the same order, no matter if it happens in a rock formation, a long plastic 'snake' or a wind instrument without keys or stops.

- 1st overtone (= partial tone No.2) is the octave
- 2nd is the fifth
- 3rd the next octave
- 4th the major third
- 5th the (next) fifth
- 6th a septime (heard as 'out of tune' with our modern, Western-tempered ears)
- 7th the next octave
- 8th the major second.

And so forth. Gradually the intervals of the pentatonic, the diatonic and the chromatic scale appear.

This system is complex and comprehensive, and many practical and aesthetic problems (not to mention cultural preferences) are involved when musicians adapt it for practical musical purposes, like building instruments and playing on them. From a historical perspective the problems have been solved through the invention of different 'tuning systems' regulating the natural interval proportions to the needs of performance practice, and through instrumental technology, e.g. by adding keys and stops to wind instruments, making it possible to play other notes than the naturally produced ones in the harmonic sequence. Man-made ideas and preferences in music have 'bent' the laws of nature and transformed them into musical practice.

Pythagoras discovered that music is based on the laws of nature. However, he went one step further. The human mind is capable of perceiving the (lawful) vibrations and tone proportions as musical notes and intervals. In Pythagorean thought, notes and intervals are also reflections of a cosmic, spiritual level. This level is inaudible, but a human being can reflect or meditate on the universal principles, which are also followed by the celestial bodies. According to the Pythagoreans, the planets vibrate in the same frequencies and proportions as audible music. This is *the music of the spheres*. The organized order of musical notes is a microcosmic reflection of macrocosmic order, including everything in the universe – body, mind and spirit. This philosophy was developed further by Plato.

We have chosen to write so extensively about this, because this theory or doctrine is the core of not only classic musicology, but also classic medical knowledge – and university education – from antiquity to the Renaissance. The medieval university was divided into *quadrivium*, including geometry, arithmetics, astronomy and music theory, and *trivium*, including grammar, rhetoric and logic (see Figure 1.1). One of the last pioneering scientists, who based his work on these principles, was the astronomer (and astrologer) Johannes Kepler. In his last treatise, *Harmonices mundi* (The Harmony of the World, 1619), his ambition is to combine the results of empirical astronomy with classical Pythagorean principles of the harmonic cosmos (Erichsen 1986). In other words, for centuries, and transversely to religious and philosophical disagreements, music was considered a phenomenon of three levels – the same levels we (re)discover or redefine today in a modern scientific context.

Medieval music philosophy (after Boethius) made a clear distinction between:

- *Musica mundana*: the spiritual level, music as a metaphysic principle – and a pathway to the experience of the deepest, universal truths.

- *Musica humana*: the level of the soul or the mind, where the moral and ethical potential of music unfolds. We are still not dealing with the sensory dimension of music, but with its potential to influence the mind in a positive direction, opening it up towards the ethical dimension.

- *Musica instrumentalis*: the physical level of the body, where the music (instrumental and vocal) sounds and can be heard by human beings. From a bottom-up perspective the experience of music is the precondition for, or a 'gate' to, the experience of the higher levels.

Parallel descriptions of levels can be found in all major cultures (for a more detailed reading of the history of music therapy theory and its connection with music philosophy, see Horden 2000; Myskja 1999; Ruud 1990).

Man was considered a 'musical instrument', which could be 'out of tune' or 'finely tuned' – indicating that the harmonic proportions of music also permeate the physical body. We find the classic philosophy elegantly formed by Shakespeare (in *The Merchant of Venice*, Act V):

Such harmony is in immortal souls;

But whilst this muddy vesture of decay

Doth grossly close it in, we cannot hear it.

'Attunement' is a favourite metaphor not only in contemporary developmental psychology (Stern), but also in the work of the Danish philosopher K.E. Løgstrup, whose concept has been adapted to contemporary music education, where 'musical attunement' signifies a self-forgetting preoccupation with music (Fink-Jensen 1997).

Humoral medicine

Music had its place in the classical syllabus of European universities. Music theory, including the Pythagorean version of the tone system and harmonic/consonant and disharmonic/dissonant proportions, was common knowledge amongst 'free men cultivating the free arts (artes liberales)'. The classical doctrine was combined with the dominating medical theories, e.g. *humoral medicine* (or *humoral pathology*) – a doctrine with great influence through many centuries. In humoral medicine health is influenced by four bodily fluids or 'humours': blood, phlegm, yellow bile and black bile. According to this theory good health was the result of a harmonic balance between the humours, while disease reflected some sort of imbalance between them. Historically the doctrine goes back to circa 400 BC, and one of its most important spokesmen was the influential medical theorist Galen in the time of the Roman Empire. It was considered foundational in medical theory right up to the eighteenth century.

Music was considered a therapeutic tool capable of influencing, even restoring, the balance between humours. A historical study of medieval treatises on music theory reveals that they often include ingenious, speculative systems correlating humours, temperaments, celestial bodies – and music.

Examples could be Robert Fludd's well-known 'Divine Monochord' (1617), or Agrippa von Nettesheim's theory (1510) correlating the three levels of music and man – body, mind and spirit – with his historical period's understanding of:

1. the physical world/the human body/the vibrations of music

2. the world of language/the human mind/the notes and intervals of music

3. the cosmos/the human spirit/the divine proportions of music.

Another fine example is Franchinus Gaffurius' *Practica Musica* (1496, see Figure 1.3).

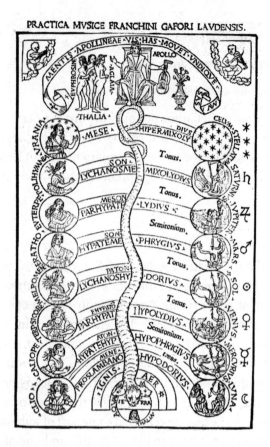

Figure 1.3: Gaffurius

In Franchinus Gaffurius' *Practica Musica* (Milan 1496) we find this representation of the affinity of the harmony of the spheres, figures from Greek mythology and Greek music theory: 'A symbolic-graphic representation of the modes.' The connection of the harmony of the spheres with the nine muses goes back to classical Greek literature, and Gaffurius follows the tradition. On top we see Apollo on his throne. He rules the harmony of the world. 'Mentis Apollineae vis has movet undique' means 'The power of the Apollonian spirit moves all muses.' Apollo's standard lyre is replaced by a (Renaissance) lute; on his right side we see the three Graces Euphrosyne, Aglaia and Thaleia. The centre axis is drawn by a creature with three heads and a snake body. It covers the whole distance from the throne of Apollo to the earth and the sphere of the four elements: water, fire, air and earth. This is the basis of the celestial harmony, unfolding to the right side of the table – the seven planets (including sun and moon) and the firmament. To the left, eight of the nine muses are portrayed; the ninth (Thaleia) is depicted below the earth. The two horizontal rows show the Greek names of the notes A-a on the left, and the names of the modes (in capitals) plus the interval (tone or semitone) between them on the right. Example: the Phrygian mode PHRYGIUS begins on e, HYPATEMESON. The correlation of notes and planets goes back to Plato and Cicero (Moon = A, Sun = D, The Firmament = a).

The ethos doctrine

The history of philosophy documents that Western philosophers (e.g. Plato, Aristotle, Augustine, Schopenhauer, Nietzsche) carefully considered the theoretical and practical role of music for the individual (the question of a person's health), for the state (the question of collective regulation of health, education and conflict), and for society (the question of social values, ethical principles and belief). Elements of the ethic of Plato and Aristotle are still alive as popular knowledge, e.g. the principle of 'the golden mean'.

The history of medicine includes many examples of health-promoting rules of conduct or doctrines, referring to classical 'dietetics' or the teaching of Hippocrates and his successors. A few doctors have created practical treatment systems or manuals including music as an integrated element (more common in Arab medicine). These manuals historically develop from more or less speculative and normative principles for the use of music to specific ailments plus general references to the classical doctrine of the vibrations of harmonic bodies, to more specific recommendations for a clinical adaptation of music, based on experiments, and medical or social experience.

Music and the mind

In a famous paragraph of Plato's *The State* (Book III) we are informed about the influence of music on the human mind. In his dialogue with Glaucon, Socrates praises the use of certain rhythms and modes that encourage man to a harmonic and brave life (the Dorian and Phrygian mode), while he makes reservations to modes encouraging indolence or sadness (Lydian and Mixolydian). Even if it is obvious that these considerations inform us more about Plato's ideals for a perfect state than about music, we still find similar ideas about the direct influence of music on the mind in music theory and medical theory through the centuries. The axiom is that music has a direct effect on the human mind and thus influences mood, character and health.

An example of this holistic, psychosomatic understanding can be found in the writings of a great Renaissance man, Marcilio Ficino (1433–1499), who was a theologian, astrologer, doctor and musician. He attempted to combine Platonic philosophy (including its music theory) with Christian dogmas by formulating guidelines for a holistic health doctrine, 'natural magic'. He regarded the soul as the mediator between body and mind, promoting a harmonic relationship between the individual person and the 'World Soul' (the mediator of heaven and earth). Ficino considered carefully selected and performed music the most effective means to obtain this balance, harmony and unity.

Eye-witnesses recall how Ficino the musician improvised, in a specific state of consciousness, a phenomenon that would be quite easy to recognize from the clinical practice of music therapists, where he was in a specific state of empathic awareness and engagement, a listening perspective allowing a flow of information between musician/therapist and listener/client (Voss in Horden 2000; Pedersen 1999). Plato called this state *furor divimus,* a condition of frenzy, when the soul is so aligned with the power of God that it becomes insensible to its embodied condition. A music therapist would speak of *countertransference* and try to maintain a bodily grounding.

The idea of influencing the body through the mind is a recurring theme, not only in the music literature, but also in clinical medical practice. The history of music therapy includes many historical reports of how music was performed regularly and systematically for the patients in somatic or psychiatric hospitals (see also Myskja 1999).

The revival of classical ideas through quantum physics

In the development of natural science, anatomy and empirically informed medicine after Renaissance music (and the theoretical framework of the three levels) gradually receded into the background. A few doctors were still experimenting with music and wrote treatises or reports (see Myskja 1999, Chapters 5 to 8), but in general medical science was occupied with different matters. It was not until the 'New Wave' of the 1960s and 1970s, especially the 'New Age' philosophy or paradigm within physics, psychology, medicine and music, that the classical themes and doctrines were revived and combined with contemporary scientific discoveries. This was done more or less carefully, and more or less speculatively, but the last decades of the twentieth century witnessed a return of many ancient ideas. It became popular to consider the human body–mind a 'musical instrument that could be tuned' (Halpern 1985), and to see a reflection of macrocosmos in the microcosmos of music (for a critical discussion, see Summer 1996).

The more serious parts of this revival are closely related to modern quantum physics with its sensational demonstration of the paradoxical relationship between the state of physical matter as wave and particle simultaneously. The implications of this paradox – going back to the discussions of Bohr and Einstein – have had enormous influence on scientific thought, epistemology as well as ontology. This is also reflected in music therapy theory (Eagle 1991). The conception of a universal order independent of man and reflected in the universe of music is proposed by Ken Bruscia, who considers the 'Implicate order' one amongst three levels of meaning (Bruscia 2000; Ruud 2000b; see also Chapter 2.4).

It is no longer unusual or suspect that a scientist may consider life a permanent journey between the different levels of human existence, from matter to spirit. He or she may also consider music a specific order – a suitable metaphor or analogy of a richer and healthier life. Music influences body, mind and spirit, and it reflects universal principles of life. This was the core of the classical theories of music and medicine. However, the basic assumptions were rarely investigated scientifically, or documented carefully. Modern music therapy theory and practice, at all three levels, makes it possible to reconsider the old ideas and give them a new framework.

We interpret the quotation from the start of this chapter in this way: the author was well acquainted with the influence of music on the human mind, and he considered it of limited duration. The systematic, scientifically based application of music in therapy and as therapy may lead to permanent change. This emerges clearly from the following chapters.

1.2 Definitions of Music Therapy

Music therapy is a profession which has emerged over the last fifty years from a variety of professional disciplines in different countries. Therefore, the process of defining music therapy both as a profession and as a discipline can vary depending on the orientation and perspective of a particular group of practitioners, or different cultures.

A general definition of music therapy needs to be inclusive, and focus on the function of music as a therapeutic medium, as well as defining for whom the therapy is intended:

> The use of music in clinical, educational and social situations to treat clients or patients with medical, educational, social or psychological needs. (Wigram 2000e)

However, the process of defining music therapy can be reflected in the way the profession itself has emerged in different countries and through different traditions. In this way, one has to take into consideration three main factors:

- the professional background of practitioners
- the needs of the clients
- the approach used in treatment.

In order to establish a more generic and all-embracing definition of music therapy, in 1996, the World Federation of Music Therapy (WFMT) produced the following definition:

> Music therapy is the use of music and/or musical elements (sound, rhythm, melody and harmony) by a qualified music therapist with a client or group, in a process designed to facilitate and promote communication, relationships, learning, mobilisation [sic], expression, organisation [sic] and other relevant therapeutic objectives, in order to meet physical, emotional, mental, social and cognitive needs. Music therapy aims to develop potentials and/or restore functions of the individual so that he or she can achieve better intra- and inter-personal integration and, consequently, a better quality life through prevention, rehabilitation or treatment. (WFMT 1996)

The disciplines from which music therapy has emerged include occupational therapy, general psychology, psychotherapy, special education, music education, music psychology, anthropology and medicine. Consequently, there are inevitable paradoxes in the way one can define the practice of music therapy:

- artistic versus scientific
- musical versus psychological
- behavioural versus psychotherapeutic
- complimentary versus alternative
- rehabilitative versus acute.

The definition of music therapy can also vary depending on the client population with whom practitioners are working. With some client populations, the process of therapy is essentially rehabilitative, and the process of restoring skills or faculties and improving functional ability is a main focus of the therapist's working practice. In work with the chronic population, one is aware that the therapeutic practice accepts the lack of potential for cure and therefore the definition of the therapy relates more to achieving potential, resolving physical, emotional and psychological difficulties and meeting the needs within the parameters of the individual's chronic disability or illness.

In contrast, music therapy is also practised with the non-clinical population, where people are seeking therapy to explore their resources, find out about themselves and achieve better health and better living. The aims of the therapy in any one of these situations will vary. However, the approach of the therapist may not. Therefore there are a variety of definitions of music therapy depending on the philosophy or approach of the practitioner or group of practitioners.

Some examples might include:

- *Behavioural music therapy*, where the therapist is using music to increase, or modify, appropriate behaviour and to reduce or eliminate bad or

inappropriate behaviours. In these situations, music may be used as a
positive or negative reinforcement.

- Psychotherapeutic music therapy, where music is used to help the client
  gain insight into their world, their needs and their life and where an
  active, psychodynamic approach will involve gaining awareness of
  issues, thoughts, feelings, attitudes and conflicts.

- Educational music therapy, where music therapy sits inside an
  educational institution where the objectives of an educational program
  have influence on the music therapy approach. Here, music therapists
  might find their objective's names relate to learning processes,
  development, realizing potential and meeting the needs of children in
  connection with their educational program.

In order to clarify the variety of definitions of music therapy and relate them to definitions of music, and therapy, separately, Professor Kenneth Bruscia has written a
book called *Defining Music Therapy*. (1998 second edition.)

In the first edition, Bruscia begins by giving a definition of music, in particular
music within a therapeutic setting. He further defines therapy and then attempts to
link these together in a definition of music therapy. Bruscia's own particular perspective on music therapy is as follows:

> Music therapy is a systematic process of intervention wherein the therapist helps
> the client to achieve health, using musical experiences and the relationships that
> develop through them as dynamic forces of change. (1998)

In the second edition, Bruscia modifies his definition slightly by changing the focus
to '… promote health …'. He then proceeds to take each element within the definition, and explain its relevance and implications.

The most important contribution in this book is that Bruscia defines the
different areas and levels of music therapy. In terms of areas of practice, Bruscia lists
the following: didactic, medical, healing, psychotherapeutic, recreational and
ecological.

Relating these to the different levels of practice, Bruscia describes four specific
levels of intervention which are also linked to the status and clinical responsibility of
the therapist:

> *Auxiliary level*: all functional uses of music or any of its components for
> non-therapeutic but related purposes.

Augmentative level: any practice in which music or music therapy is used to enhance the efforts of other treatment modalities, and to make supportive contributions to the client's overall treatment plan.

Intensive level: any practice in which music therapy takes a central and independent role in addressing priority goals in the client's treatment plan and, as a result, induces significant changes in the client's current situation.

Primary level: any practice in which music therapy takes an indispensable or singular role in meeting the main therapeutic needs of the client and, as a result, induces pervasive changes in the client's life. (1998)

As was stated at the beginning of this section, the approach in music therapy, or the method of intervention, is closely related to the client population, and Bruscia's important contribution at a theoretical level is to define different approaches and then identify the process and goals of the therapy involved.

In connection with our overview of models of music therapy (Chapter 4), we will correlate the models with Bruscia's four levels of clinical practice.

A complementary model has been developed by Dileo, who proposes three discrete levels of clinical practice (Dileo-Maranto 1993b):

1.   supportive

2.   specific

3.   comprehensive.

An illustration of this model can be made using the area of pain management. Here we have modified Dileo's three levels in application to this specific area of treatment:

Levels of music therapy	Practice in pain management
1. Supportive Level	
Needs of Client:	Temporary relief from pain
Level of Therapist:	Beginning, intermediate
Depth:	Distraction, provision of *coping* skills
Function:	Supportive of medical intervention
Common Music Therapy	
Intervention:	Music and biofeedback, music-based relaxations, *vibroacoustic therapy*

2. Specific Level

Needs of Client:	Understanding of pain
Level of Therapist:	Graduate studies (Master's level)
Depth:	Dialogue with or confrontation with pain
Function:	Equal with medical intervention
Common Music Therapy Intervention:	Improvisation, music and imagery techniques

3. Comprehensive Level

Needs of Client:	Resonance by therapist with pain
Level of Therapist:	Primary
Depth:	*Entrainment, guided imagery and music*
Function:	Resolution of pain
Common Music Therapy Intervention:	Advanced level / specialized training
	(NB 'Supportive' must not be confused with 'supportive', the specific supportive style in psychotherapy)

(Adapted from Dileo 1999 and reprinted with the kind premission of the American Music Therapy Association)

Figure 1.4 Music therapy levels of intervention compared with levels of intervention in the treatment of pain

As we have mentioned earlier, music therapy interventions are closely related to the client population, taking into consideration their needs and their potentials. The important theoretical contribution of Bruscia is the definitions of several discrete procedures, related to the consequences in attending to the process of therapy and related therapeutic objectives.

Music therapists working within the health system frequently establish collaborative professional relationships with doctors, nurses, paramedical professionals including physiotherapists, occupational therapists, speech and language therapists and others, and psychologists. Working in health systems, music therapists frequently find that their approach and treatment objectives are directed towards improving the general health of the patient, working with specific pathological problems and disorders, and maintaining quality of life and stability in the more chronic population. Work is undertaken in collaboration with the multidisciplinary team, and the music therapists find that they are approaching patients within the context of an overall plan for the patient's treatment.

Music therapists also work in the field of special education and in schools. Here, music therapists are often standing alongside music teachers and music pedagogues and there can be some confusion over the different roles involved. Generally, music teaching is a process which involves teaching children to acquire skills in the use of instruments and knowledge of music. This generally involves performance, composition and abilities to analyse music. The objectives for music teachers are frequently to work with students towards the achievement of skills in music, either at instrumental performance, singing or knowledge of music. The music therapist, on the other hand, is primarily working with the non-musical needs of the client at the centre of the treatment or remedial program, their therpeutic needs.

In special education, children present with a variety of learning difficulties, behavioural problems, social problems and psychological disabilities. The music therapist takes these problems as the primary focus for intervention and the function of the music is to act as a medium for meeting the needs of the client. Therefore, the acquisition of musical skill is not a primary objective, nor is it a requirement for the child to respond to therapy that they have achieved musical skill or even an aptitude for music. The music is a tool by which therapy occurs.

Nevertheless there is a grey area between the music therapist orientated within an educational setting and a music teacher who has adapted his/her working practice for children with special needs and has included remedial therapy objectives within his/her work. The main difference remains that a music teacher primarily focuses on promoting the development of musical skills, while a music therapist is focused on meeting therapeutic needs which nevertheless still need to be linked with the school's educational programs, and the individual educational program (IEP) of each child. In this method, the objectives of therapy can be connected to a child's overall development and may also be connected to his/her specific social or pathological problems.

It is appropriate to understand music therapy and (special) music education as poles in a continuum. Differences are important, but similarities and common goals and problems must not be underestimated (Bonde 1998; Bruhn 2000; Robertson 2000). Figure 1.5 may illustrate the continuum and the most important differences, similarities and transitions.

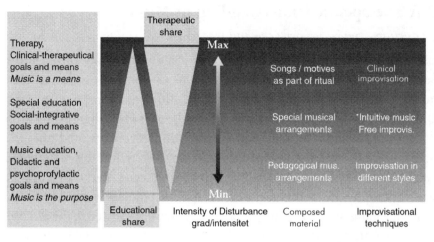

Figure 1.5 The relationship between music therapy and music education – a continuum model (Bonde, adapted from Bruhn, 2000)

Robertson (2000) has proposed a different continuum model. He suggests four main categories on a continuum from left (music therapy) to right (music profession):

1. clinical music therapy (surviving – coping – functioning – reacting)

2. educational music therapy (subconscious learning – contributing – growing – responding (aesthetic))

3. music education (conscious learning – refining – focusing – responding (artistic))

4. music profession (training – working – informing – performing).

In conclusion, while the definition of music therapy that has at present been formulated by the WFMT is a very inclusive and all-embracing definition, variability is inevitable within different cultures and according to different traditions. In Denmark, for example, music therapy is practised at psychotherapeutic level and the definition of music therapy here relates specifically to meeting the therapeutic needs of the clients to the psychodynamic development of a relationship and the place of music within that relationship. Further discussion regarding the application of music therapy in relation to a definition will be undertaken in subsequent chapters where more specific techniques are explained.

1.3 A Therapeutic Understanding of Music

Introduction – music, experience and meaning

Music can be experienced, understood and analysed in many different ways. As music history has fostered many different theories on the essence of music, the history of music therapy has embraced many different concepts of music and its meaning. Theories of music aesthetics reflect the ever-changing historical, cultural and social framework of music production and reception, and the changing concepts of music in the history of music therapy also reflect the changing ideas of music and healing in medical theory. This can be seen when different aspects of music philosophy are observed from a historical point of view. The idea of the inherent meaning of number and proportions in music is related to the philosophical idea of harmonic proportions in the relationship of body and soul in Greek philosophy. The idea of 'ethos' ('how to live a good life') is connected to humoral medicine (or *theory of humours*: the classic philosophy of how biological processes (health and disease) are related to the internal balance of the four body fluids: blood, phlegm, yellow bite and black bile). The theory of musical effects in the baroque period is related to the mechanical physiology of the same period. The concept of music as a psychophysical stimulus is related to positivism and its notion of errors in the apparatus of the human body and the idea of objective cause-and-effect within medicine, etc. (Ruud 1990, p.326).

Therefore, it does not make sense to have the ambition of presenting a general and valid definition of music in therapy, however, it does make sense to present some of the problems related to the question of the essence and meaning of music – as discussed in contemporary music therapy theory.

The understanding of music in music therapy theory is closely related to the understanding of human nature and health, and in most cases the three elements form a coherent and logical whole (Ruud and Mahns 1991). As music therapists take the clinical application of music as their starting point, they rarely understand music as an abstract or autonomous phenomenon, but rather as a unique means of self-expression and communication.

Basically there are three different views on the question of meaning in music (Pavlicevic 1997):

The absolutist position (also called the theory of autonomy, or absolute formalism). Music has no other meaning than the music itself. It is non-referential and independent of objects or emotions in the external world, and its 'meaning' is a matter of specific aesthetic events or processes governed by unique musical laws.

The referentialist position (also called the theory of heteronomy).

Music represents, expresses or symbolizes phenomena outside the realm of music itself, but within the world of man: emotions, ideas, narratives etc. The meaning of music is closely related to those who produce and perform it, and music is a testimony of human life.

The expressionist position is a compromise between or a synthesis of the two positions already mentioned. Music is considered an aesthetic phenomenon with its own principles, but the elements of music are related to and share important qualitites with basic human experiences. The aesthetic experience of music is a key to the understanding of human existence – and vice versa.

Many music therapists – especially therapists working within a psychodynamic or humanistic-existential framework – reject the idea of music as an autonomous aesthetic object and maintain that music is a representation and expression of the psychological world of their clients. Music is often considered a symbolic language allowing the therapist to explore its meaning for the client in improvisations followed by verbal therapeutic dialogue and/or hermeneutic ('morphological') interpretation (Priestley 1994; Tüpker 1988). The specific musical expression of the client and musical interaction in dyads or groups may also be interpreted as an analogy to the expression and interrelationships of the client in general (D. Aldridge 1996a; Smeijsters 1999 – see below).

This means that music therapists are confronted with three classic questions in music theory and music psychology:

1.   Is music a language? If it is, how does it differ from verbal language?

2.   Does music have meaning beyond internal musical principles and 'laws'? If it has, how does the musical expression or narrative relate to the external world?

3.   Can music have a meaning even if it cannot be expressed in words? If it can, is this 'inexpressible' or ineffable meaning a specific form of knowledge, recognition or awareness?

These are very complex questions, and any attempt to give an answer to them will depend on the ontological and epistemological position of the theorist or clinician. In this chapter we will consult two major figures within contemporary music therapy theory: Professor Even Ruud (University of Oslo, Norway) and Professor Ken Bruscia (Temple University, USA).

Even Ruud rejects all attempts to define music as an unambiguous, objective or universal phenomenon. If music has a healing potential it cannot be explained by any simple cause-effect relationship or by universal, metaphysical principles. Ruud considers health a multifactorial phenomenon (and music as one of many factors in this complex) – and music can be understood as an ambiguous, 'polysemic' phenomenon: the meaning of music is always constructed in a specific context, be it private, local, regional or national. Social, cultural, biographical and therapeutic factors will always influence the production and reception of music. Music is 'communication and social interaction' (in Norwegian: 'kommunikation og samhandling'), and the meaning of music grows out of complex processes of context-bound communication.

This is the standpoint of relativism and constructionism, critically opposed to positivist objectivism as well as speculative theories and metaphysical dogmas. Through the application of theories of communication and interaction this has also become a very influential position within music therapy theory (Ruud 1990, 1998a). Ruud elaborates his standpoint in an essay which also discusses the development of context-bound 'code competency' and culture-bound music discourses (Ruud 1998a).

Ken Bruscia represents a different position. Based on his research in the meaning of therapeutic music improvisations (Bruscia 1987) as well as music experiences in *receptive music therapy* (Bruscia 1995) he has come to this conclusion: music is fundamentally a matter of music experiences – of meaning and beauty expressed in music. Music is both a specific historical and cultural phenomenon – and a universal phenomenon. Meaning in music may on the one hand be a construction in a specific context (local, relative, subjective, stylistic etc.); on the other hand meaning may be inherent in the music in a universal, objective, context-independent way.

In a recent interview (Bruscia 2000) he pointed out that meaning in music may be understood either as a *result*: meaning is produced as a result of therapy; as *process*: therapy is a process of creating or transforming meaning; or as *communication*: the meaning of music is negotiated in interaction and dialogue.

Bruscia has also identified three sources of meaning:

1. *Meaning as implicate order*, which is independent of human perception and the absolute order of the world.

2. *Meaning as experience* of the implicate order, which is the often ineffable experiences of human consciousness (in normal or altered states) of being alive, in harmony with itself and the world – through music.

3. *Meaning as variously constructed* – the communication of these and other music experiences in a verbal language that reflects the context: culture, society, geography and biography.

Bruscia elaborates his description of these sources, especially aesthetic and transpersonal experiences in music therapy, in the same interview:

These experiences are truly ineffable. They are impossible to capture in words, and they are impossible to reconstruct musically. (Bruscia 2000)

In other words, Bruscia's position embraces an objective, universal and metaphysical as well as a subjective, local and relative understanding of music and meaning. He is both essentialist and relativist, and one of his points is that theorists as well as clinicians must always make their choice between several possible and legitimate constructs and perspectives.

We consider the positions of Ruud and Bruscia to be very important, and before we take a closer look on how the two professors define music and music experience, we will formulate our own answers to the three questions mentioned above:

1. Yes, music is a type of language – in the sense that music is an art of expression that follows certain perceptive and syntactical rules. It has its indigenous notation system (musical notation), and it has meaning for most people. However, music is not an unambiguous, discoursive language and it can never represent or designate phenomena of the external or internal world with the exactness of verbal, categorial language. Music can be characterized as an ambiguous, presentative symbolic language (Bruscia 1998a; Langer 1942).

2. Yes, music can contain and express meaning – beyond the pure musical or aesthetic content. This meaning is constructed in a complex interplay between the participants involved, e.g. composer–performer–listener or client–therapist. Music can be a direct expression of a client's emotions, or a musical representation – symbolic or metaphorical – of spiritual or complicated psychological states and conditions, or the musical expression can be an analogy to the client's being-in-the-world (D. Aldridge 1996a; Bruscia 1994, 1998a; Pavlicevic 1997; Smeijsters 1999).

3. Yes, music can have meaning even if it cannot be expressed in words. This 'tacit knowledge' or 'inexpressible meaning' can be found at different levels. At a structural level it is often impossible to formulate an even very precise musical experience in words. At a level that may be called the 'level of nuances' (Raffman 1993) the rich, dynamic and nuanced experiences of music listening or performance are perceived at a pre-verbal stage of knowledge that can be very precise and conscious even if verbal concepts are not at hand (this is probably what Mendelssohn meant when he claimed that music is not less precise but more precise than verbal language). At a transpersonal level the dualism

between subject and object (e.g. between a 'listener' and a 'musical object') is dissolved, and this experience transcends verbal language, even if it is conscious and clear (Bruscia 2000; Raffman 1993; Ruud 1998a).

Some disagreements and differences between theorists can be understood by observing that different concepts or discourses on music are related to different qualities and properties of music. Again we let Even Ruud and Ken Bruscia (re)present two relevant theoretical models.

Ruud (1990) has presented a model of four levels of music, distinguishing between four basic properties and four levels of experience, understanding and analysis:

- The physiological level – corresponding to music as a physical sound phenomenon: the 'material' properties. An analysis on this level has focus on the physiological effects and medical potential of music. *Music as stimulus.*

- The syntactical level – corresponding to music as an aesthetic phenomenon: the organized or structured musical elements. An analysis on this level (traditional academic musical analysis) has focus on a precise description and interpretation of musical elements, their role in the musical process, their interplay and functions in the therapeutic interaction. *Music as therapy.*

- The semantic level – corresponding to music as expression and meaning: the 'message' of the music or its references to an external or internal world. An analysis on this level has focus on the interpretation of the music as metaphor, icon, index or symbol, and the meaning of the music for the client, the interplay and the therapeutic relationship. *Music in therapy.*

- The pragmatic level – corresponding to music as a social, interactive phenomenon: the role of music in the theraputic process or the social context. An analysis on this level has focus on the potentials of musical interaction and its effects in treatment. *Music as communication and social interaction.*

According to Even Ruud an analysis can never be 'neutral' or 'objective'; it will always be influenced by the orientation, axioms and bias of the theorist or clinician. The 'meaning of the music' will always be (re)constructed in the context of the analysis, and this will influence the results. A human being constructs the narrative of himself/herself and his/her life, and music can play a very important role in the construction of identity. How this role is played can be researched by investigating how the person attaches meaning to specific music selections, and how music is related to important life events (Ruud 1997, 1998a Chapter 3).

A different view on meaning in music is advanced by Ken Bruscia who has presented a systematic overview of what he calls 'The six dynamic models of Music Therapy' (Bruscia 1998a, Chapter 15). His point of departure is that 'to analyse the dynamics of music therapy is to analyse the various ways in which the client experiences music' (p.132), and the needs of the clients are typically met by their therapists in one of six 'design models', each focusing on one of six basic properties of music: objective, universal, subjective, collective, aesthetic, transpersonal (see Figure 1.6). Bruscia has based his model on Wilber's quadrant model (see Chapter 2.2). The first

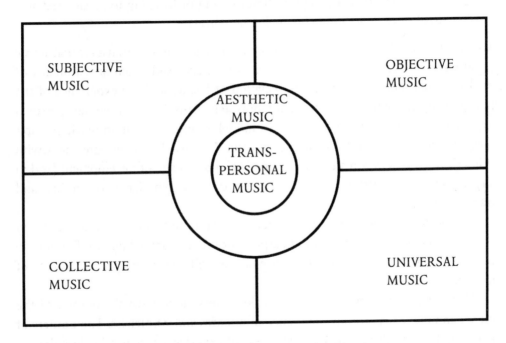

Figure 1.6 The six dynamic models of music therapy (Bruscia 1998)

four dynamic models are directly referring to Wilber's quadrants:

1. 'Music as objective experience' refers to practices using music's properties to 'directly influence the client's body or behaviour in an observable way' (following stimulus–response patterns documented by research).

2. 'Music as universal energy form' refers to practices using music as a 'living energy form' (universally appraised sounds and vibration patterns

with healing properties and/or music as a manifestation of organic principles of order and balance found in nature).

3. 'Music as subjective experience' refers to practices using musical processes and/or products as representations of the client 'and how s/he relates to the world of self, other, and object' (improvising or listening to music as an exploration of the client's values, relationships to self and others in a meaningful way).

4. 'Music as a collective (or socio-cultural) experience' refers to practices where the choice and use of music is placed within a larger, socio-cultural framework, in order 'to provide a shared identity of people who belong to a community' (improvising or listening to music used as a ritual or re-enacting archetypal experiences).

The last two models – 5. aesthetic music experiences and 6. transpersonal music experiences – refer to types of musical experience accessible from or within any of the four other models: both the appreciation of beauty and the experience of the transpersonal realm transcend the quadrant system. Bruscia has placed transpersonal experiences of music at the centre of his model 'to indicate that, in music therapy, they are accessed through the aesthetic realm' (p.134). This is in agreement with Wilber's theory, as he stresses that any person at any stage of development (and in any of the quadrants) can have a profound peak experience of higher and transpersonal states.

The *aesthetic properties of music* make it possible for the client to experience beauty and meaning, in the music itself or in aspects of life represented by or referred to in the music (in all four quadrants). An analysis will focus on specific aspects of meaning and its musical context.

The *transpersonal properties of music* make it possible to cross the borders of the model and move towards an experience of oneness and wholeness. The borders of music analysis are also crossed: this modality of experience can only be described to a limited extent.

In this context we will not make an evaluation of the two models, their similarities and differences, advantages and disadvantages. We regard them as two highly qualified suggestions for theoretical and analytical levels of meaning. A clinician may use them to reflect on his/her personal concept of music and music experiences and eventually use one of the models as a theoretical framework for clinical practice or research.

We shall continue the discussion of meaning in music in Chapter 2.4. Here we present two very important and helpful approaches, in our opinion, to music as/in therapy: music as analogy and music as metaphor. Both approaches have their limitations, and they do not systematically cover all four levels in Ruud's model or all six types of experience in Bruscia's model. The investigation of music as analogy and metaphor has focus on the relationship between what Ruud calls the syntactic and the semantic level. In Bruscia's model it refers primarily to subjective and aesthetic music experiences.

CHAPTER 2

Theoretical Foundations
of Music Therapy

2.1 The Psychology of Music

Knowledge of music psychology is essential for music therapists. Knowledge concerns basic processes in the ear and in the brain, which are the physiological preconditions of music perception, as well as the psychological preconditions of music experience and musical preferences. Erdonmez (1993) has formulated it this way:

> I believe that we, as music therapists, can add to the knowledge of brain functions in that we work with a highly creative art form, which activates many areas of the brain. We need to work alongside psychologists and neuropsychologists in order that we are better informed about the effects of music on brain functions, and so we can better inform other professionals about our clients' non-verbal functioning level. (1993, p.123)

The psychology of music is a relatively new area of study, and is not established as a profession or a research field in all European countries, but from an international perspective the psychology of music can be characterized as an exciting interdisciplinary science at the point of intersection between musicology, psychology, acoustics, sociology, anthropology and neurology. Important topics within this area include:

- the function of music in the life and history of mankind
- the function of music in the life and identity of a person
- auditory perception and musical memory
- auditory imagery

- the brain's processing of musical inputs

- the origin of musical abilities and the development of musical skills

- the meaning of music and musical preferences for the forming of identity

- the psychology of music performance and composition.

There is no international consensus concerning the classification of the areas and topics of music psychology. This becomes obvious in a comparison of the contents in different recognized handbooks. Deutsch (1982, 1999 second edition), who has edited one of the few handbooks within the cognitive tradition, emphasizes topics in music perception. The same can be said about Hodges (1980, 1996a second edition). However, the German literature is very different from the American. Bruhn *et al.* (1985) place the basic questions of music psychology in a cultural and social context, while Motte-Haber (1985) makes knowledge of music a central category. She also breaks explicitly with the positivistic tradition in music psychology, and her handbook is based on a humanistic view of man and music.

Natural science and humanistic views exist side by side, and we consider them complementary and equally important. Within the tradition of natural science, music psychology research is characterized by experimental studies, structured observation of behaviour, standardized inventories and tests etc., while research within the humanistic tradition prefers the use of interviews, participant observation, self-inquiry, narratives and hermeneutic interpretation.

It is possible to make a distinction between a psychological understanding of a *single tone* and *music*. The first type is concerned with the study of human response to delineated and carefully defined stimuli (tones, rhythms, sounds), while the latter studies the experience of complex, often naturally produced phenomena (melodies, musical interaction). Contemporary cognitive music psychology is predominantly concerned with *music*, while *single tone stimuli* historically formed the core of music psychology (see below). Theories and research results emerging from studies in the psychology of music have had, and still have, significant influence on music education and music therapy.

In this chapter we shall present a sketch of the history of music psychology and then narrow the focus to five important areas that are foundational for the study of music therapy, irrespective of whether the reader's inclination goes to natural or humanistic science:

1.   psychoacoustics and the auditory system

2.   music and the brain: neurological aspects of musical experience

3.   music faculty and hemispheric dominance

4.   early responses to music and sound in child development

5.   emotional effects of music.

Other important areas of music psychology have separate entries in the book: the physiological effects of music are discussed in Chapter 3.6, and the relationship between music and language in Chapter 2.4.

The chapter ends with a commentary on the status of contemporary cognitive music psychology.

The history of music psychology

As an independent area of theory and research the psychology of music developed in the last decades of the nineteenth century, when the first laboratories were set up. The major names of this early phase are Helmholz, Stumpf, Riemann and (in the USA) Seashore, who established the psychology of music as a recognized scientific discipline in its own right. This first phase (1880–1920) was characterized by experimental research based on a positivistic paradigm: music was considered an objective, empirical phenomenon, and the aim of research was to observe and measure human responses to selected sound stimuli, with special focus on the basic parameters of any tone or sound – frequency, amplitude, intensity and wave form. This was the foundation of the empirical study of auditory discrimination skills (*tone* psychology) and the later development of musical tests (Seashore) and behaviouristic music psychology (Lundin). The basic theoretical assumption was that sensory perceptions are stored in memory in a way that can be mapped and described exactly.

The development of tests of musical skill, aptitude, preference and many other aspects of musical behaviour was a crucial step for the practical application of music psychology in music education. Together with observational methods they made it possible to study the effect of music teaching and practice, measuring positive or negative change (or lack of change) over time in selected dependent variables. Early research in musical aptitude was based on the distinction of musical capacities in sub-domains that could be studied and evaluated separately. This classical cause-effect paradigm was later replaced by a more pragmatic, interactive understanding of music perception and cognition. Contemporary research studies focus on naturalistic conditions, e.g. practising by high level students, situated music learning in different cultures or the development of representation in the process by which a child perceives and interprets music. The developments of and controversies within the history of music psychology are reflected in the understanding of *musi-*

cality (musical aptitude etc.) in different paradigms (positivistic, Gestalt, behavioural, anthropological etc. – see Jørgensen 1988).

In the 1920s and 1930s new theories were developed from a Gestalt point of view, in USA by Mursell (1937) among others, and in Germany by Kurth, who pioneered a shift of paradigms with his holistic *Musikpsychologie* (1931). Kurth did not reject classical *tone* psychology; however, he wanted to see it in a new context: sub-components and single perceptions should be understood within the 'flowing' totality of *'music as experienced'*. Kurth's psychology of music is in fact a general theory of music, a systematic theory of musical phenomena and the psychological experience of 'power, energy, tension, volume and mass' in music.

After World War II behaviourism had a decisive influence on the psychology of music, e.g. Lundin's *An Objective Psychology of Music* (1967), in which the scientific study of musical behaviour became the core of music psychology. Also, within the psychoanalytic tradition, a more or less coherent understanding of music was developed, using the theoretical framework of Freud and later ego psychology (Feder *et al.* 1990, 1993; Kohut 1950).

The latest important 'wave' is the so-called cognitive psychology of music, today represented in Europe by the European Society for the Cognitive Sciences of Music (ESCOM), supporting theory and research through international conferences and the interdisciplinary journal *Musicae Scientiae*.

The majority of recent important European contributions to the literature on music psychology belong to this tradition (Hargreaves 1986, Hargreaves and North 1997; Sloboda 1985, 1988, 1995).

Relevant areas for music therapy

PSYCHOACOUSTICS

An understanding of psychoacoustics, or one's perception of music, is important in considering variability in how people hear and perceive musical sounds. Psychoacoustics includes a number of elements such as timbre, volume, pitch and duration. Timbre defines the quality of the sound. For example, a sinusoidal sound wave is the simplest and purest sound and, apart from sound waves produced by function generators, the closest we achieve by non-electronic means to a sinusoidal sound wave is a note played a flute, or a young child's voice. Most sound waves are far more complex than a single pitch. All naturally produced sounds are made up of the following elements: 1. the fundamental pitch, 2. the harmonic series (other pitches that are related in direct ratio to the fundamental pitch), 3. other pitches (pitches that are not directly related to the fundamental pitch) caused by acoustic factors e.g. in a conical shaped pipe (oboe, bassoon, trumpet etc.), as the sound wave travels along the gradually widening bore, new pitches arise, 4. subjective pitches, 5. noise (random frequencies including the transient).

Sound travels in waves not unlike the ripples on the surface of a pond when one throws a pebble in. The difference is that the waves of a sound travel in three dimensions not two – so one could imagine ever-increasing spherical ripples radiating from the source. The ripples in the pond are caused by an original displacement of water; in sound it is air molecules that are displaced causing ripples of air density. These ripples, as they spread out at a speed of approximately 1100 feet per second (720 mph), eventually die down with the friction of the 'still' air molecules being displaced. If the air ripples should meet any other molecules the ripples will attempt to displace these too. So, for instance, if the ripples come into contact with a stone wall, they would attempt to make the stone wall molecules ripple as well but, because the molecules of stone are of a different construction, there is so much *resistance* that a considerable amount of energy is lost and the remainder bounces off.

Sound waves that contact a human body attempt to do the same thing and we can perceive these ripples or vibrations as tingling sensations on different parts of our body. The thinner the layer of molecules, the easier it becomes for sound waves to displace them at the same rate. Therefore, the most sensitive receptor to the movement of air compressions is the very thin membrane in the ear called the tympanic membrane or eardrum. It is interesting to note that eyelids and fingertips are among the most sensitive receptors to certain frequencies of sound reported by people with hearing loss. This is partly explained by the thin membrane in the eyelid, but in the case of fingertips by the dense concentration of nerve endings found here.

Intensity represents the loudness of the sound. Intensity is measured in decibels, a measure that represents the actual loudness of the sound, whereas the subjective experience of the loudness of the sound varies depending on how individuals perceive it.

Pitch can be measured in two ways: 1. how many waves occur in a given distance or 2. how many waves occur at a given time. It is the second method that is usually used. Therefore there are 440 cycles (of waves) per second in the modern concert A – the faster the vibrations, the higher the pitch, and therefore the shorter the waves (the slower the vibrations, the lower the pitch, and therefore the longer the waves).

Duration is an important element in sound as the medium in which intensity, pitch and timbre are expressed. The measurement for the length of time it has taken to hear these elements begin and end is called duration. Intensity, pitch and timbre can all change in the duration of sound. These elements can be fairly consistent in a forced vibration such as a held note on a string or wind instrument. Otherwise, they can be changeable as in a guitar or piano.

THE EAR

In music therapy training and practice, an understanding of the ear, its function and malfunctions related to it is of significant relevance as the medium of therapy is primarily sound. Hearing loss caused by ear disorders and diseases in the outer, middle and inner ear such as otitus media, inflammation, otosclerosis and tinnitus are potentially present in many populations with whom music therapists work, and an understanding of the range and type of hearing tests is also relevant and necessary. Many music therapists have worked with children and adults with hearing impairment, most notably Claus Bang from Denmark, and Clive and Carol Robbins from New York. The value of music to hearing impaired people cannot be underestimated, especially when they achieve the highest levels of musical skill, as is the case with the world famous percussionist, Evelyn Glennie, who has a reported 95% hearing loss. Music therapists also have to be aware of problems associated with hearing, where sound is distorted, and people develop hyperacusis, or a hypersensitivity to certain frequencies and sounds. This is increasingly evident, for example, in children and adults with autistic spectrum disorder.

The ear is a complex part of the body, where the reception and interpretation of sound stimuli is a remarkable process. The outer ear (pinna) is there to catch sounds, and certain frequencies (2 kHz to 5 kHz) are boosted by the outer ear. This is an important area for speech sounds. We hear binaurally and the distance between our two ears helps us to locate the direction of sound and calculate its distance from us. We can also distinguish foreground sounds from background sounds. As the sounds travel down the ear canal, which is shaped like a funnel, they are concentrated onto the tympanic membrane or eardrum.

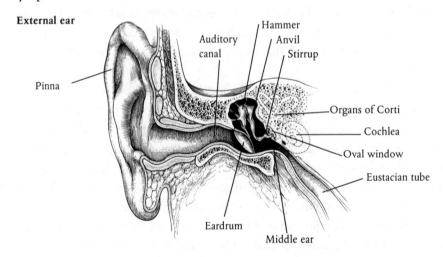

Figure 2.1 The outer and middle ear

The tympanic membrane is a translucent piece of elastic flesh, a quarter of an inch in diameter and three thousandths of an inch thick. It is remarkable that it can receive and process every vibration from an large orchestra, choir or audience and it can vibrate as a whole or in segments in order to fully perceive the complex array of sounds. It is a very complex form of vibration and it is a mystery how it can collect so many vibrations. Sound is transmitted into the middle ear in which three small bones, the hammer (malleus), anvil (incus) and stirrup (stapes), convey the sound through the middle ear. Without these bones, the sound would go straight to the cochlea and 97 per cent would bounce back and be lost. These bones are in constant action, and perceive sound even during sleep. The louder the sounds, the greater the movement of these bones. At birth, these bones are fully formed (they are the only bones in the body which don't grow) and as we age, they deteriorate and grow more rigid. Therefore one can experience a loss of hearing in upper frequencies with increasing age.

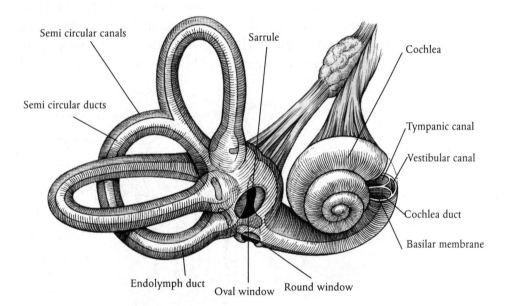

Figure 2.2 The inner ear

The sound moves through into the inner ear where the cochlea receives the sounds. Vibrations pass through the fluid in the cochlea and stimulate hair cells which fire and transmit the signal through afferent cells (i.e. cells going to the brain). Frequencies of the sounds are encoded by whichever hair cells are firing. Our actual discrimination of frequency is less than one fiftieth of a semitone. The auditory nerve transmits the sounds which are now converted into electrical impulses to the thalamus, and therefore into the cerebellum. The thalamus integrates all incoming data and relays it to appropriate areas of the cortex, in this case to the auditory cortex.

MUSIC AND THE BRAIN: NEUROLOGICAL ASPECTS OF MUSICAL EXPERIENCE

Many parts of the brain are involved in the appreciation of music and the performance of music. In studies on the responses of the brain to music, neurologists are particularly concerned with components of musical life in relation to a person's capacity to read, comprehend, compose or perform music. Modern neurology emerged from around 1850, with the development of concepts around the localization of function in the brain. Some German neurologists analysed disturbances of musical function in patients with brain disease and attempted to find the responsible lesions. Knoblauch introduced the term 'amusia', which means an impaired capacity for musical activity. Sensory amusia is the inability to hear, read or understand music, while motor amusia is difficulties in singing or writing music, or instrumental performance. These amusias were initially attributed to lesions in the left, or dominant, hemisphere of the brain. However, research has shown that it is not that simple, and different aspects of musical activity will be impaired by either right, left or localized

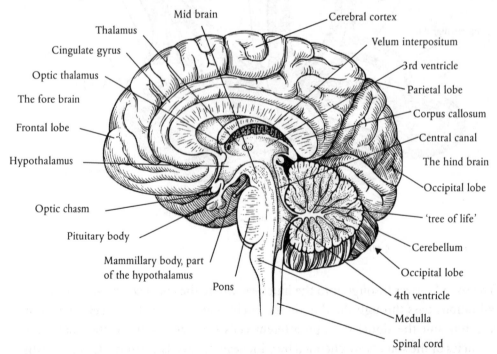

Figure 2.3 Medial view of the brain, showing brain stem, limbic cortex and cerebral cortex

cerebral damage. Experiments involving the temporary paralysis of function in the right hemisphere resulted in defects in singing, and the perception of melody, while speech remained intact. Conversely, temporary paralysis to the left side of the brain (or permanent damage as in the case of a stroke) revealed that people could sing much better than they could speak. This has been utilized in music therapy by music therapists working with stroke victims (Taylor 1997; Tomaino 1998).

It is not possible to localize creative activities such as composition or performance within the brain. Only elementary physiological activities can be assigned to different areas of the cortex. More complex activities depend on several appropriate parts of the brain, linked together by subcortical and interhemispheric pathways. Composition, performance and listening all require the senses of sight and hearing, intellectual and emotional functions, and sensory motor activity. This tells us that these activities involve the cerebral cortex, the subcortical motor and sensory nuclei, and the limbic system. We combine the more structuring, mathematical and organizing functions of our left brain with the creative, emotional and 'spiritual' right brain to balance all the elements in musical activity. We now know that the theories of hemispheric specialization at least don't apply to music activity, although damage or impairment in a specific area of the brain can reduce an important component of musical function. For example, a case was reported of a female music teacher who suffered a right side stroke. In rehabilitation, she found that while she could still play scales and arpeggios, she had lost the creative capacity to extend a melody. Another case was of a man who had lost his aesthetic appreciation of classical music. Investigations using a Positron Emission Tomography (PET) scan revealed that there was a shortage of blood supply approaching 10 per cent to the right temporal lobe of the brain, perhaps indicating that this area is important in the appreciation of complex art forms.

The auditory system, visual system, somatic motor and sensory systems and memory all play an important role in the appreciation and performance of music. For example, auditory imagery, the ability to hear with one's 'inner ear' the music you want to play or compose, is highly developed in musicians. Beethoven must have had a remarkable capacity, considering early onset of hearing impairment in no way reduced his capacity for increasingly complex music, as he carried musical composition from the classical style into the romantic style.

Memory is also well developed, and you cannot undertake a simple musical task without using memory. The enjoyment of any listener in hearing a piece of music is conditioned by his memories of similar melodic and harmonic passages. Sensory motor and visual memories are particularly necessary for performance.

There are many examples of amazing skills in musical memory. When he was only 14 years old, Mozart wrote down the whole of Allegri's *Miserere* (an elaborately ornamented choral work composed in nine parts for two choirs) after hearing it in the Sistine Chapel. Mendlessohn also did the same thing, and on one occasion, when the score of *A Midsummer Night's Dream* was left in a taxi, he wrote it out again from memory. There are many examples of musicians' ability to memorize and play music without the score. Even more remarkable is a person's capacity to memorize and play music just from hearing it, without ever seeing a score. This skill was found recently in a 16 year old man with autism. He could listen to music in sections, played on a tape recorder, and then reproduce it almost exactly after only hearing it once. He had a mental age of eight, and would be described as an *idiot savant*.

MUSIC FACULTY AND CEREBRAL DOMINANCE

As has already been stated, dominance for one skill, such as visual and tactile processing or verbal skills, can no longer be attributed to one hemisphere of the brain alone. Although singing appears to be a function of the right hemisphere, songs have lyrics – language – which is controlled by functions of the left hemisphere. One question raised by Critchley in his book *Music and the Brain* (1977) was: 'If we talk with our major (left) hemisphere and sing with our minor (right) hemisphere, by what method do we cope with intermediate vocalisation [sic], such as chanting?' Music differs from verbal language in its intimate structure as a code, and the way it is used by human beings in society. The fact that music is not used as a primary language or means of communication explains why people show such differences in their ability to appreciate music, or in the way performances of music reflect different interpretations. Music therapists have to pay particular attention to this point. While the concept of the 'language of music' providing a framework for communication is a core idea in music therapy, it has to be understood more as a framework, not as a precise language with consistently understood meaning.

The argument about hemispheric localization in terms of music function continues, and there are a number of contradictory studies. Earlier studies indicated that there was a connection between amusia and aphasia (loss of speech). However, recently other case reports have contradicted this. In the research on music perception, Milner (1962) suggested that the right hemisphere is overwhelmingly concerned with musical activity. Perhaps a good compromise is found in the study by Bever and Chiarello (1974), who found that naive listeners perceive melody in a Gestalt fashion, while musically experienced listeners tend to look at relationships between musical elements. Therefore they produced the hypothesis that a holistic appreciation is carried out by the right hemisphere, whereas the detailed analysis of the musical 'patchwork' will be carried out by the left.

Conclusions from the research can be summarized in this way:

- We don't have enough data for a good theory regarding musical ability and cerebral dominance.

- Musical faculty and cerebral dominance for verbal language are not intimately related.

- There is evidence of a developing cerebral dominance for certain features of musical faculty:

  1. a right hemisphere dominance in musical performance, independent of knowledge and training
  2. variable dominance for musical perception – mainly right hemisphere for untrained or naive people, developing into left hemisphere dominance in the case of more musically sophisticated people.

EARLY DEVELOPMENT OF MUSICAL RESPONSES AND SKILLS IN CHILDREN

Some traditions in music therapy are based on early mother–baby interaction, and the therapeutic relationship can be perceived as involving elements of vocal and gestural behaviour from this early stage. Our early experiences of sound are very formative. For example, singers find that their unborn babies are quieter when they are singing, and mothers who play instruments notice that their unborn children become more active while they are playing. There is an increase in body tension in crying babies, and while low frequencies seem to have pleasant associations, high frequencies have unpleasant ones. It has also been suggested that one attraction of 'beat', pop or very rhythmic music is the emotional link with the security of the mother's womb. Tapes have been produced of the sounds of the womb, including the sound of the placenta and the blood movement in the pulses from the umbilical chord. They were used with newborn infants prone to long periods of crying to try and calm them. Babies only react to about a third of the available acoustic stimuli in their first hours of life, but this rapidly increases, and the first six months is the period of 'learning to hear'. After 11 to 12 weeks babies prefer human voices to other noise. At 12 to 14 weeks they can discriminate between their mother's voice and a stranger's, and between 14 to 16 weeks they can stop crying when they hear their mother's footsteps.

Helmut Moog wrote a lot about the early development of musical responses, noting the attention of infants to music at four to six months, and the beginnings of repetitive movements to music after six months. He described the emergence of 'musical babbling' after speech babble has started, but that children sing their first 'babble song' before they say their first word. In tests on babies of six months, he found that rhythmic tests attracted little attention, whereas songs and instrumental music attracted the most active attention and movements. Babbling songs of 12-month children begin to show aspects of musical organization with pitched glissandi, downward melodic lines and four note figures (Moog 1976).

Singing has received more attention in children than any other aspect of musical development. In the last 30 to 40 years much has changed as televisions, tape recorders and CD players have replaced home-based music-making, and it is even questionable how many mothers still sing to their children. In a recent study on premature infants in Germany, only three out of a sample of 200 mothers said that they felt comfortable singing to their baby (Nöcker-Ribaupierre 1999).

Children produce two types of vocal music – chants and songs. Chants appear to evolve from speech, and the rhythm of the chant is the same as that of speech. The famous 'children's chant' – g g e a g e involving the minor third interval – is very characteristic. Children create chants and songs during play, and chanting is also a primitive musical art form used in tribal and religious ceremonies, not to mention modern day football matches and political rallies. The construction of simple songs begins at 12 months, with children gaining some concept of form in the music, developing phrases. At two years, spontaneous songs are emerging with repetitive phrases, clear pitches, melodic contours and rhythmic patterns. By three and a half, there is evidence of harmonic organization, and from four to six children make spontaneous 'pop' songs with original words. By the age of five, children have a wide repertoire of standard 'nursery' songs of their culture, and can perform recognition memory tasks better with these songs than with unfamiliar musical material (Hargreaves 1986).

There is some difference of opinion as to whether rhythmical skills develop before or after melodic skills, or independently. According to some researchers, rhythmic skills are probably the first to emerge and develop in the infant's response to music as seen in the early stages by different types of physical movement – rocking, nodding etc. Most studies of rhythmic development have investigated children's ability to produce regular patterns by tapping or clapping. Increasing levels of skill develop naturally with age, and are associated with rhythms in speech and songs.

For music therapists it is important to have some awareness of these early stages of development in music. For example, when working with people who are mentally handicapped, despite the fact that their chronological age may be anything between 10 and 80, if their mental age is at a pre-school, even pre-verbal level, one has to adapt expectations of their skills and abilities in producing or creating melody and rhythm. In interpreting musical engagement from the point of view of the therapeutic relationship, the fact that a person may perseverate or lose attention to maintaining a steady pulse or rhythm may not be due to emotional or interactive negativity, but is perhaps more linked to their musical stage of development.

EMOTIONAL EFFECTS OF MUSIC

Inherent in any approach or theory of music therapy is the concept of the emotional effect of music. Although music has the power to cause mental, physical, emotional and spiritual responses in us, beyond a few generalizations we don't completely understand how and in what way different types of music will affect us. Not everyone responds to music in the same way, and an individual does not necessarily respond to one composition the same way twice. Responses can be extremely intense, and depend on the likes and dislikes of certain types of music or the composer or performer.

Most research shows that the effects of music are greater when the music has more meaning for the listener. Because of its dynamic quality, our primary attraction to music is both physical and emotional. In a physical way, the music causes pressure waves that are felt bodily, and for the emotional effect, music creates mood environments to which we respond at a subconscious and non-verbal level. Our emotional reaction to music creates in us physical reactions – the goose-bump effect or when we feel the hairs on the back of our neck rising, tears coming into our eyes, our heart beating faster, and our breathing temporarily stopping. Physical reactions to certain types of music, in some of the same ways as just described, also cause us to experience emotional feelings. So what comes first when we are listening? The answer is that these reactions happen very fast, one after the other, and before we have had time to process the experience in our analytical brain. One thing is certain: you can't have the emotional response to music without the physical response – and vice versa. Music therapists can therefore observe and evaluate these reactions as part of their understanding of the client.

Emotional reactions are often due to associations, memories and past experiences that may have been good or bad. The English psychologist John Sloboda found that people's memories of their early experiences of music could be unpleasant – such as being told they can't sing by the school music teacher – or nice – the first time they heard Mozart's Clarinet Concerto and fell in love with the sound of the clarinet (Sloboda 1987, 1991). Music often has special significance between people when they fall in love, and songs or pieces hold treasured memories – what Sloboda described as the 'Darling, They're Playing Our Tune Again' phenomenon. In music therapy work with the elderly, they may often ask for children's songs, or Christmas carols. When played, tears of sadness or happy memories come, allowing the person to remember events in their life – happy or sad – and work through their feelings of loss as they come to the end of their life.

Whereas emotions result from responses to specific objects, situations or persons, moods have been called 'metaphysical generalisations [sic] of the emotions' which create feelings. Hevner's 'Mood Wheel' (1936) was a design to see how we can move through a sequence of moods to get, for example, from solemnity to excitement. The process of moving from one mood or emotion to another is part of the skill of the musician, composer, and certainly the music therapist. The mood of the music often needs to reflect the emotional state or mood of the patient to begin with before a subtle process of movement can occur. You can't suddenly change the mood in a depressed person by introducing light, fast, syncopated and amusing music into the improvization. Contrary to popular belief, music cannot express emotions with any degree of success, but rather creates moods to which we respond at an emotional level. This is mainly referring to instrumental music, because songs do express emotions, but do so primarily through the lyrics. Stravinsky once said 'music is, by its very nature, essentially powerless to express anything at all, whether a feeling, attitude of mind, psychological mood, or phenomenon of nature'. However, Mendelssohn suggested the opposite view that 'the thoughts which are expressed to me by a piece of music which I love are not too indefinite to be put into words, but on the contrary are too definite'. Music essentially expresses mood qualities upon which we project a specific emotional meaning.

Conclusion: the relevance of the psychology of music for music therapy

Many music therapists' first associations to 'the psychology of music' are probably still 'tests of isolated perception skills' or 'controlled experimental studies of limited relevance for clinical practice'. Brain research using PET scanning and other compli-cated high-tech procedures may also come to their mind. Of course all three areas of research mentioned are included in the repertory of modern music psychology. However, it is also important to say that contemporary studies have a much more holistic and naturalistic outlook, including a diversity of music experiences in all sorts of contexts. For the same reason these studies are very often relevant for music therapy clinicians. Let us give a few examples of this.

For decades the developmental psychology of music was dominated by the stage theories of Piaget (Hargreaves 1986), but now there is a variety of theories on the musical development of the child understood as a complex and interactive process (Briggs 1991; Hargreaves 1986, 1992; Swanwick 1994). Current developmental psychology of music relates to general developmental psychology, especially the theories of Daniel Stern (1985, see also Hannibal 2001) and Colwyn Trevarthen (Trevarthen and Malloch 2000). These researchers have documented that 'musical patterns of behaviour' are inborn and have the function as a biological and psychological basis of human communication. Studies of musical development are no longer limited to childhood and youth; man's relationship to music is a lifelong developmental process, as reflected in 'life span music psychology' (Bruscia 1991). Bruscia also demonstrates how the disturbance of normal development in specific phases leads to phase-specific problems or pathologies, which again require specific music therapy interventions.

The study of the emotional effects of music goes back to some of the classical experiments of music psychology. Already, in 1936 Hevner developed her systematic model of emotions, or rather moods, that can be expressed in music in a way that a listener can recognize it. Hevner's 'Mood Wheel' (Figure 2.4) has been criticized, but it still plays an important role in music therapy.

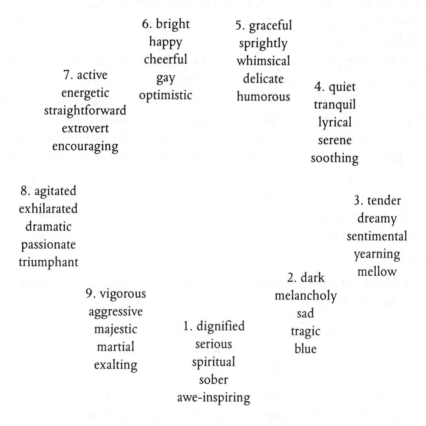

Figure 2.4 Hevner's 'Mood Wheel' (revised version). Category 7 is an addition that allows the inclusion of forms of popular music (Bonde 1997)

It is used as a tool to classify music in Guided Imagery and Music (see Chapter 3.1.), where it is useful to match the mood of the client in the first music sequence of a session (the 'ISO principle'). New research gives us a growing body of knowledge on the relationship between feelings, emotions, moods and music (Gabrielsson 1993, 1995, 1999; Pavlicevic 1995, 1997).

Musical preferences, their foundation and development and their role in music education and music therapy are a rather new research area. However, it is clear that especially the preferences (and 'code confidentiality') of adults set a practical limit to the choice of music in a clinical context (Bonde 1997).

Jørgensen (1988) has defined the 'psychology of music experience' as a specific area. In this book a great number of research studies are reviewed, and many of them are relevant for clinical practice. One of the most interesting topics is the study of 'strong (or peak) experiences of music', relating to Maslow's concept 'peak experience' (see Chapter 2.3).

The role of music in the formation of personal identity has been studied extensively by Ruud during the last decade. The most important results are presented in the book *Musikk og identitet/Music and Identity* (Ruud 1997, English summary in Ruud 1998).

The cognitive psychology of music is the dominating trend in current music psychology. It includes, and has renewed, the classical area of music perception studies, and it has developed a whole range of new research areas. Amongst the most important of these are the psychological aspects of music performance, improvisation and composition – as reflected in the title of one of the many publications of the British music psychologist John Sloboda. We will end this chapter by quoting 'five basic assumptions' presented by Sloboda in the preface to the book *Generative Processes in Music. The Psychology of Performance, Improvisation and Composition* (Sloboda 1988). In our opinion these assumptions are equally important in music education and music therapy. Sloboda writes that cognitive music psychologists agree that:

1. Music generative capacity is inherent in all human beings, although it may be developed to a greater or lesser extent.

2. The capacity to generate any but the most primitive musical sequences is based on the ability to derive sound sequences from higher-order structures or rule systems.

3. These rule systems have some universal constraints on them (arising from general facts about human cognitive capacity) but incorporate specific constraints picked up from the prevailing musical culture.

4. Specific instruction is not necessary for skill acquisition, but practice is. Through practice, and possibly through general developmental changes, similar stages in skill acquisition can be observed in several generative domains.

5. Many aspects of skill become partly automated, and not open to conscious introspection. Their nature must therefore be elucidated by observation and analysis of generative behaviour rather than (or in addition to) verbal self-report. (Sloboda 1988)

2.2 Theory of Therapy and Psychotherapy

Music therapy has been significantly and diversely influenced by the historical development of therapy, where therapy is defined as a form of treatment administered by a therapist. Over the years, three main therapeutic schools have emerged for the treatment of mental illness, emotional disturbance and psychological disorders:

*   Psychoanalytic/psychotherapeutic: this model of therapy incorporates a wide variety of approaches which place the 'unconscious' as the source of emotional disturbance. Therefore, exploring and understanding hidden or 'unconscious' drives and feelings provides the main focus for therapeutic intervention.

*   Behaviour therapy: this approach generally regards only obvious behaviour as significant, and therapeutic approaches tend to focus on the treatment and modification of behaviour.

*   Traditional neuropsychiatry: this approach considers physiological or chemical disorders to be the primary cause of emotional disturbance and as a consequence uses medication or primarily physiological methods as the therapeutic intervention.

In the development of music therapy, the first two models have formed the primary, therapeutic foundation for the development of music therapy theory and music therapy practice. The early development of music therapy in the USA was predominantly linked with theories of behaviourism and behaviour therapy although, in recent times in certain areas, particularly the East Coast, psychotherapeutic and psychoanalytic approaches are also common. However, the main foundation for many therapists trained in the American school of music therapy is behavioural.

In Europe, psychotherapeutic and psychoanalytic approaches have become more dominant. There is not a clear division, and therapists are significantly influenced by both their teachers and the forms of therapy that they have experienced.

There are some schools which advocate an eclectic model, teaching a variety of therapeutic theories which can be applied depending on the client group with whom one works. The arguments in favour of this are that the needs of patients differ widely, and while the complex emotional and psychological problems presented by clients in acute psychiatry may be well served through a psychotherapeutic model of intervention, clients with severe learning disability and challenging behaviour might respond better to a more behavioural approach. Activity-based music therapy, with reinforcement and positive reward-based programs, is very different from depth psychology, involving the exploration of the past and a development of understanding where the current behaviour and personality of the client has emerged from.

However, some argue that it is impossible to be an eclectic music therapist, whereby one might switch one's therapeutic approach from one client to another depending on their profile and needs. The development of the therapeutic method with which one feels comfortable and which suits one's own individual personality and style of work often starts when students select the course of study which they wish to follow, and they can't be 'behavioural' one day and 'psychoanalytic' the next. Some music therapists recognize this early on, and will refer on clients for whom they feel their particular approach may not be suitable. Others may not immediately recognize the need for an alternative therapeutic approach to meet the needs of the client and may attempt to use their own particular method irrespective of the primary needs of the client.

On music therapy courses, it is valuable for students to have a clear understanding of different models of therapeutic approach, based on the theory of therapy, even though they are typically being trained in a particular style of work. In addition to that, psychotherapy is a very 'broad church' ranging from a spectrum of cognitive behaviour therapy through to analytical, existential and person-centred therapy. The approach used can very clearly be differentiated by two main parameters:

- the nature of the relationship between the client and the therapist

- the goals or expectations of therapy.

Behavioural approaches

Behaviour therapy is a relative newcomer on the psychotherapy scene and did not emerge until the late 1950s as a systematic approach to the assessment and treatment of psychological disorders. Originating with the work of Ivan Pavlov, contemporary behaviour therapy now includes *applied behaviour analysis*, neo-behaviouristic mediational stimulus-response models, social learning theory and cognitive behaviour modification.

Applied behaviour analysis promoted by the work of Skinner (1953) relies on operant conditioning, where the fundamental assumption is that behaviour is a function of its consequences. Techniques such as reinforcement, punishment, extinction and stimulus control are derived from laboratory research.

Neo-behaviouristic mediational stimulus-response therapy comes from the learning theories of Pavlov and others, and involves the use of intervening variables and hypothetical constructs. Central importance is assigned to anxiety, and many treatment techniques involve 'systematic desensitization' and 'flooding' in order to reduce or get rid of underlying anxiety that is assumed to maintain phobic disorders.

In social learning theory, the person themself is the agent of change and the theory emphasizes the human capacity for self-directed behaviour change as a result of cognitive processes which control what environmental influences are responded to, how they are perceived and how the individual interprets them.

Finally, cognitive behaviour, coming from the work of Ellis and Beck, is also based on a cognitive process where the person's interpretation of the experience can produce a psychological disturbance. The therapy therefore is orientated towards the alteration or modification of irrational ways of thinking or belief systems which affect a person's interpretation of the world and as a result, their behaviour within the world. Personality theory is also very important in the development of behaviour therapy, and many of the associated batteries of personality tests rely on a complex analysis of behaviour and ways of thinking in order to identify personality characteristics or traits that control or influence the way a person is behaving.

Almost all behavioural therapies have some common characteristics which can be summarized as follows:

1. Abnormal behaviour which provokes psychological illness is primarily related to 'problems of living' which might include anxiety reactions, sexual deviance or conduct disorders.

2. Abnormal behaviour is developed in the same way as normal behaviour and therefore can be treated through the application of behavioural procedures.

3. Assessment in behaviour therapy looks at what is happening now, rather than any historical antecedence. (This is not entirely true when relating to cognitive therapy and rational emotive therapy, where the

development of irrational ideas and belief systems has occurred over time since a very young age.) The person is best understood and described by what they do in particular situations. Understanding the origins of a psychological problem is not essential for producing behaviour change, and if you achieve success in changing or eliminating a problem behaviour, it also doesn't mean that knowledge has been gained about its origins or etiology [sic].

4.   Treatment involves the careful and detailed analysis of the different parts of the problem and then developing procedures to work on different elements. They are individually tailored to different problems for different individuals.

5.   Behaviour therapy is a scientific approach which includes a clear conceptual framework, a treatment drawn from experimental-clinical psychology, and therapeutic technique is something that can be measured objectively and replicated. (Wilson 1989)

The arguments in favour of behaviour approaches in therapy are that it can be measured, it solves the problem without going into a deep exploration of the origins of the problem or the history of the patient and that it is faster and more effective. In many ways, it is a process by which symptoms are treated but the cause is regarded as either irrelevant or chronic and therefore unchangeable. In psychoanalytic approaches, a patient may spend 20 years exploring the origins of his/her personality and way of being, but still be faced with the everyday problems that have emerged as a result. Behaviour therapy, especially cognitive behaviour therapy, has become increasingly popular in psychiatry and psychology over recent years in hospitals and clinics in Europe and the USA because it is seen to effect change, particularly in clients who have very limited capacity to gain insight into the reasons why they are the way they are or behave as they do.

Psychotherapeutic and psychoanalytic approaches

The emergence of psychotherapy, since the work of Freud in the latter part of the nineteenth century and early twentieth century, has been exciting and diverse. Theories and methods have been built upon each other and styles of work have splintered off into a multiplicity of methods, many influenced by cultural influences and the state of society at a particular given moment. Psychotherapeutic approaches in therapy can be parochial, and ignorance or isolation can emerge because each different school knows little about the others. However, whichever school therapists are trained in, they will typically go through their own therapy. Therefore they succumb to a very strong influence which is more powerful than just being taught a theory or clinical methods. They believe in their therapeutic approach because they have experienced it themselves.

The main models that have influenced music therapy are psychoanalysis (Freud), analytical psychotherapy (Jung), person-centred therapy (Rogers), Gestalt therapy (Perls), existential psychotherapy (May and Yalom), transactional analysis (Berne) and, coming from this, the humanistic psychology group including Maslow and also Perls, and to some extent personal construct theory (Kelly), which has been used in music therapy research.

PSYCHOANALYSIS

Psychoanalysis is a process which continues the main tenet of Greek philosophy which is to 'know thyself'. It is a system of psychology derived from the discoveries of Sigmund Freud, and was developed as a method for treating particular psychoneurotic disorders. It has come to serve as a foundation for a general theory of psychology and has also been very important in understanding and treating many psychosomatic illnesses.

Psychoanalysis perceives the mind as the expression of conflicting forces and it is this element of conflict which emerges within human beings during their early development. The functioning of the mind is also related to events in the body and basic responses to stimuli are controlled by a natural human tendency to seek pleasure and to avoid pain (the 'pleasure principle' described by Freud in 1911). Freud constructed his theory in terms of a structural organization of the mind, and mental functions were grouped according to the role they played within this process of conflict.

ANALYTICAL PSYCHOTHERAPY

Carl Gustav Jung was a contemporary of Freud and shared many of his ideas. He developed a perspective of a relationship between the conscious and the unconscious through a symbolic approach. The psyche was perceived by Jung as a self-regulating system whose function is directed towards a life of fuller awareness. Therefore in analytical psychotherapy process, the dialogue that emerges uses dreams, fantasies and other unconscious products in order to explore the dialogue between the conscious state of the client and his/her personal as well as collective unconscious.

In his work Jung wrote extensively about the process of imagery and symbolism and these were brought into the therapeutic process in a very practical and important way. He formulated the idea of archetypes after a patient reported a hallucination in which the sun had a phallus that moved from side to side causing a wind. He related this to imagery from ancient times, a period of which the patient in question could have had no knowledge, and therefore he created a level of primordial imagery in the unconscious which could be common to all humanity. He called this the *collective unconscious*, and the images within it were described as archetypes. Freud could not accept this theory, and this was one of the reasons why these two pioneers parted and went their separate ways. Jung developed concepts such as the personal unconscious, the persona (the word originally meant the actor's mask), the shadow (understood as our 'other side' – which could be defined as a compensatory side to our conscious ego, as was seen in the case of Stevenson's *Dr Jekyll and Mr Hyde*, or Hans Christian Andersen's fairytale *The Shadow*), the animus and anima (central elements in the Chinese philosophy of yin and yang – the feminine and masculine elements) and the self (the archetype of the self as a god within ourselves).

Jung had a revolutionary approach to therapy and was ahead of his time with his insistence on a creative dialogue between the client and his/her unconscious. This therapeutic procedure is not limited to free associations (as in Freudian psychoanalysis); in Jung's *active imagination* the client amplifies and explores important symbols using creative writing and painting. A few articles report on Jung's view of music as a therapeutic modality. Contrary to Freud, who was negative towards music because he could not explain why he was influenced by it, Jung was able to see the therapeutic potential of music. Apparently, in Jung's consultation room, people danced, sang, acted, mimed and played musical instruments. The pianist and music therapist Margaret Tilly was invited to give Jung a music therapy session in 1956. She reported that Jung went deeply into the musical experience and that he recognized the possibilities in this non-verbal modality, considering it to be of very significant importance in reaching into the unconscious world of the patient.

PERSON-CENTRED THERAPY

Person-centred therapy, sometimes called client-centred therapy, was developed by the psychologist Carl Rogers as early as 1940. It has become very popular as the foundation for music therapy interaction and the music therapy relationship, as it relies on an equal term relationship between therapist and client and the development of trust. It allows clients considerably more power and decision-making in the therapy process, such as choosing the frequency and length of their therapy, whether they want to talk or be silent, what they want to explore and enables them to be the architects of their own lives. A primary concept is 'unconditional positive regard' for the client, where the therapist respects and accepts from the client whatever they wish to explore.

The development of this quality by the therapist towards the client is a process of genuine regard through empathy, and the importance of being empathic reflects the therapist's concern and interest in the client's world and the feelings of the client. A person-centred therapist greatly values the therapeutic relationship, encourages the client to determine the direction both in and out of therapy, accepts and respects the client's ways of thinking and perceiving, and relates to the client on a feeling level.

GESTALT THERAPY

Gestalt therapy was developed by Fritz and Laura Perls in the 1940s and teaches therapists and patients the phenomenological method of awareness in which perceiving, feeling and acting are distinguished from interpreting and rearranging pre-existing attitudes. The goal is for the clients to become aware of what they are doing, how they are doing it and how they can change themselves, while at the same time learning to accept and value themselves. It focuses much more on the process (what is happening) than content (what is being discussed) and so it involves a concept of here and now (*hic et nunc*). Gestalt therapy involves the phenomenological perspective which helps people stand aside from their usual way of thinking so that they can tell the difference between what is actually being perceived and felt in a current situation and what is coming from the past.

Field theory underlies Gestalt phenomenological perspectives, which is a method of exploring that describes the whole field of which the event is currently a part, rather than analysing the event in terms of a particular class to which it might belong by its nature.

The aim of Gestalt therapy, as stated by Laura Perls, is the awareness continuum – the freely on-going 'Gestalt' formation – where something that is of importance comes into the foreground where it can be fully experienced and coped with, so that when it goes back into the background it will leave the foreground free for the next relevant Gestalt.

This 'here and now' process is very congruent with music therapy practice, particularly in Europe (Frohne-Hagemann 1990; Hegi 1988), where through improvisational methods (e.g. *musical psychodrama*, Moreno 1999), experiences can be highlighted and the feelings experienced in the present.

The main goal of Gestalt psychotherapy is awareness – a greater awareness of a particular area, awareness of other people, awareness of the situation within which one is coping, awareness of problems and how to solve them and, at the end, the development of a greater and more enlightened self-awareness.

HUMANISTIC PSYCHOLOGY AND PSYCHOTHERAPY

Abraham Maslow labelled psychoanalysis and behaviourism 'the first and the second wave of modern psychology'. He was among the founders of the 'third wave'; together with, amongst others, Victor Frankl, Rollo May and Carl Rogers, who were all practising psychotherapists. Humanistic psychology criticised the positivist view of human nature – that man can be understood completely as a biological and social creature. Specific human features and phenomena like (peak) experiences, values, the search for meaning and psychological growth were highlighted and put on top of the psychological research agenda. A humanistic and anthropological view of human experience was formulated as an alternative to controlled experiments and statistical methods.

The rejection of determinism, as found in psychoanalysis and behaviourism, is a fundamental stance in humanistic psychology and therapy. Importance is attached to the 'here and now' situation (like in Gestalt therapy), to the therapeutic relationship and to the understanding of the client's problems. Free will is a free will to choose and change – no-one is determined forever by childhood traumas or conditioned responses. Humanistic psychotherapy is growth oriented and directed towards mild psychological problems and personal development (self-realization). The great 'therapy wave' that washed over the Western world from the 1960s is inextricably linked with the growth of humanistic psychology. Many music therapy models are growth oriented and founded on humanistic principles, and the understanding of the client–therapist relationship as an 'encounter' and an 'I–Thou' situation plays an important role in music therapy theory (Garred 1996).

TRANSPERSONAL PSYCHOLOGY AND PSYCHOTHERAPY

The fourth and last 'wave' in psychology is the so-called transpersonal psychology. In this tradition the focus is on the last element in the triad body–mind–spirit. Its spokesmen are inspired by Eastern spiritual and Western esoteric traditions and their procedures to (re)integrate the levels of the soul and the spirit in psychological theory and psychotherapeutic practice. In many reference books Ken Wilber (see Chapter 2.2) is labelled 'transpersonal psychologist', but the scope of his quadrant model (see Chapter 2.3) illustrates clearly why this is not the case. Already in 1983 Wilber announced his departure from transpersonal psychology – and today he considers 'the fourth force' of psychology as dead a phenomenon as 'psychology' itself. Wilber (2000) mentions four traditions or schools within transpersonal psychology:

1.   the magic-mythic group

2.   the altered states group

3.   the post-modern group

4.   the integral approach – which is no longer affiliated with transpersonal psychology (counting names like Roger Walsh, Frances Vaughan, Don Beck, Francisco Varela – and Wilber himself).

Thus we can say that integral psychology grew out of transpersonal psychology, but is no longer part of this movement or tradition (some of whose most important current representatives are Grof, Tarnas, Rothberg, Washburn and Lawlis).

Influences on music therapy – an overview

The development in music therapy in many countries in the world has been influenced by these theories and methods of therapy. In the USA, the pioneers of music therapy, E. Thayer Gaston and William Sears (Gaston 1995; Sears 1996) defined music therapy very much within the behavioural concept. Juliet Alvin, a concert cellist who developed a process of both remedial and psychotherapeutically based work, relied on developmental concepts, to some extent behavioural, but also strongly advocated the psychotherapeutic and psychoanalytic model of work. The course which she developed at the Guildhall is one of the so-called eclectic courses in music therapy. Mary Priestley, the main founder and pioneer of *analytical music therapy*, used both Freud and Jung in her development of therapeutic theory for music therapy. Nordoff and Robbins relied on the fields of anthroposophy and humanistic psychology and related more to existential and transactional therapeutic theories. They cite particularly the concepts of Abraham Maslow, including self-actualization and peak experiences, in their therapeutic process. Gestalt therapy is the basis of the theory and practice of Isabelle Frohne-Hagemann's and Fritz Hegi's work in central Europe and is also closely related to Moreno's musical psychodrama. Helen Bonny, the founder of Guided Imagery and Music, bases her model on a therapeutic foundation related closely to Jung's concept of symbolic representation and active imagery, to Stanislav Grof's theory of perinatal experiences and matrices and to transpersonal psychology. Latterly, the theories of post-Freudians such as Melanie Klein, Donald Winnicott, Margaret Mahler (*object relations theory*), Heinz Kohut (self-psychology) and Daniel Stern (psychology of intersubjectivity and interrelationship) have influenced and still influence the music therapy practices and theories in Europe.

Helen Bonny, the founder of Guided Imagery in Music, also founds her method on a therapeutic foundation related closely to Jung's concept of symbolic representation and imagery.

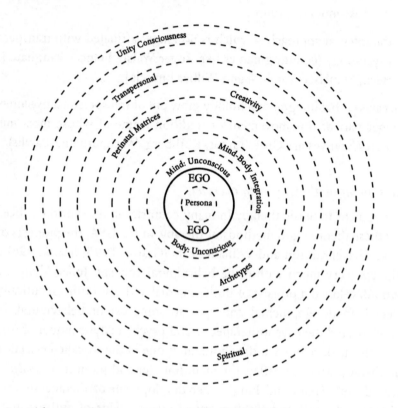

Figure 2.5: Helen Bonny's 'Cut Log' diagram. Bonny's model can be read from the centre. It illustrates how Freudian layers are overlayered by layers from the theories of Jung, Grof and Assagioli.

Several of the models and traditions mentioned are now introduced in greater detail in Chapter 2.3, as it is important to clarify the influence of psychoanalytic, psychotherapeutic and transpersonal theories on music therapy. There is evidence that music therapy theory has kept pace with modern development in these theories, and this is the object of discussion in Chapter 2.3. Further reference to these theories emerges in Chapters 3 and 4, which address clinical models and areas of clinical practice.

2.3 Analytical, Psychodynamic and Transpersonal Theories

Introduction

It is characteristic for many music therapists in Denmark and other European countries to base their professional identities on a humanistic, psychodynamic and music-psychological foundation. From this foundation the Aalborg University music therapy program teaches students basic skills and knowledge in the areas of music, psychotherapy and special education, as well as basic scientific tools for undertaking their work.

The theoretical background for understanding clinical work includes psychodynamic theories, theories of communication and theories of learning, as music therapy always involves work with contact and communication, whether or not the therapy is focused on training more specialized functions. For this reason music therapy includes, uses and develops theories from psychoanalysis and its offshoots in developmental psychology, Freudian-based psychoanalysis, ego psychology, object relations theories, self-psychology and transpersonal psychology. In addition, music therapy has found inspiration and models for understanding from many different theories of therapy and from the psychology of music. Depending on the client population receiving therapy, it can also be relevant to understand and describe clinical practice through communication theory and theories of learning.

Thus, music therapy theory and the growing science of music therapy rest on a compound theoretical foundation. The profession of music therapy must continually apply, critically regard and develop from existing theories in psychology, psychoanalysis, education, musicology, medicine and communication. Music therapists work and identify professionally within a field that is both art and science, a fact that can make establishing an identity as a music therapy 'scientist' complicated and multi-faceted.

In this chapter we will address some of the theories applied and developed by the music therapy profession.

Classical psychoanalysis

Music therapy in Denmark and Europe has been inspired by psychoanalytical and psychotherapeutic theories in the attempt to understand and describe the complex processes in music therapy with clients who are diagnosed with psychological and psychiatric problems.

Freud's description of the unconscious and his division of the psyche into id (containing drives and primitive wishes), ego (directing drives outwards in an acceptable form) and superego (controlling morals and values) has helped create a basis for the further development of psychoanalytical and psychotherapeutic theories.

Music therapy, however, has primarily used the *technical rules* and *clinical concepts* developed within classical psychoanalysis, rather than Freud's theories on the structure of the psyche. Within music therapy theory an attempt has been made to adapt these *technical rules* and *clinical concepts* to the reality of the music therapy setting, where the main instrument is music.

The aim of classical psychoanalysis (as originally described by Freud) was and is for the patient to discover himself/herself. The model of the therapist as helper is taken from the medical models of that time. The therapist is compared to the surgeon, who must be able to act in a neutral way in order to discern clearly and determine when and how to intervene. Psychoanalysis is primarily described and documented through these *technical rules* and *clinical concepts* and to a much lesser degree through psychological/theoretical concepts.

Technical rules such as *neutrality, abstinence, free-floating awareness* and *active listening* are the basis of the practice and understanding of classical psychoanalysis. Music therapy can be characterized as analytic, because these original *technical rules* and *clinical concepts* underlie the music therapist's questions concerning his/her role as therapist, and the therapeutic relationship – especially when working with psychological and/or psychopathological problems.

TECHNICAL RULES

One of the fundamental *technical rules*, the rule of the therapist's *neutrality*, is emphasized in psychoanalysis as a precept, whereby the analyst can create the right conditions for the analytical process to begin. The therapist must be without ambitions on his/her own or on the patient's behalf, in order to be available for the patient's needs, and he/she must maintain an objective, non-judgemental attitude and value-neutrality in relation to the patient's material. According to the psychoanalytical view, the therapist is expected to keep an emotional distance, showing at the same time an attentive and aware, non-involved interest in the patient. The analytical view is characterized by a balance between closeness and distance. The reason for the rule of neutrality is that the therapist should be able to create a projection screen for the patient's *transference*. The therapist must maintain a clear identity and autonomy and must not let himself/herself be drawn into the patient's disturbed object relations, but consistently represent reality to the patient.

In music therapy this rule of neutrality has to be redefined. The music therapist is an active participant in improvisational duets, and therefore cannot maintain neutrality in the same sense as in psychoanalysis. Instead, the music therapist must be aware of the way in which he/she is drawn into the patient's patterns of relationship and into his/her fantasy world. In music therapy there is a different form of balance between closeness and distance, as the music therapist is active – he/she reacts to the patient's music and at the same time participates in creating the shared musical expression. The music is not the patient's music alone. Distance is therefore not created by 'holding oneself outside of' appeals or emotional outbursts from the patient, but rather by listening attentively to what is happening at each moment in the music, and by structuring the music, so that it can accompany and make clear the patient's patterns in building and sustaining relationships.

Examples:

1. A patient plays fragmentally and moves quickly from one musical key to another on the piano. There is very little cohesion between the notes and the patient seems uninvolved in the music. Here the music therapist can create a fixed point in the music (a repeated rhythm, a note or a short melodic phrase) and try to 'lure' or 'call' musically, so that the patient becomes aware of the music. At the same time the therapist can vary the dynamics in order to reinforce the music's centerring function around the fixed point. In this way the patient can experience feeling more connected to the music and to the therapist while playing together. The patient's pattern of interaction, characterized by a fear of relatedness, can be changed through the non-verbal contact of the musical situation.

2. A patient is afraid of powerful expressions/outbursts (for example loud or angry-sounding music) and always plays softly in a slow walking tempo. The music therapist can gradually increase the tempo and the volume and thus confront the patient with the difficulty of keeping a slow tempo while someone else plays in a faster tempo. The patient can experience frustration and stop playing, which can then become the object of analysis and negotiation, or the patient can be seduced to play louder or faster and discover that it isn't dangerous to express oneself powerfully in a musical improvisation. This pattern of relating in a patient is most often characterized by a reluctance to express feelings and a fear of being rejected or of violence towards others if he/she expresses emotions. This pattern can change as the patient gradually has the courage to express himself/herself more dynamically in the music and discover that it isn't as dangerous as he/she believed.

3. A patient plays a melancholy melody on an instrument. The therapist can play sad, minor-sounding chords that give the music weight and

substance, while at the same time amplifying its emotional intensity and ability to contain and accompany sorrow and pain. In this case the patient can transform a feeling of resignation (everything is depressing, and I don't know what to do – I feel so small and powerless) into a feeling of having more 'inner space' to contain emotions (I can allow myself to contain suffering and can feel strong by taking part in a more complex and grand expression of these feelings). This patient's pattern of relating is characterized by a lack of belief in own self-worth and a failure to find the support of others meaningful. The musical involvement of the therapist can help the patient to transform his/her resignation into a feeling of substance and meaning – being able to contain and express difficult emotions in an aesthetically acceptable manner.

As can be seen in the above examples, the second original *technical rule* in classical psychoanalysis is *the rule of abstinence*. Here, the therapist must refrain from satisfying the patient's infantile needs and demands of love, and let needs and longings remain with the patient as a motivation for therapeutic work and change. This is also modified in music therapy. Again, it is rather the awareness of *how* the therapist satisfies the patient's needs that is the focus of analysis, as well as a clarification of the development in the relationship.

The third and last of the original technical rules, *the rule of free-floating awareness* (where the therapist remains in a *free-floating awareness* and refrains from prioritizing certain themes) is also modified in music therapy as it is in many other types of psychotherapy, especially short-term therapies. In music therapy there is generally an agreed upon objective or aim, and often partial aims during the process. Often *playing rules* are the starting point for the free improvisations. The improvisations originate from inner images, connected to memories or to emotions and moods that emerge in the moment. The musical improvisation can, however, also cause new images, emotions or moods to emerge, so the musical improvisation can be said to both express the theme/problem and at the same time work through and change the problem through the musical process and performance. The music therapist, just as the analyst, must be aware of which themes give way to new ones and which themes are repeated. The music therapist can often direct and hold the patient's attention to musical themes – by using the patient's themes in the shared improvisation and by further developing them.

Pedersen (1997, 2000b) has attempted to describe the music therapist's balance between closeness and distance with the concepts *listening perspectives* and *listening attitudes*. She describes listening attitudes and listening perspectives as tools for orientation and information.

A listening perspective can be described as listening simultaneously to:

- a foreground – the patient's 'here and now' presence and expression, and

- a background – the patient's *split reality* (often a reality with very strong emotions).

For the therapist this involves listening to the field of tensions and movement (or the lack thereof) between these two polarities – the foreground and the background. The therapist can move between two different listening attitudes. The therapist can, for example, assume an *allocentric* attitude. Here the therapist listens with his/her full awareness directed towards the patient and resonates deliberately and authentically with the patient's physical presence in the room (the foreground). Gradually he/she then makes it possible for small 'sparks' of emotion from the patient's split reality (the background) to become a part of their relationship (both within the music and outside of it).

The second listening attitude can be identified as an almost embodied, flowing, inward and more primitive state of listening that ensures more distance from the patient, while at the same time making relatedness possible on a more primitive level. The distance created here is different from the distance created when the therapist assumes an observing attitude, making the patient the object of observation from a neutral therapeutic position. The therapist is in a state of acute sensitivity and 'heightened readiness', and strives to be open to all nuances of vibrations that might flow between the therapist and the patient. This listening attitude can make it easier to be resonant to the patient's need for closeness and distance.

For some patients, it can be especially important that the therapist perceives their need for distance. Listening in the primitively organized way described above can give the therapist the means to create the necessary closeness or distance – without invading or rejecting the patient. The balance in each particular case is defined by the patient's presence.

The technical rule of neutrality in music therapy is best defined as disciplined subjectivity – described here through listening attitudes. Disciplined subjectivity is defined as:

Being subjectively present and at the same time resonant to the patient's universe. This means that the therapist is acutely sensitive and attentive, and can move in and out of the transitional space. This sensitivity is necessary, for the therapist to:

- actually perceive the vibrations (non-verbal sensations) of which she is a part
- take responsibility for not being overwhelmed by the vibrations/emotions/ experiences of which she is a part
- be aware of and take responsibility for the *transitional space* of which she is a resonant part
- be committed to continuously finding ways of understanding the processes that take place in the *transitional space* of which she is a part. (Pedersen 2000b)

In this way many fields of awareness are activated simultaneously, and it appears that there is a similar focus on the therapist's technical way of being present in music therapy as in psychoanalysis with its rules of neutrality, abstinence and free-floating awareness. In music therapy as a whole, one can say that movement and actions are an important part of the therapist's presence, and that a distanced form – as described here through neutrality – is only one of many possible forms. The context determines the music therapist's way of being present.

CLINICAL CONCEPTS

Transference and Countertransference

The technical rules of classical psychoanalysis are logically associated with *clinical concepts* such as '*transference, countertransference, resistance, and repetition compulsion*'. Music therapy also uses these clinical concepts to a great extent – here related to the fact that music is the main therapeutic agent, balancing and alternating with verbal parts of the therapy.

'Transference' is Freud's radical discovery and the pivotal point of psychoanalysis. The forerunners of the original concept of transference are hypnosis and the power of suggestion – where subconscious wishes for specific objects are actualized in the analytic relationship, which is perceived as reality. However, the term transference no longer holds the same meaning as it did originally. This change has happened gradually, as psychoanalysis has moved from being perceived as purely monadic (all conflicts take place intrapersonally within the patient's psyche) to being perceived as dyadic. In dyadic therapy the premise is that early experienced relationship patterns, object relations, defence strategies etc. are played out here and now in the patient/therapist relationship. Countertransference refers to the therapist's way of being present and his/her reactions to the patient, and needs to be taken into account in understanding the therapeutic process.

Today most therapists see transference as a phenomenon to do with relationships, to which both patient and therapist contribute. Transference, as a clinical concept, is still crucial in understanding the therapeutic process – both in the verbal and the musical parts of the therapy. Therefore the therapist should be aware of the emotions that the patient projects on him/her. However, he/she must not always directly express the emotions that emerge.

The therapist must 'contain' or 'carry' these emotions and in this way understand the patient at a deeper level. According to Heimann (1950), these countertransference reactions and feelings can guide the therapist in his/her interventions. Heimann describes how the therapist should use not only free-floating awareness and active listening, but also a spontaneously awakened emotional sensitivity. She states that emotions often are closer to the heart of the matter than intellectual reasoning, and that countertransference can be used as an instrument of orientation in overdetermined material. The countertransference represents a product that is not only connected to the therapist's personality, but also to that of the patient. The therapist's conscious and active use of countertransference can help to counteract his/her subconsciously becoming an actor on the patient's 'stage'.

Transference is a very central concept in the treatment of psychological problems through music therapy. It can guide not only verbal interventions and clarifications, but also musical interventions and the therapist's way of relating to the patient generally.

The music therapist often contains and carries primitive projected feelings from the patient through the music. He/she is trained to listen with great sensitivity. Music as a means of contact and communication aids the music therapist in developing a spontaneously awakened emotional sensitivity. The music makes it possible for the therapist to feel the emotions and at the same time use them consciously as a tool for orientation. The music therapist can then 'return' the emotions to the patient, because they are made audible. He/she can present the emotions in a 'processed' form through the improvised music.

The therapist must be able to sense when the patient is ready to see the *split-off elements* – in an altered form – and to integrate them into his/her consciousness. In this way he/she aids the patient's development and integration process. He/she must also be aware of how long it is necessary to be the *'container'* for the emotions in the relationship.

In psychoanalysis and psychotherapy, the focus of the therapist's observation has changed from being directed purely towards the patient. It has moved to being directed partly towards the patient in relation to the therapist, and also partly towards the therapist himself/herself in relation to the patient. This is another way of studying the unconscious.

Transference and countertransference in music therapy theory

Priestley (1994) has defined transference from a music therapy perspective, where she distinguishes between two kinds of countertransference – empathic

countertransference (E-countertransference) and complementary countertransference (C-countertransference).

She describes E-countertransference as a psychological awareness that emerges
in the therapist through an empathic identification with the patient. This empathic
identification can be understood as a resonance from something outer to something
inner – just as the music of a vibrating string (the patient) is amplified by the sympa-
thetic vibration of the string instrument (the therapist). Priestley describes the therapist's experience of gradually, during interaction with the patient, or suddenly like a
bolt from the blue, becoming aware of this empathic resonance with the patient's
emotions through his/her emotional and physical presence. These are often
repressed emotions, not yet accessible to the patient's consciousness, but they can
also be emotions that are close to becoming conscious. In the latter case, the
emotions can be very dynamic and almost 'flow through' the therapist, especially
when he/she is improvising with the patient.

Priestley emphasizes further that the therapist's countertransference is
dependent on his/her sensitivity and openness to experiencing the emotions that
emerge. But the ability to articulate these emotions consciously and to use them in
the therapy is dependent on clarity of thought. She warns against letting the therapy
process unfold through intuition alone, as it can easily lead to the therapist being
overwhelmed by emotion, or having to 'block off' the patient's emotions (as they
aren't made conscious and articulated verbally as an important part of the process). It
is important that countertransference experiences be transformed from an intuitive
sense in the therapist or patient to information that can be shared with the patient,
making it possible for the patient to internalize the emotion and take responsibility
for feeling it and living with it.

Priestley describes C-countertransference as something that occurs when the
therapist identifies with one of the patient's close relationships (for example a shel-
tering mother or a strict father). It is a subconscious process that the therapist can
make conscious by continually asking himself/herself, 'Why am I speaking/
playing/acting as I am?', and by being aware of being put in another role than
he/she would normally take. This countertransference can be played out consciously, when it is recognized (role-play), and can gradually be dissolved, as the
patient becomes ready, or it can be played out with reversed roles (the therapist reacts
in a way contrary to the patient's expectation).

Lindvang (1998) emphasizes the importance of letting the two countertransference reactions work together. The therapist often acts out a complementary
countertransference (nurturing, for example), while at the same time feeling an
empathic identification with the patient's emotions – sorrow or loneliness, for
example. The empathic identification can strengthen the therapist's capacity to be

nurturing, and it can also be a tool for orientation, as to which kind of nurturing is necessary. Lindvang compares this to Stern's theoretical description of the way in which parents attune to and identify with the small child in order to understand how the child feels and thereby fulfil his/her needs (Stern 1995). Lindvang points out that by studying communication between child and primary care-givers it becomes clear that these two ways of identifying are closely connected and mutually support each other.

Resistance and repetition compulsion

Two other original clinical concepts from psychoanalysis, later adopted by other psychotherapists and music therapists, are the concepts of resistance and repetition compulsion. In classical psychoanalysis, resistance is understood as the forces in the patient that subconsciously resists treatment. Resistance is a central phenomenon in psychiatric illness – the patient wishes to be well, but works at the same time against his/her own treatment.

The concept of resistance has developed theoretically since Freud. It is assumed that resistance is born of the same forces that caused the disturbance, and that now maintain the repression. Resistance is no longer seen as a 'dangerous drive from the id', as originally defined by Freud, but also as a force related to the ego. The dangers to which the ego is exposed come not only from the libido, but also from the ego, the superego, and from the outer world.

In psychoanalysis it is assumed that resistance emerges as a reaction to danger, and that the original source of danger is the child's helplessness. This helplessness can manifest itself in subconscious anxiety and fantasies of annihilation (if others reject me, I won't exist), or fantasies of not being worthy of others' love (if others don't express their love for me, I am worthless) or a feeling of being 'paralysed' and unable to act (I can't live out my energy or act as I feel, without being harmed by my surroundings) – fantasies that can colour any danger experienced in the moment. These forms of anxiety can be seen in serious psychiatric illness. In psychosis, annihilation anxiety dominates, while in neurosis it is the fear of being harmed, if the client lives/acts out his/her desires.

The ego mobilizes resistance against the emergence of anxiety. One can only understand the power of resistance if one understands the anxiety behind it. If fear of annihilation is the cause of the illness, then it is also the cause of the patient's resistance to change. The therapist must identify empathically with this locked position that is often the patient's only security. The suffering related to the illness is less than that of the patient's imagined alternative, if he/she were healthy. The patient is, in this way, bound to his/her illness. The therapist must at the same time realize that the patient's closed world isn't impenetrable, and that there is a reason for the patient's participation in treatment.

In music therapy, because of the therapist's active participation in music-making with the patient, it is often difficult to distinguish between transference, countertransference and resistance. A resistance to change can, for example, show itself in the following way: the therapist is stuck in a characteristic style of playing – so much so that the patient refuses to play if the therapist changes his/her style of playing. In this case there is a merging of the conscious use of complementary countertransference on the therapist's part with the clarification of the patient's resistance. As exemplified in vignette no. 2 (see p.85), the therapist here has one possibility – allowing the patient's resistance to act as a structuring factor in the musical improvisation, as long as the patient's fear of change is greater than his/her desire for change. At the same time, the music creates a framework, within which the patient can experience being heard and 'met' – with his/her resistance as an essential element of the musical expression. This acceptance of the resistance and the therapist's conscious gratification of the patient's needs can contribute to reducing the patient's anxiety sufficiently, so that he/she can be coaxed to change his/her style of playing and in that way gradually 'loosen' the resistance.

Often the concept of resistance is accompanied by another clinical concept – repetition compulsion. According to classical psychoanalysis, repetition compulsion describes a phenomenon whereby the patient re-enacts the traumatic experience, rather than remembering the original trauma. In new relationships and in therapy the patient acts subconsciously in a way that seems to bring about the same interpersonal problems again and again. The patient relives the experience unknowingly and this constant repetition blocks the memory of the original trauma. The psychiatric illness is seen not as a historical development, but as a demonic force the patient is subjected to. Repetition compulsion is a force that, according to Freud, lies beyond the 'pleasure principle' and is connected to the *death instinct* (Thanatos) – the patient re-enacts the experience even though it is unpleasant. The patient exercises self-punishment, which becomes very pronounced in the self-destructive behaviour of psychotic patients. Repetition compulsion has become a pivotal point in the later development of theories on psychic structures, especially theories that integrate aspects of developmental psychology.

In this way, music therapists have made use of newer developments in psychoanalytic theory – from object relations theory and dynamic psychotherapy theory to cyclic dynamic theory. This means that present life events and relationships have gradually begun to play a larger role in theory building and therapy than they have previously. The patient's actions are not only understood as a product of his/her early history and possible traumas, but also as connected to later developmental phases and to current interactional patterns where each person continually influences each other. This means that the patient's presentation of subconscious material in the specific context is just as important as identification of repressed material from childhood. This view differs from more traditional psychodynamic theories primarily in the way in which early experiences are seen to form current experiences, emotions and behaviour. Early experiences are significant because they put the person on a life-path, where the force of movement is strong, and this makes certain types of experiences more probable than others. It is the accumulative effect of many such experiences that eventually results in maladaptive patterns of interaction – and in this way becomes the cause of the psychological problems in a cyclic dynamic perspective (Høstmark Nielsen and von der Lippe 1996; Pedersen 1998b). Stern further develops this idea (that the accumulative effect of early experiences influences present patterns of interaction) from the perspective of developmental psychology (see p.85–88).

In a music therapy context, it is important that verbal as well as non-verbal interactions are made audible, and that they, in tangible form, can become the object of analysis of interaction. This is currently a focus for many music therapists, in clinical practice as well as research.

Is music therapy psychoanalytic?

There has been a great deal of discussion within psychotherapeutic circles on whether or not a therapy can be described as psychoanalysis or analysis, when interpretation and insight no longer are central curative factors, and when the structures of the mind are no longer understood through Freud's libido theory. According to Wallerstein (1988), it is the *clinical theory* (the combination of technical rules and clinical concepts) rather than the metatheory that is the decisive factor for whether or not therapeutic work can be seen as psychoanalytic. What is crucial is whether or not the clinical work builds on fundamental concepts such as transference, countertransference and resistance – phenomena that can be observed and described with reasonable clarity. According to Pine (1990), four psychological theories have been developed that can underlie psychoanalysis: libido theory, ego psychology, object relations and self-psychology.

Interpretation or empathy?

During the last twenty years there has been a growing interest in developing psychoanalytic treatment for more *regressive illnesses*. Here it is clear that interpretation as the main intervention cannot stand alone, and in many cases cannot be used at all. It must be supplemented with, or replaced by, a more empathic way of relating on the therapist's part. At the same time he/she must clarify and confront – in order to remedy the patient's tendency to divide the world into black and white, and in order to strengthen the primitive ego function.

This has caused many psychoanalysts to suggest that classic psychoanalytic understanding should be supplemented with a developmental psychological frame of reference, and direct itself towards an understanding of the therapist/patient relationship as a healing potential. Interventions are called for that are either ego-supportive or directed towards development of the self. Interpretation is not the main technique, but rather 'containing' (Bion), 'holding environment' (Winnicott) or 'affirmation and empathic identification' (Killingmo).

It is difficult to observe and clearly define these techniques, and to grasp their therapeutic meaning, because these methods are not only directed towards the patient's symptoms, but towards the patient as a whole person. For the major part of the therapy, the therapist needs to take an affirmative approach and to direct the treatment towards establishing the patient's identity through stabilization of the ego and development of the self. The patient must first achieve considerable development in this area before the therapist can continue with more insight-oriented therapy, where the patient obtains insight into his/her own participation in the psychodynamics – through ways of relating and subconscious playing out of primitive wishes.

Music therapy has great potential for offering 'containing' and a 'holding environment', as the sounding music often can act as a facilitating co-therapist. Consequently, music therapy is primarily directed towards the patient as a whole, rather than towards the patient's symptoms. What we are talking about here is the further development and definition of the technical rules – through description of the therapist's way of relating – and of clinical concepts such as transference and countertransference, as they are played out in music therapy. Winnicott emphasizes that when the patient's ego function is not intact, no transference neurosis (as originally described by Freud) will develop. The patient's primary condition is absolute dependence. In this case transference is characterized not by the degree of irrational emotions on the therapist's part, but by the degree to which the therapist can allow the patient's past to be present in the relationship (a symbolic realization). On these grounds Winnicott believes that the theoretical and technical modifications in therapy with regressive disturbances are fully compatible with the analytic frame of reference.

In the treatment of regressive disturbances, the third clinical concept *resistance* is used in a modified form. Every relationship strategy that the patient chooses must be considered the best solution, if he/she is to survive the threat of total annihilation.

Generally one can say that the clinical concepts and technical rules in classical psychoanalysis, as described and delimited in relation to regressive disturbances, are more applicable and directly transferable in music therapy than in verbal psychotherapy. The relationship between the reality of the moment and the originally experienced interactional patterns (that guide the patient's choices and relationship potentials today) merge together and are less separated in musical interaction than in verbal psychoanalysis/psychotherapy. In this way there is often a 'regressive' aspect connected to the music therapy process.

This also means that music therapists can use newer psychoanalytic theories more easily – theories developed through a gradual paradigm shift via object relations theories, ego psychology, self-psychology, interpersonal theories and interactional theories. This development reflects the fact that psychoanalysis has moved from a monadic to a dyadic form. It also reflects a change in the understanding of mental structures and psychopathology, and in the significance of the early mother/child relationship as a metaphor for the therapist/patient relationship. Libido theory has therefore no importance in modern music therapy theory.

Two prominent psychoanalytic schools of thought were developed in work with *regressive disturbances*: Kernberg's expressive psychodynamics and Kohut's self-psychology.

The development of psychoanalytic theories via egopsychology and self-psychology

Kernberg (1975) did not follow the psychoanalytic trends in the 1960s and 1970s concerning the use of affirmative techniques, especially in treatment of *regressive disturbances*. He developed a metatheory based on Freud's libido theory, but with a more differentiated view on psychological development. For example, he did not believe that there was a linear development from id functions to ego functions. He believed that there was a hierarchical development within each function – a development that wasn't necessarily related to the other functions. During the time that this theory was developed there was an increased focus on other types of personality organization than neurosis and psychosis – borderline and narcissistic disturbances, amongst others. These personality types did not fit into a classical, linear understanding of development.

Neurotic, borderline or psychotic organization is reflected in characteristics that dominate the personality concerning:

- degree of identity integration
- type of defensive strategies

- capacity for reality testing.

Neurotic personality organization is characterized by an integrated identity – contrary to the other two types of organization – and resistance is actualized primarily in repression of reality. In the two other types of organization, there is a deep 'split' in the experiencing of reality, that is seen as alternately black or white. Reality testing is intact in neurotic organization and in borderline organization, but not in psychotic organization.

The aim of therapy with borderline patients is to integrate *split-off* object relations while at the same time neutralizing libido-related effect, which strengthens ego functions. In the transference situation the therapist will be seen as alternately good and evil. According to Kernberg, the therapist's task is to identify these projections and interpret the dyads that occur in the moment. Kernberg (1975) emphasizes the importance of the therapist's authentic interest in the patient's emotional reality. The therapist's interest is a healing factor in the therapy. Kernberg does not believe that supportive therapy or traditional psychoanalysis are suitable for these patients. He believes that affirmation must be imparted as a precise and well-timed interpretation of the patient's basic conflict. An intervention of this type shows the patient that the therapist has understood something very important about him/her. Kernberg, therefore, does not use affirmation as an intervention in itself. Quite a few music therapists from Germany, Holland and other mid-European countries have described cases where this theory is brought into practice in music therapy.

In contrast to this is Kohut's self-psychology. Self-psychology departs radically from the metapsychology of Freudian psychoanalysis by disputing the theory that drives are the basic elements of a child's experience. Heinz Kohut (1984) believes instead in basic mental functions that are related to the creation of self and to the first experience of a sense of self. The basic mental functions are defined as 'healthy self-assertion in relation to the mirroring self-object and healthy admiration for the idealised [sic] self-object'. Moreover, a continuous sense of identity over time is an important characteristic of the healthy self.

In Kohut's hypothesis on the restoration of the damaged self, disintegrated structures disappear and a healthy self is recreated. Childhood memories are revised, because recalling the past in a therapeutic context helps to re-establish continuous sense of the self in time. The purpose of memory in this context is not to make the subconscious conscious, but to strengthen the cohesion of the self. In analysis, the genetic roots of the self are sought, the way in which the core self originally was consolidated (or not consolidated) is reactivated, and the patient's capacities and skills are re-experienced. The core self is defined as a delimitation of the self – creating a basis for a sense of being an independent centre for initiative and perception. This sense of independence, along with the person's most central ambitions and ideas and his/her experience of body and psyche, creates a unit in time and space.

During musical improvisation clients often experience that they can express themselves from a level of inner resources that seems healthy and assertive despite many other 'layers' of self-devaluation in the personality. In long-term music therapy it is often meaningful to see personal growth as establishing contact to 'healthy self-assertion', though this can only be stabilized through mirroring and repetition over time. In the 1950s, Kohut wrote two (now classic) articles, about the psychological and therapeutic functions of music (Folker 1994; Kohut 1994, Kohut and Levarie 1994), showing how musical activities can nourish 'healthy narcissism'.

Stern also uses the term 'the core self', as one of the 'domains' of development in his interpersonal theory. His understanding of the mental structures differ however, as they are based solely on observations of mother/child interactions. Because ways of relating and experiencing in musical improvisation are sometimes similar to those of early mother/child interaction, and because Stern writes in language similar to musical description, his theories have often been used in describing processes in music therapy. It is therefore relevant to look in more detail at Stern's theories and how they relate to music therapy.

DANIEL STERN'S INTERACTION THEORY

Daniel Stern is an American psychologist, psychoanalyst and researcher, who, in 1985, presented a theory describing the development of the interpersonal world of the infant (Stern 1985). Stern's work is considered an essential contribution to the on-going debate in the field of developmental psychology. Based on empirically grounded research, he has revised the psychoanalytic view on development. Stern's most significant contribution is a coherent theory describing how the infant from birth actively builds and develops its sense of self. The sense of self is based on the experience of actual interactions and incidents. This means that the development of a sense of self is seen more as a product of real experiences than of unconscious drives and fantasies. There is a focus on the relational aspects of development and on the mechanisms that characterize early interaction between mother and infant.

The development of the child's sense of self consists of five levels: the first three are pre-verbal and the last two are verbal. The new element in Stern's theory is that these developmental levels are seen as 'layers' of maturation and experience that exist side by side (and not phases the child moves through, as in traditional psychoanalysis). These layers of development are related to different senses of the self, and to different ways of experiencing 'how-to-be-with-another'.

This means that the experiences and knowledge that the child attains pre-verbally are different from knowledge based on words and symbols. Stern uses the terms 'implicit' and 'explicit' knowledge. Implicit knowledge is subconscious, action-based and 'tacit/silent knowledge', while explicit knowledge is conscious, and can be expressed potentially in symbolic or verbal form.

Stern describes psychological development as follows:

- The child already actively interacts with its surroundings from birth.

- Development is characterized by different senses of self and different ways of being with another.

- The child builds a fundament of implicit knowledge about the world before language is developed.

- The emergence of language makes more precise communication possible but at the same time it inhibits access to the pre-verbal sense of self.

This theory has contributed greatly to the understanding of relational processes in psychotherapy. Stern's theory about pre-verbal interaction has especially contributed to the understanding of what happens in the therapist/client relationship (see Dosamantes 1992; Reyner 1992). Stern describes how the child builds an implicit and procedural knowledge of his/her ability to act, to have feelings, to have a coherent sense of the body and a sense of time. These sensations re-emerge in the therapeutic situation, where clients, for example, can feel unable to act, have difficulty recognizing emotions, experience a 'dissolving' of the body's boundaries or lose their sense of time. In other words, their difficulties lie in the domain of the sense of self that Stern calls 'the core self'.

Stern also describes how children develop the ability of 'inter-subjectivity', and how they learn which emotions can be shared with others and which cannot. This process has great significance for the way in which the person later in life is able to share his/her inner world with others. In therapy, the process of showing and sharing emotions can often cause great problems and, because of this, the client has a limited capacity for inter-subjectivity. These problems are related to the sense of the self that Stern refers to as the 'subjective self'.

From the point of view of music therapy, Stern is especially interesting, because he describes basic pre-verbal interaction as containing many of the same elements as music. For example, he states that elements of communication such as tempo, rhythm, tone, phrasing, form and intensity are necessary for the child, in order to 'decode' and organize sensory experiences of interaction into generalized mental structures. Stern describes how the child forms Representations of Interactions that have been Generalized (RIGs) – mental structures also referred to as 'schemas'. In this process, according to Stern, the child obtains implicit schematic knowledge of 'how-to-be-with-another'. In other words, Stern's theory seems to support the view that interaction, communication and music are fundamentally made up of the same elements. This supports, therefore, the assumption that musical improvisation and music listening can reflect and activate relational patterns and the senses of self connected to these. The aim of psychotherapy and music therapy is exploring, working through and changing dysfunctional relational patterns. Therefore it is obvious that Stern's theory is important in understanding the origin of these patterns and their dynamics in the 'here and now' therapy situation.

Since he presented his developmental theory, Stern has attempted to integrate the developmental aspect of his theory with the therapeutic aspect, especially in two areas. One of these areas has to do with theories on motherhood and mother/child therapy (Stern 1995). Here Stern translates his developmental theory and his understanding of the relational dynamics between the child and its surroundings directly into therapy with dysfunctional families.

The second area concerns a theory on the meaning of the non-interpretative mechanisms in psychotherapy that Stern proposed with a group of researchers (Stern et al. 1998). This proposal is considered important, because it focuses on implicit experiences in therapy. Experiences that cannot be verbalized, but only felt, are found to be central to the development of the client's ability to know, recognize and share emotions. In the therapy setting this means that the therapist and client share experiences without verbalizing them in the situation. The reason for this is that language, in the therapeutic situation as well as in a developmental context, often creates a distance to the pre-verbal sense of the self.

Music in music therapy often unfolds in a non-verbal context. Clinical experience shows that musical improvisation can enhance the implicit dimension of an experience. Musical interaction is therefore considered a means of making clear the fundamental elements of interaction and thereby the basic ways of relating.

The resemblance between pre-verbal relationships and transference patterns in musical interaction has been supported by recently conducted research (Hannibal 2000). In this case, transference is seen as the client's repetition and re-experiencing of emotions that originate in experiences with significant others. This repetition and re-experience can be observed in relational patterns in the musical interaction. The study shows that Stern's theories on pre-verbal relationships can be used to describe relational themes in both the verbal and the musical context with adult clients, and that these relational themes and patterns have the quality of transference. Stern is less direct in his description of clinical concepts such as transference, countertransference, defence and repetition compulsion, but he argues that the unconscious, implicit level of the therapeutic relationship is related to these psycho-analytic concepts.

Stern's theories have greatly influenced our understanding of how we relate and interact. His theories confirm that relational patterns, which are the focus of the therapy process, contain non-verbal knowledge about relationships, and that this knowledge seems to be expressed in the musical interaction. The theory also implies that transformation of these basic patterns can also take place without words. We believe, in addition, that in some cases these patterns may actually be clearer in a non-verbal or musical context.

TRANSPERSONAL AND INTEGRAL PSYCHOLOGY

In the history of psychology, transpersonal psychology is considered the 'fourth force' (behaviourism being the first, psychoanalysis the second, and humanis-tic-existential psychology the third). Abraham Maslow is often considered the initiator of the third as well as the fourth force, and Ken Wilber – whose *integral psychology* is introduced below – represents an important development of the fourth force (the transpersonal 'school') which focuses on the vast field of spiritual, non-ordinary experience and knowledge in Eastern and Western philosophy and psychology that should be considered as particularly relevant for music therapy.

The 'transpersonal field' – encompassing concepts such as spiritual, religious and transrational, and often associated with the 'eternal philosophy' ('philosophia perennis') – has been considered 'unscientific' during most of the decades since psychology established itself as an experimental, natural and social science in the late nineteenth century. However, gradually research has approached and settled in this controversial area.

RESEARCH INTO STATES OF CONSCIOUSNESS

The research of Freud and Jung already put 'the unconscious' on the agenda of psychology in the early twentieth century, as they developed their theories of the personal and collective unconscious. Within psychodynamic thinking it has been assumed that there are transitional states between conscious and unconscious states of consciousness (e.g. primary, secondary and tertiary processes). These transitional or altered states have been used in different psychotherapeutic models (see Chapter 2.3). In the 1960s Maslow, Assagioli and others added 'super- (or supra-) consciousness' to the map of human consciousness, and with his concept of 'peak experience' Maslow formulated a new psychotherapeutic goal: the self-actualization of man – the realization of the full potential of body and mind.

Biomedical researchers have done parallel studies in the 'vigilance' of the brain in different states, and they have identified four frequency spectra or bands of brainwave activity:

1. the Delta band, which is physiologically connected to deep sleep (and pathologically to the coma state)

2. the Theta band, which is related to states of deep introspection (e.g. meditation) or light sleep

3. the Alpha band, connected to states of relaxation

4. the Beta band, which is the frequency band of the waking state, alert conscious activity and awareness. Using advanced techniques of brain scanning (e.g. PET) researchers have gathered further information on the activity of the brain in different states, and this has led to what may be called the neuro- and psychophysiology of consciousness.

During the last four decades psychologists, neurophysiologists and psychotherapists have studied the so-called 'altered states of consciousness' (ASC), which give access to experiences beyond the normal, alert state (Beta band activities). ASC can be induced by pharmacological stimuli (hallucinogens like LSD), by psychological stimuli (sensory deprivation or overstimulation, e.g. through autogenic training, meditation, trance dance or hyperventilation) or by a combination of techniques. Within music psychotherapy this knowledge of entering ASCs is also used. The physiologically stimulating (ergotropic) type is represented by Grof's holotrophic breathwork, in which hyperventilation and powerful rhythmic music is used to induce ASC; the relaxing, introvert (tropotropic) type is represented by Guided Imagery and Music, in which autogenic training or other relaxation techniques are used (Bonny 1999, see also Chapter 3.1). Music can in itself induce and stimulate ASC.

WILBER'S INTEGRAL PSYCHOLOGY

Since the 1970s the American philosopher Ken Wilber has written a number of books and numerous articles and prefaces to other authors' books (now re-edited as his collected works in eight volumes, see Bonde 2001c). He is often given a prominent, and somewhat controversial, position within psychodynamic and transpersonal psychology. This controversial position is based on his strong desire to integrate Eastern and Western traditions, and also to integrate scientific and religious thought. Wilber is beyond doubt an important figure in modern psychology and philosophy. He is one of the scholars who has done most to (re)integrate the transpersonal field in the scientific discourse of psychology and philosophy, based on intense studies in Western as well as Eastern psychology, philosophy and religion (Wilber's publications on psychology encompass development psychology, psychopathology, psychotherapy and meditation practices).

The provisional result of Wilber's work-in-progress is what he calls 'integral psychology' (Wilber 2000) – graphically summarized in the All Quadrants, All Levels (AQAL) model (see below). This is a synthesis of all the most important and (more or less) well-known theories of the human mind, levels of consciousness and the scientific study of five basic levels: matter (physics), life (biology), mind (psychology), soul (theology), and spirit (mysticism). In this chapter it is only possible to outline the framework and central components of Wilber's world of ideas, and a good starting point could be his definition of psychology – the first paragraph in his latest book:

> Psychology is the study of human consciousness and its manifestations in behaviour. The functions of consciousness include perceiving, desiring, willing, and acting. The structures of consciousness, some facets of which can be unconscious, include body, mind, soul, and spirit. The states of consciousness include normal (e.g., waking, dreaming, sleeping) and altered (e.g., nonordinary, meditative). The modes of consciousness include aesthetic, moral, and scientific. The development of consciousness spans an entire spectrum from pre-personal to personal to transpersonal, subconscious to self-conscious to super-conscious, id to ego to spirit. The relational and behavioural aspects of consciousness refer to its mutual interaction with the objective, exterior world and the socio-cultural world of shared values and perceptions. (Wilber 2000, p.433)

All concepts and categories mentioned in this definition are relevant for the theory and practice of music therapy, but here we shall focus on Wilber's theory of psychological development – his so-called 'spectrum theory' of the developmental 'fulcrums' of consciousness – and the related psychopathologies and psychotherapeutic models.

Development is not one, but many processes

Wilber understands development as several parallel lines (or 'streams') that are fairly independent of one another: cognitive, emotional, moral, interpersonal etc. It is possible and quite common that a person has reached a high level within one area (e.g. emotional, empathic) but a lower in another area (e.g. cognitive, intellectual). The different areas are not causally linked, and a development within one area may be a necessary, but not a sufficient, condition for development within another. This understanding of the lines as (to some degree) independent modules is, in some aspects, similar to Howard Gardner's theory of multiple intelligences, and Wilber shares the educational optimism connected with Gardner's perspective on development.

Development is differentiation: the fulcrums and the spectrum model

Wilber's idea of the self is that it is the functional system ('the navigator' or the 'centre of gravity') responsible for balancing and integrating the many different developmental waves, streams, levels and states. The self has its own developmental sequence, and Wilber makes a distinction between an 'I' ('the proximal self') and a 'Me' ('the distal self').

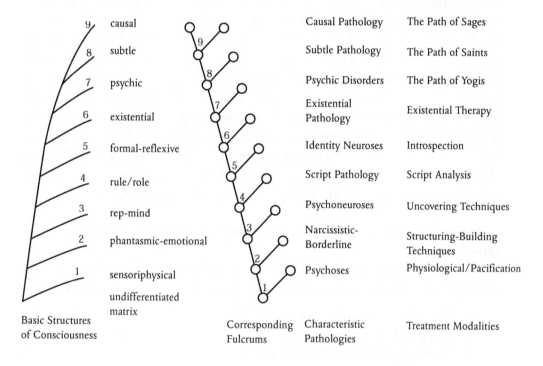

Basic Structures of Consciousness	Corresponding Fulcrums	Characteristic Pathologies	Treatment Modalities
9 causal		Causal Pathology	The Path of Sages
8 subtle		Subtle Pathology	The Path of Saints
7 psychic		Psychic Disorders	The Path of Yogis
6 existential		Existential Pathology	Existential Therapy
5 formal-reflexive		Identity Neuroses	Introspection
4 rule/role		Script Pathology	Script Analysis
3 rep-mind		Psychoneuroses	Uncovering Techniques
2 phantasmic-emotional		Narcissistic-Borderline	Structuring-Building Techniques
1 sensoriphysical		Psychoses	Physiological/Pacification
undifferentiated matrix			

(from GRACE AND GRIT by Ken Wilber.© 1991, 2000 by Ken Wilber. Reprinted by arrangement with Shambhala Publications, Inc., Boston, www.shambhala.com)

Figure 2.6 Wilber's spectrum model. Position between mental structure, fulcrums, psychopathology and forms of treatment.

Independent of a theoretical platform, development can be described in three phases which the self goes through each time it encounters a new level of consciousness:

1.   identification or fusion (the unclear confluence or symbiosis of subject and object)

2.   gradual differentiation or separation (of subject and object)

3.   integration ('reflexive' consciousness of the differentiation).

These three phases cover just one round in the long developmental span. When one round is over, a new can begin, with a new agenda of differentiation and integration. The combination of nine levels and three sub-phases of each fulcrum gives a typology of 27 major self-pathologies, described in detail in *Transformations of consciousness* (or Collected Works Vol. IV, pp.117–133). Within psychiatry it is well known that psychological disturbances are connected to problems of differentiation. Psychotic disorders are related to a disturbed differentiation on the physical level, narcissistic and borderline disorders are related to problems on the emotional level of differentiation, and neurotic problems to the mental level. This corresponds to the first three levels of differentiation – or 'fulcrums' – in Wilber's theory (he also uses the metaphor 'milestones', 2000, p.467). As in fulcrums 1 to 3 the processes and the problems follow the same principle in fulcrums 4 to 6 and 7 to 9: if the differentiation process – learning to discriminate between self and other(s) within different 'developmental agendas' – does not succeed, pathological problems may develop and these may require a treatment finely attuned with the level or 'agenda'.

The prepersonal, the personal and the transpersonal level – and corresponding pathologies

Wilber's spectrum model has three basic levels (or 'waves'), each divided into three sub-levels or fulcrums. A characteristic pathology corresponds to each level:

- The *prepersonal* level (fulcrums 1 to 3):
  1. sensory-motor/psychosis –
  2. emotional/narcissistic-borderline –
  3. rep-mind (c: consciousness with psychic representations of the outer world)/psychoneuroses

- The *personal* level (fulcrums 4 to 6):
  4. rule-role/'script'-disturbances –
  5. formal-reflexive/identity neuroses –
  6. existential/existential disturbances

- The *transpersonal* level (fulcrums 7 to 9):
  7. psychic/psychic disturbances–

    8. subtle/subtle disturbances –
    9. causal/causal disturbances.

This systematic account makes it – among other things – possible to make a precise positioning of the different psychotherapeutic models: they are related to one or more of the specific levels. Supportive, structuring therapy models thus relate to Fulcrum 2, the uncovering process of psychoanalysis relates to Fulcrums 3 to 4, transactional analysis to Fulcrum 4, existential psychotherapy to Fulcrums 5 to 6. Fulcrums 7 to 9 have not been addressed much in Western psychotherapy models; they have been the domains of experienced and advanced teachers and gurus within religious, spiritual and transpersonal traditions.

The four quadrants
Wilber uses different models with a different number of levels in his books, which can be confusing. His own explanation of this (and of the coherence of the different models) is this:

> The overall spectrum of consciousness, as outlined in The Atman Project, containing almost twenty-four basic levels (which are simply an elaboration of the Great Nest of Being, matter to body to mind to soul to spirit). I usually condense these into nine or ten major levels, and sometimes use even fewer, such as the traditional five I just gave (which are essentially the same as the Vedanta uses), and sometimes only three: body, mind, and spirit (or gross, subtle, and causal). (Collected Works Vol. III, p.11)

Only some of Wilber's books are (presented as) genuinely scholarly achievements (*Transformations of Consciousness, 1986; The Marriage of Sense and Soul, 1998; Sex, Ecology and Spirituality, 2000d; Integral Psychology, 2000a*). In the last three books Wilber explores his – until now – broadest model (or 'template') of consciousness: the 'quadrant model'.

Wilber developed this model as a graphic and comprehensible combination of four different and equally important perspectives on development and consciousness: the inside and the outside, the singular and the plural (also called the dimensions of I, it, we, its). The 'we' quadrant for instance contains the developmental levels of world-views shared by a collective (from family to nation). The major point is that each of the levels, lines and states of consciousness has these four quadrants. This 'all-quadrants, all-levels, all-lines, all-states' model (AQAL) … Opens up the possibility of a more integral approach to education, politics, business, art, feminism, ecology and so on.' (Wilber 2000, p.4). The AQAL model is a classification of the many different developmental theories in Western and Eastern psychology. The upper, 'Northern' half of this model deals with individual processes while the lower,

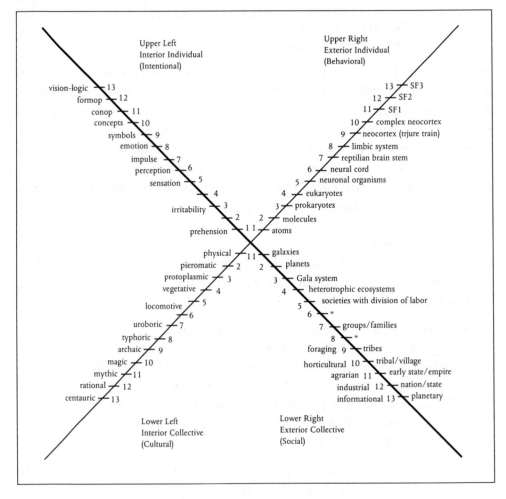

(SEX, ECOLOGY, SPIRITUALITY by Ken Wilber. © 1995, 2000 by Ken Wilber. Reprinted by arrangement with Shambhala Publications, Inc., Boston, www.shambhala.com)
Figure 2.7 Wilber's quadrant model

'Southern' half deals with collective processes. The left, 'Western' half deals with inner, subjective processes of consciousness; the right, 'Eastern' half with outer, objective processes of matter and materials.

This means that 'developmental psychology' (the area of Wilber's fulcrums) belongs to the upper left quadrant, while the corresponding upper right shows the development of the human brain. The lower left quadrant is the home of the cultural development of human societies and their value systems, while the lower right shows the development of social and societal organization systems.

The quadrant model can also be used to distinguish between therapeutic models in a broad sense: medical therapy in upper right, psychotherapies in upper left, and environmental therapies and rehabilitation programs in lower left and right quadrants.

Transpersonal experiences

An important point in Wilber's theory is that transpersonal experiences may occur at any level of development – no human being is excluded from the transpersonal field. The cultural history of the human race bears numerous witnesses of these often short and intense experiences of something mystical, sacred or 'numinous' (a concept coined by Rudolf Otto). Even though these experiences have been studied systematically, mostly within Eastern traditions, they are also known in some Western philosophical, religious and mystical traditions (as meditative states or experiences attainable through spiritual practices). Wilber makes a very important additional point. A human being inevitably needs to interpret a transpersonal experience, and this interpretation will be influenced and limited by the developmental stage, or horizon, available. This is also well known, but not always properly recognized in psychotherapy and self-developmental work. It may even explain some of the enigmas of religious fundamentalism, so sadly prominent during these difficult months and years in the life of our planet.

The psychotherapeutic and music therapeutic relevance of Wilber's theory

In a developmental perspective it is useful to have a theory integrating the different 'lines of growth' described by well-known theories, i.e. Piaget's cognitive operations development, Erikson's ego and psychosocial development, Kohlberg's moral development, and Fowler's faith development, as observed by Clark (1999). What Wilber provides is a contemporary theory based on 'orienting generalisations' [sic] about the nature of body, mind and spirit. For music therapists his system or model may be especially relevant, because it addresses the most important ontological and epistemological questions they face as clinicians and theorists:

- What is the nature and potential of consciousness?
- Can science be integrated with art and religion?
- How can we understand spirituality and the transpersonal realm?
- Is truth always culturally situated?
- Are hierarchies always oppressive and marginal?
- How can the roles of music(king) be described within a larger epistemological and ontological framework?

'An archaeologist of the Self' is Wilber's metaphor for 'the full-spectrum therapist' (Collected Works Vol. IV, p.541). Clients bring problems to therapy, and these problems may be identified as belonging to one or more fulcrums. Thus the therapist must be able to work with differentiation or integration problems of the body, the shadow, the persona, the ego, the existential self, the soul and the spirit – when relevant – and help the client bring these aspects of the self into consciousness as a whole. According to Wilber himself this is not eclecticism, as it is not a question of incommensurable or competing paradigms or value systems; integral psychology has the noble and daring ambition of dealing with all the aspects and forms of human existence.

The few references to Wilber's books in the music therapy literature are one of the following types:

1. general and unspecific, more or less announcing a leaning towards the ontology and epistemology – 'universal integralism', not to be confused with classic essentialism – of Ken Wilber, also suggesting the importance of metatheoretical understanding of transformation processes in music therapy (Bruscia 2000; Bunt, Burns and Turton 2000; Kenny 1989)

2. specific references to the fulcrums (or other versions of Wilber's spectrum of consciousness model) in analyses of client experiences, suggesting that a client's specific pathology or problem can be correlated with a specific developmental stage (Bruscia 1991; Lewis 1999; Rugenstein 1996)

3. specific reference to, or elaboration of, Wilber's evolution theory (the quadrant model) in a music therapy context (Bruscia 1998a)

4. the use of Wilber's theory to underpin the understanding of transpersonal experiences in therapy (Clark 1999; Lewis 1999).

It is not a coincidence that Wilber's theory serves as a good theoretical framework within Guided Imagery and Music (GIM) and is required reading in the GIM training. Client experiences in GIM are so manifold that a psychodynamic, a human-istic-existential or even a Jungian framework is not always sufficient. GIM needs a metatheory including archetypal as well as spiritual and transpersonal experiences (Wilber's fulcrums 7 to 9). Imagery within this realm is very different from imagery within the personal, psychodynamic spectrum (fulcrums 4 to 6) (Bonny 2001). Laurie Rugenstein has described case examples where clients in their imagery expe-rience 'oscillate' between different levels of consciousness, in and between sessions (Rugenstein 1996).

Bruscia has based his 'six basic models for designing the client's musical experience' on Wilber's quadrant model (Bruscia 1998a, Chapter 15). The model is discussed in Chapter 2.3. Bruscia also refers to Wilber in Chapter 10 of his book, on how music therapy can 'promote health'. Health is defined as 'the process of becoming one's fullest potential for individual and ecological wholeness' (Bruscia 1998a, p.84). In his further discussion of wholeness and how to reach this, Bruscia uses Wilber's concepts of holons and holarchies, because he finds them more inclusive and adaptable to music therapy than other definitions of the relation between parts and wholes: 'Webster's dictionary cites the main parts of the person as mind, body, and spirit, whereas Wilber divides the person into object (exterior holons), and subject (interior holons), both of which include spirit.' The same goes for ecological wholeness, and Bruscia is also clearly referring to the quadrant model here.

2.4 Music as Analogy and Metaphor

Every illness is a musical problem –
Its cure a musical solution.

(Novalis)

We shall continue the discussion of meaning in music from Chapter 1.3. We now present two important approaches to music as/in therapy: music as analogy and music as metaphor. Both approaches have their limitations, of course. For instance, they do not systematically cover all four levels in Ruud's model of music's properties, or all six types of experience in Bruscia's model (see Chapter 1.3). The investigation of music as analogy and metaphor has focus on the relationship between what Ruud calls the syntactic and the semantic level. In Bruscia's model it refers primarily to subjective and aesthetic music experiences.

The concepts of 'metaphor' and 'analogy' cannot be found in any standard music lexicons or handbooks (e.g. Decker-Voigt 1996). Nevertheless, many music therapists talk and write about music based on the (more or less conscious) axiom that the client's music, expression or experience is closely related – an analogy – to the client's personality or pathology. In an even broader sense, music is analogous to a human being's way of thinking, feeling and interacting. This is expressed in the improvisations of *active music therapy*, and in the listening experiences of receptive music therapy.

Music as analogy

One of David and Gudrun Aldridge's papers bears the title 'Life as Jazz' (Aldridge and Aldridge 1999), and David Aldridge has often used similar analogies or metaphors in his characterization of the relationship between music and human body, mind and spirit. In a chapter entitled 'Health as performance' (Aldridge 1996a, Chapter 20) he suggests that the creative act (especially musical improvisation) is a core element in the question of how health is achieved or promoted. Thus Descartes' classic motto *'Cogito, ergo sum – I think, therefore I am'* should be replaced by *'Ago, ergo sum – I perform, therefore I am'*. In a wider perspective he suggests that personal identity should be understood as a dynamic expressive act, very much like a musical improvisation – or, with a metaphor, man is a composition, and the composed self is an improvised order. Based on principles from phenomenology, neurology and music psychology Aldridge emphasizes the close affinity between musical and human processes:

> The perception of music requires a holistic strategy where the play of patterned frequencies is recognized within the matrix of time.

> People may be described in similar terms as beings in the world who are patterned frequencies in time. (Aldridge 1996a, p.31)

Smeijsters has written extensively about the affinity between musical processes and expressive properties on the one hand, human life processes and pathological characteristics on the other hand. He has developed a comprehensive theory of analogy that will be introduced briefly in the following section (Smeijsters 1998, 1999).

The core axiom is that psychological/psychotherapeutic knowledge and therapeutic knowledge of music are interdependent, and that a music therapist develops his/her professional competence by integrating them. Smeijsters writes:

> … analogy in itself resembles the object it refers to. In analogy there is no dualism between symbol and object, and therefore there is no need for interpretation. In analogy there always is a resemblance with the object, but this is not a concrete visual representation.

> When there is analogy, the person expresses his being in an object, in the same way he expresses himself in other behaviours, in other contexts and by other objects. For instance, the soft dynamics of a shy person's musical play are expressions of his personality. They are analogous to the way he expresses himself in verbal communication. Playing pian(issim)o in musical improvisation is analogous to staying in the background during a verbal discussion, not talking at all, or talking softly. Because the musical behaviour is not the original

verbal behaviour, because it is 'same and different' (Ansdell, 1995, page 180), it is called an analogy. (Smeijsters 1998, p.300)

There are many non-specific analogies between pathological problems and patterns of behaviour, e.g. if a client feels isolated from the surrounding world and is unable to engage in the therapeutic process (be it a talking cure or arts therapy). Smeijsters' theory sets the stage for an identification of specific analogies in music therapy, because valid and useful indication criteria demand this specification. He thinks that musical elements like melody, rhythm, tempo, dynamics, timbre, form, interaction etc. are specific symbolic equivalents of non-musical elements of human behaviour and interaction. An example: a client who is unable to express his feelings improvises without any noteworthy variation in tempo, rhythm, dynamics etc.

Smeijsters thinks – proposing an equivalent analogy – that specific musical processes corresponding to psychological processes may gradually set the client free, enhance development and promote new life quality, for example when a client struggling with boundaries learns to distinguish her own music from the therapist's and/or other clients' contributions in a group, develops the courage necessary to take the space of a soloist or to find a clearly defined role in the music of a group. Many other examples can be found in Chapter 2.2.

Smeijsters has coined the double conceptualization of 'pathological-musical processes' and 'therapeutic-musical processes'. They refer to the two core analogies in clinical music therapy. He underlines that comprehensive experience with and knowledge of these analogies makes it possible to decide whether music therapy is an indicated treatment or not, and in *Grundlagen der Musiktherapie* (Smeijsters 1999) he unfolds the theory within two clinical core areas of music therapy – 1. psychiatry (schizophrenia, depression) and 2. special education (autism, developmental disability). The very close affinity of analogy, diagnosis, indication and goals, procedures and techniques of the treatment is carefully worked out.

The analogy between the elements of music and the existential themes and qualities of human existence is also a core construction in the Improvisational Assessment Profiles (IAP) of Ken Bruscia (1987, 1994). When developing this method for description and interpretation of clinical improvisations Bruscia looked for concepts that would give the six 'profiles' – each a specific listening perspective – also psychological relevance. What he came up with was:

- *salience* (with five scales forming a spectrum: compliant, conforming, attending, controlling, dominating)

- *integration* (with the spectrum: undifferentiated, synchronized, integrated, differentiated, overdifferentiated)

- *variability* (rigid, stable, variable, contrasting, random)
- *tension* (hypo-tense, calm, cyclic, tense, hyper-tense)
- *congruence* (unengaged, congruent, centred, incongruent, polarized)
- *autonomy* (dependent, following, partner, leader, resistor).

In the preface to the Norwegian translation of the IAPs, Bruscia (1994) writes that the method gives guidelines for how the musical elements and the process of an improvisation can be interpreted, based on psychoanalytic and humanistic-existential theories. The IAPs are an assessment tool based on two basic assumptions:

1. improvised music is a sound reflection of the improviser's way of 'being-in-the-world', not only in the here and now world of the improvisatory

PARAMETER	Salient elements
FORM	*Theme:* a metaphor for entity Being = a gestalt, a metaphor of wholeness Form is composed of entities in a mutual relationship (similarities/differences)
TEXTURE Monophonic/ homophonic - polyphonic	*Melody with acc.:* metaphor of cooperation with a leader *Solo with orchestra:* metaphor of an individual versus group/community
TIMBRE	*Spectrum of overtones:* the identity of the entity *Tone formation:* related to a body area *Mixture:* contrast versus complementation
VOLUME	*Power:* metaphor of giving and taking space over time *Intensity:* metaphor of the quality of the experience of the entity
PULSE/RHYTHM METER AND TEMPO	*Pulse:* holding and supporting (or not) *Rhythm:* metaphor of the independence of the entity as related to the pulse *Tempo:* metaphor of the flexibility of the entity as related to material *Meter:* regulation system
MODALITY	*Modus/key:* metaphor of the basic emotion: belonging to a matrix with a center. The mode/key is an emotional matrix, the home base
MELODY	*Melody* is a specific model Gestalt (like an Aria): mataphor of an emotion being formed and experienced. The melody caries the message and relieves the feeling.
HARMONY	*Harmony:* gives the melody colour, direction, and context *Consonance/dissonance:* creates and releases tensions *Complexity:* the differentiation of the melodic expression

Figure 2.8 Musical Parameters as Metaphor

moment itself, but also of the more expanded context of the person's life world
(…)

2. each musical element provides a universal metaphor – or perhaps archetype –
for expressing a particular aspect of 'being-in-the-world' (…) Thus each
musical element has its own range of possibilities for expressive meanings
which are different from the other elements. (1994, p.3)

The first assumption is basically identical with Smeijsters' analogy concept, and we
consider it an axiom of psychodynamic music therapy. The second assumption is
unfolded in the IAP method, but here we will try to give a short overview of
Bruscia's metaphoric interpretation of the musical elements on the basis of psychoanalytic and existential psychology.

Metaphor of:	Metaphorical questions
BEING IN TIME	Is the entity identifiable? Does it develop? How? Is it in balance? If not: How? Is it dynamic or static?
BEING IN SPACE	Is it characterised by cooperation, competition or conflict? Is there a leader? How many voices are involved? Are they grouped?
THE SPECIFIC QUALITY OF BEING IN SPACE	Who, what, how is it? How is the sound produced, where does it enter the body? Is it in balance, harmony – or the opposite?
THE SPECIFIC QUALITY OF BEING IN TIME	Is it convincing? Is it present and intense, also when soft and/or loud? Does it leave time and space for me?
THE ORGANISATION OF LIFE ENERGY IN TIME (physical/temporal relationships)	Can I follow it(s development)? Can I count on it(s support)? Is it flexible? Free or frozen?
THE ORGANISATION OF LIFE ENERGY IN SPACE (emotional/spacial relationships)	Does it speak clearly to me? Does it speak freely and in a differentiated way? Is it centered or chaotic (unreliable)?
THE EXPRESSION OF THE SELF	Do I understand, what it is saying to me? Does it understand, what I am saying? Does it talk precisely and in nuances? "How does feelings feel?" (Langer)
THE SPECFIC CHARACTER OF SELF EXPRESSION	Do I understand, what it is up to? Is it banale or adventurous? Challenging? Is it organic? Is it complex?

Bruscia considers metaphoric interpretation or psychogical analogies as two of many possible and available perspectives or modes of consciousness – the clinician or researcher may choose them when relevant. The use of the concept 'archetype' must not be misinterpreted as an ontological claim that the elements described as such exist as universal or context-independent entities. According to Bruscia 'archetype' is a Jung-informed construct that may be used to describe how a client experiences 'the implicate order' (see Chapter 2.4).

This is not the place for a discussion of Bruscia's IAPs (see Stige 1995, 1996; see also the contributions in the Web Forum of the *Nordic Journal of Music Therapy* 2000–2001). However, we are convinced that many music therapists share the basic assumptions of the IAPs, and that music therapy theory needs these types of concrete, detailed suggestions for the interpretation of the relationship between music and human existence.

Music as metaphor

With his theory of analogy, Smeijsters has formulated a general theory of music therapy, with the purpose of 'bridging the gap' between music in psychotherapy and music in special education. The theory of music as metaphor is a more narrow and specific clinical theory describing the psychological equivalence of musical elements, how clients present their music experiences verbally using metaphors, and how these metaphors have clinical value and significance as information on the client's sense of self (Bonde 2000; Jungaberle 1999).

Until recently, metaphors of the type 'the eyes are the mirror of the soul' or 'music is the language of emotions' were considered mere decoration, an ornamentation or embellishment of language. Aristotle was sceptical towards the metaphor, which he considered 'dark' and manipulative. For this reason it was not awarded any epistemological or argumentative value. For centuries metaphor was left to poets, dramatists and other people with a talent of verbal imagination. Contemporary scholars have a quite different understanding of the metaphor. The French philosopher Paul Ricoeur studied how metaphor creates tension within discourse and in this way contributes to the development of cognitive strategies (Kemp 1994; Ricoeur 1978). Within the field of contemporary cognitive semantics (the study of the epistemological functions of language) metaphor is considered a basic tool of cognition, closely related to the body and the development of body schemata. It is connected to physical experiences of being-in-the-world, for example: joy = 'up', while sadness = 'down'.

The metaphor contributes to the image of a person's life world, its elements and dynamics ('If your husband was a car, what car would he be?'), and it helps us to understand the surrounding world and ourselves better. Metaphor bridges mind and body, and the theory of metaphor transcends the classic dualism of emotion of cognition. This is underpinned by contemporary neuropsychology in the documentation of the close affinity of emotions/body and reason/consciousness (Damasio 1994; Lakoff and Johnson 1999). From a psychological perspective metaphor gives us an opportunity to (re)create and (re)interpret our life world by adapting meaning from one area of life and transfering it to another. The metaphor is a specific 'transfer of structure' used by man to grasp his world better (Jensen 2001).

For the same reason many psychotherapists have studied metaphors in therapy (Siegelman 1990; Theilgaard 1994). They assign special importance to the inherent tension and ambiguity of the metaphor, which enables significant moments of awareness and insight. The metaphor 'reveals and hides' at the same time, and this makes it well suited to being a therapeutic tool, not least because it is based on the client's personal imagination and language.

In active music therapy metaphors are extensively used in the verbal dialogue on the improvisations. Examples: 'It was like being in a witches cauldron', 'I felt beyond time and space', 'The melody hit me right in the heart'. An analysis of these metaphors not only shows very clearly how clients experience the music, but also how they experience themselves, and how they may (not) benefit from music therapy.

Jungaberle, Verres and DuBois (2000) has studied musical metaphors extensively, first through an analysis of music reviews, next through an analysis of clients' verbalizations of their therapeutic experience of music. In the review a series of core metaphors was identified, like 'Music is xyz' (e.g. 'Music is space', 'Music is a landscape', 'Music is water'). These metaphors were also found in the clients' verbal reports on their music experiences, but they were even richer, containing several new core metaphors (or 'metaphor families' in Jungaberle's words).

Examples: one family is 'Music is energy and power' with subgroups like 'Music gives access to the inner world' or 'Music moves me'. Another family is 'Music is language' with subgroups like 'Music can hide truth' or 'Music makes the ineffable understandable'. Jungaberle attaches special importance to the family 'Music is a landscape', because it expresses the spaciousness of music – there is 'room for everyone', and most people can 'find their place' in the music.

Based on his study, Jungaberle has formulated a theory of 'the metaphorical circle'. Extramusical structures influence the music experience, when we hear or project into the music specific qualities from our life world. And intramusical structures (the music experience) have an impact on our life experience, when we extract or project qualities from the music that give meaning to our life. Structures are transferred both ways – through the metaphor. And thus metaphors provide clients and therapists in improvisational group music therapy with 'maps' of musical experiences.

But metaphors also play an important part in receptive music therapy. The client's 'music travel' in Guided Imagery and Music is often composed of metaphors in different modalities (even if the client's eyes are closed, he/she 'sees', 'hears', 'smells', 'tastes', 'feels' and 'moves with' the music). In the dialogue with the therapist (metaphorically the 'guide') the client's inner world stands out as imagery – reported verbally as metaphors. Example: If the therapist/guide suggests the opening image of 'a garden' to the client/traveller, and chooses Beethoven's Emperor Concerto (second movement) as a travel accompaniment, the client may experience the garden as anything from a vast open park with flowers in all colours, to a small, narrowly delimited backyard with burnt off grass and a dead pear tree. This of course invites an interpretation – based on the principle that only the client knows the meaning of the image/metaphor. (The German psychotherapist Hanscarl Leuner, who had some influence on GIM in its starting-up phase, used specific induction images diagnostically, based on a classic psychoanalytic interpretation of their meaning. This position is no longer considered appropriate in GIM.) The crucial element in GIM (and other metaphor-based therapies) is how the metaphors are configured and transformed over time – in the single session and through a complete therapeutic process.

Based on a substantial amount of empirical GIM material Bonde (2000) has suggested that the metaphors are configured in narrative units, and he has identified three levels of metaphoric thinking in GIM, which, in the light of narrative theory, have profound implications for psychotherapy:

1.   The narrative episode, configured round one or more core metaphors of the client. The configuration often follows specific structural patterns, e.g. the victim, the butcher, the spectator, the abandoned child.

2.   The narrative configuration of metaphors of the ego and the self (in therapy). This configuration makes the client's personal voice audible and clarifies his/her psychological position, e.g. the client takes responsibility for his/her own story, or dares to be the protagonist of the story.

3.   The full narrative, where the imagery and metaphors of the client are configured into a narrative with a plot (in one session or over time). This narrative often resembles myths or fairytales, e.g. the plot of the 'Hero's Journey' or the myth of 'Amor and Psyche').

Of course there are no causal relationships between music, metaphor and narrative. The imagery of the clients cannot and must not be directed. On the other hand, a music selection cannot stimulate or support any (random) kind of imagery and metaphor. The affinity of musical elements and metaphoric potential is discussed in the following part.

Three levels of music – or a metaphorical listening to four selections of baroque music

THREE PSYCHOLOGICAL LEVELS OF MUSIC

In Chapter 1.3 we introduced three levels of music application in therapy – an auxiliary, an augmentative and an intensive level (an adaptation of Bruscia's four levels). Here we will suggest three levels of music itself, in a process of metaphorical listening referring to the theories of music as analogy and metaphor described earlier.

When talking about 'music' in the context of pain management, alleviation of stress or anxiety and psychotherapy, we must be specific. Not all music has the potential for pain or stress relief, and when music is used in psychotherapy we must differentiate. Music can be labelled supportive, explorative, regenerative etc. However, it would be sad if the music of Mozart, Mahler, Messiaen, Mendelssohn or Miles Davis should be considered primarily on the basis of their medical or psychotherapeutic potential, and not on their experiential, existential and aesthetic qualities. Music can be arousing, hypnotic, anxiety provoking, mind healing or shattering, a source of inspiration or spiritual vision – it is like a magic mirror enabling the listener, be it a client or a therapist, to find answers to deep existential questions. No clear distinction can be made between the aesthetic (non-therapeutic) and the psychological (psychotherapeutic) potential of music experience and awareness.

As an alternative we will try to identify *three psychological levels of music*. One of the professional qualifications of a music therapist is to assess and evaluate the medical, social or psychological potential of improvised or composed music – based on the following or equivalent systematic criteria. Of course it is a theoretical construction to label three levels of music, and we think that some examples may help the reader to a clearer understanding of the idea. We have chosen to focus on four selected examples of composed music from the baroque period. The argument is that in baroque music it is fairly easy to isolate one musical feature (variable) which is held stable, while other features (variables) change. However, we think that in principle the considerations presented here are valid within a psychodynamic, metaphoric interpretation of music, independent of style, genre and origin (improvisation or composition).

A favorite musical principle in the baroque period is called *basso ostinato* (with cognate names like *canon, ground, chaconne* or *passacaglia*). The basic idea is well known from (but not quite identical with) the canon *Frère Jaques*, where each of the three parts are identical and introduced with a certain time interval. (In the third movement of Mahler's first Symphony the first section is such a *Frère Jaques canon*, however in minor and with a special orchestral colour, endowing this simple canon with an uneasy, almost surrealistic quality.) A typical baroque canon or chaconne has a bass part that is repeated unchanged from the beginning to the end of the piece/movement. The upper parts imitate each other with specific time intervals, presenting the primary melodic material of the composition (more or less like *Frère Jaques*). A composition of this type is:

   PACHELBEL: Canon in D (four string parts with basso continuo) – CD cut 22.

The bass introduces the ostinato in a solo over two bars. The meter is 4/4, and the ostinato is composed of eight notes of the same length (crotchet), beginning on tonic d and ending on dominant a – a new round can begin. The ostinato is repeated over and over without changes, while the upper string parts unfold a three-part canon. Violin 1 introduces the melody, two bars of stepwise melody progression in crotchets (like the bass), then Violin 2 begins on the same melody while violin 1 proceeds with a new phrase. Two bars later Violin 3 enters, following the same procedure. The most catchy characteristic of the composition is that the canon melody becomes more and more lively and varied, while the ostinato remains the same, in its steady and stable 'rocking'.

   Is it possible to find a suitable analogy to this composition in (developmental) psychology? Is it possible to experience this canon as a metaphor for interaction principles? We think so.

   The bass conducts itself like any 'good enough' father or mother would behave towards a child – it creates a perfect 'holding environment' (Winnicott 1971). No matter what the child comes up with, it will be held and contained. When listening to Pachelbel's *Canon* it is obvious that the three 'canonic parts' unfold more and more lively and 'independently'. They 'dare' do this exactly because their base is safe and predictable. This is a perfect metaphor for what developmental psychologist Margaret Mahler calls 'the rehearsal phase', where the child by turns tests itself in experiments in the surrounding world and returns to 'fill the tank' and be confirmed by a significant other. Within Guided Imagery and Music numerous client experiences confirm that Pachelbel's *Canon* is 'holding music', a safe and predictable composition enabling a safe 'arrival' after a long and maybe frightening journey in the world of imagery.

   We label this level of experience *the supportive and image stimulating level 1.*

   Now, the question is, do all compositions based on an ostinato have this 'holding' quality? A closer investigation of other selections will demonstrate that it is not so. A provisional explanation is that music is a multi-layered composition (or configuration) of many elements, which play their specific role in the construction of meaning. When a composition is more complex, the ostinato may change its metaphoric potential. This is evident when we take a closer look at two ostinato-based compositions by Johann Sebastian Bach.

J.S. BACH: Passacaglia and fugue in C minor, BWV 582 – CD cut 23.

(Composed for organ, but also arranged for orchestra by (among others) L. Stokowski.)

The bass ostinato of this passacaglia is twice as long as Pachelbel's, and Bach's composition has a much larger scope. The melodic, canonic parts are ever-changing in timbre and character (which is emphasized in the orchestral arrangement), and there are many contrasts in the passacaglia alone. From a musical point of view this ostinato is not as predictable and stable as Pachelbel's. Even if the actual notes remain the same, duration, rhythm, timbre and volume do not. The first half of the ostinato is preserved in the fugue (as the 'dux' theme), and according to the principles of a fugue it is heard in all (four) parts respectively. In the fugue version the ostinato has a stable and more extrovert, powerful character. Taken as a whole it is a majestic and quite overwhelming composition.

Experienced metaphorically the ostinato is a voice-in-command. No matter what other (parts) may say or do, it maintains its 'dictum', it cannot be persuaded or 'moved' to 'change its mind'. This may be experienced as a dominating, patriarchal voice (the father, boss, even God), and it makes the passacaglia a genuine psychological challenge. Many brave GIM clients have fought against such an antagonist, a commanding authority or a superego figure.

We label this level of experience *the explorative and uncovering level 2.*

The example makes it clear that an ostinato may be anything but supportive and calming. We meet a third and completely different type of ostinato in a movement from Bach's Mass in B minor.

J.S. BACH: Crucifixus from the Mass in B minor, BWV 232 – (The following analysis is based on the recording by the New Philarmonia Orchestra/Otto Klemperer, EMI: 7633642, which is not included on the CD with this book).

This movement is based on a four-bar ostinato in E minor, which is repeated 12 times. One of its specific characteristics is that it features a descending chromatic line with five halftone steps from the fundamental e to the dominant's b. With a certain knowledge of symbolic meaning in Bach's compositions it is possible to identify this chromaticism as an expression of the utmost agony and its passionate mystery. The agony is amplified by the four vocal parts, not only due to the text (*'He was crucified for us …'*), but also because the music exposes a variety of extreme dissonances.

There is tremendous tension between the four parts internally, but also between the vocal parts and the ostinato. The parts 'cross' one another; Bach has composed a 'tone painting' of the crucifixion. No matter if the listener experiences this as pure music, as religious litany or metaphorically, it is music of an oppressive character. Death on the cross is inevitable, and the music takes an iron grasp of the listener. This is not the voice of a stern father or superego, it is rather the voice of absurdity, the unescapable destiny bringing death or loss of ego and self. Bach has composed this existential zero point in absolute contrast to the exaltation and joy of the following movement – *'et ressurrexit/and was resurrected from the dead'*.

In the GIM music program *Death-Rebirth*, the *Crucifixus* is the turning point in a life-giving journey, a descension into the symbolic land of shadows, which is followed by a slow ascension to a new beginning (Mahler: excerpt (the last ten minutes) of *Abschied* from *Das Lied von der Erde*).

This music can only be used for special clinical (or self-experiential) purposes, and we label this level of experience *the intensive level 3*.

The bass is fundamental. In the baroque period this so-called 'thorough bass/Generalbass' symbolized the very harmonic order of the universe, on which the expressive melodic parts depended. This is very clear in:

J.S. BACH: Air, second movement of Orchestral Suite No. 3 in D major BWV 1068 – CD cut 25.

This bass part is firm and stable, almost like Pachelbel's ostinato. However, this is not an ostinato, rather a 'walking bass', moving untiringly forward in stable and slow major or minor seconds. The composition is in two sections (the second twice as long as the first), and both sections are repeated. Most listeners experience this composition as very relaxing and comforting, not the least because the tempo is close to 60 beats per minute – the pulse of a slow and steady heartbeat. But how does this relate to the salient contrasts and tensions between the calm progression of the bass and the expressive melodic lines of the upper parts?

The movement is an 'air' – i.e. 'a song without words'. However, it is possible to interpret the 'words' or the meaning of the song. The baroque doctrine of 'musical affects' makes it possible to identify the emotions (or affects) expressed in Violin 1 (and to a lesser degree in Violin 2). The melody is complex, irregular, characterized by large melodic intervals and 'sighing' accents ('Seufzers') or suspension that create a harmonic tension between melody and bass. This is a symbol of suffering. There are also melodic episodes characterized by a striving upwards, in syncopated rhythms and with increasing volume. This is a symbol of passion. Heard as a whole the passionate voices express longing – a longing of the heart.

Experienced and interpreted in this way, Bach's Air is a musical expression of the passionate human being, integrated in a higher order. This (divine) order is (re)presented by the bass and its accompanying harmonic chords, proceeding in a solemn progression undisturbed by human suffering, passion, longing and mistakes. In our post-modern era it is not common to understand man as 'enfolded' in a higher order. However, the experience of 'coming home', 'belonging' and 'being accepted' is accessible through music listening, and many GIM 'travellers' have experienced this during their imaginal journey through Bach's Air. The music is therefore identified as belonging to level 1.

If you listen to the music selections on the CD (and the Crucifixus from the Mass in B Minor, J.S. Bach from another recording) it becomes obvious that Pachelbel's Canon and Bach's Air may potentially be used in pain management and supportive psychotherapy. The other two Bach selections would be inappropriate for these purposes; however, their potential can be unfolded in intensive psychotherapeutic, existential or spiritual processes.

(If the reader wishes to compare the four selected examples with other ostinato-based movements we can suggest a few. An example of a fast, merry and reassuring ostinato movement is the final *Halleluja* of Buxtehude's cantata *Der Herr ist mit mir*. The Death of Falstaff from Walton's suite *Henry V* is based on an ostinato of the same length and melodically is quite close to Pachelbel's. However, as it is in a minor key and the mood is very different, this rather simple composition belongs to level 2 or 3. The title of Bach's cantata BWV 12 is 'Weinen, klagen, sorgen, zagen'. This is also the text of the first chorus, based on the same music as the *Crucifixus*. Through the text we gain information on the nuances of pain and suffering expressed in the music, and if the interpretation accentuates the many advanced dissonances, the music will probably function at level 2 rather than level 3. Much of the same can be said about 'Dido's Lament', the final aria 'When I am Laid in Earth' from Purcell's opera *Dido and Aeneas*. A movement with a chromatic descending ostinato may also have a lighter character. An example of this is the instrumental 'Ground' from Blow's opera *Venus and Adonis* (a predecessor of Purcell's more popular work). Melodically this ostinato is very close to the *Crucifixus* ostinato, but it is in triple time, the tempo is relatively fast, and so together with the poignant rhythm this makes the movement noble and light at the same time. The function level will therefore be 1 or 2.)

The selected recordings of baroque music in GIM and on the CD accompanying this book are all more than 30 years old, in arrangements for full orchestra or a fairly large string body, and the performances follow the romantic style of performance and recording that dominated in this repertoire until 1980. Contemporary baroque performances are very different, including the use of period instruments and based on scholarly studies of baroque performance practice. However, many of these excellent recordings cannot be used in GIM because they do not have the absolutely necessary 'holding quality' of the romantic performances, enabling the client to let go and delve into the music experience.

In summary, we will present some general characteristics of level 1 music that may be applied in pain and anxiety management, in deep relaxation and in supportive psychotherapy (called *sedative music* by Helen Bonny):

- medium or slow tempo (60 bpm or slower)
- steady, predictable rhythm (matching the breathing and pulse of the client)
- simple structure with recognizable melodies or themes (instrumental or vocal)
- simple, consonant harmony without sudden shifts or modulations
- stable dynamics without sudden shifts or contrasts.

Even though Bonny recommends classical music, it is obvious that these characteristics can be found in almost any musical style or genre. We also know that some people achieve relaxation and wellbeing using *stimulating* music, which differs from the above by a faster tempo and a more active rhythmic drive. Two different principles may be followed when music is selected for modification or transformation of mood:

1. Following the ISO principle, music must be selected that matches the mood of the client in the beginning, and then gradually induces the intended mood.

2. Following the compensation principle, music must be selected that contrasts the mood of the client and thus gradually (re)attunes the client's mood.

The two principles are not mutually exclusive, as they can be related to two different aspects of the music. The ISO principle works on a vegetative level where the musical sequence corresponds to the listener's bodily sense of tempo (slow/fast; accelerando/ritardando), excitement and relief, tension and release. The compensation principle works on the emotional level where there is a complex interaction of the mood expressed in the music and the client's mood and emotional state.

Music at level 2 or 3 cannot easily be characterized in the same way. Not only is the music more complex in itself, but the combination of selected movements is like a psychologically informed composition itself. It is part of the qualification of a GIM therapist to make clear distinctions between the three levels in clinical practice (using the 30-plus music programs and their, in principle, unlimited combination potential). This expertise is developed not only through traditional music analysis of structure, melodic material, harmonic progression etc., but also through self-experience (the music as heard in an altered state of consciousness) and phenomenological description of the music sequence – what is salient in the listener's experience of the music as it is unfolding – and of the imagery potential, based on personal and client imagery.

In other words: a GIM therapist is systematically trained in *metaphoric music listening*. However, music experienced as metaphor is not the privilege of experts or therapists. Open and attentive listening is the (only) gate to a thorough understanding of music's enormous existential and therapeutic potential.

CHAPTER 3

Models and Methods
of Music Therapy

Introduction: Music Therapy Models from an International Perspective

How can a music therapy model be defined – as different from a 'school', a 'method' or a 'technique'? This question is important if you try to establish an international overview of music therapy in theory and practice. In 1993 Cheryl Maranto edited a comprehensive anthology with chapters on music therapy in 38 invited countries from all continents (Dileo-Maranto 1993b). It was impressive (and also somewhat confusing) to be informed about the many different ways of practising and understanding music therapy. Maranto identified 14 models or 'schools' in the USA alone, and more than 100 different techniques, all carefully documented in the book. Before we begin this chapter's introduction to a few selected models and approaches, we will outline our understanding of some core concepts. Bruscia's definition of what is a method, variation, procedure, technique and model is relevant here in connection to understanding terminology in theoretical descriptions (Bruscia 1998a):

> A *method* is here defined as a particular type of music experience that the client engages in for therapeutic purposes; a *variation* is the particular way in which that music experience is designed; a *procedure* is everything that the therapist has to do to engage the client in that experience; a *technique* is one step within any procedure that a therapist uses to shape the client's immediate experience; and a *model* is a systematic and unique approach to method, procedure and technique based on certain principles. (p.115)

In some countries and languages, especially European, there is no sharp distinction between 'method', 'approach' and 'model', and this often causes linguistic confusion and communication problems. However, what we describe in this chapter are five internationally well-known and acknowledged *models* of music therapy (Chapters 3.1 to 3.5), and three traditional *methods* of music therapy (Chapters 3.6 to 3.8).

The 9th World Congress of Music Therapy in Washington (1999) presented 'five internationally known models of music therapy' as a concurrent theme. These five models were introduced and illustrated from many different perspectives: history, theory, clinical practice, research and training, and they included Guided Imagery and Music (developed by Helen Bonny), Analytical Music Therapy (developed by Mary Priestley), *Creative Music Therapy* (developed by Paul Nordoff and Clive Robbins), Benenzon Music Therapy (developed by Rolando Benenzon) and Behavioural Music Therapy (developed by, amongst others, Clifford K. Madsen).

Four of the five model founders were present in Washington; only Mary Priestley was absent (but her paper was presented by others). In this chapter we have chosen to give a concentrated introduction to four of these five models – those most relevant in northern and central Europe. We have chosen not to include Benenzon's model, even though it deserves attention (which it receives mainly in South America and, to a limited degree, on one or two courses in southern Europe), more because of its eclectic character, with theoretical elements, procedures and techniques inspired by many different psychological and psychotherapeutic models. This makes it unsuited to a text like this. However, many of Benenzon's most important texts are available in English (Benenzon 1982, 1997).

Many other models are internationally well known and deserve attention. We have chosen to include Juliette Alvin's *Free Improvisation Therapy*, which meets the same criteria as the four models mentioned above and seems more relevant in this guide to music therapy.

Each model is presented in the same format:

1.   a historical outline and one or more definitions

2.   the session format, its elements and characteristic procedures and techniques

3.   clinical applications

4.   documentation: in most cases preferred documentation formats and research examples are included

5.   the model is identified using the categorization system of levels of clinical practice suggested by Bruscia (1998a). However, we have modified this

categorization in the following way. Bruscia identifies four levels of practice: *auxiliary, augmentative, intensive* and *primary*. We find three levels sufficient: *auxiliary, augmentative* and *intensive* – where *intensive* includes *primary*.

Bruscia also identifies six areas of practice: didactic, medical, healing, psychotherapeutic, recreative and ecological. However, this categorization will not be further discussed in this chapter, and can be more comprehensively understood from *Definins Music Therapy* (Bruscia 1998).

After the survey of five selected models, other important methods and procedures are presented. We do not consider them *models*, as they are typically *methods* for specific clinical areas with more or less connected procedures, variations and techniques: physiological responses to music (Chapter 3.6), *music in medicine* (Chapter 3.7), and music and healing (Chapter 3.8).

3.1 Guided Imagery and Music – The Bonny Model

In receptive music therapy the most important procedure is active music listening. There are several models and procedures within receptive music therapy, for example 'regulative music therapy' developed by Dr Christoph Schwabe in Germany (*Regulative Musikterapie*, Schwabe 1987). However, the most internationally renowned model is the Bonny Method of Guided Imagery and Music (GIM). GIM has practitioners in North and South America, in Oceania and in ten European countries. In Denmark there is one certified training program, led by Torben Moe, and five GIM therapists. Level one of the GIM training is included in the Music Therapy program at Aalborg University, and the Danish training program is open to other Scandinavian trainees.

The official definition of GIM informs us that 'GIM is a music centered [sic] investigation of consciousness' (Association of Music and Imagery 1999). However, this is also the case with other models of music psychotherapy, and it may be more precise to use the definition of the founder of the model, Helen Lindquist Bonny, who states that 'GIM is a process, where imagery is evoked during music listening' (Bonny 1990). A more comprehensive definition is that GIM 'is a depth approach to music psychotherapy in which specifically programmed classical music is used to generate a dynamic unfolding of inner experiences ... (it is) holistic, humanistic and transpersonal, allowing for the emergence of all aspects of the human experience: psychological, emotional, physical, social, spiritual, and the collective unconscious' (Goldberg 1995).

The history of GIM

In the 1960s Helen Bonny was trained as a music therapist and researcher in the behavioural tradition, but her background as a musician (violinist) and a minister's wife, working for many years in pastoral counselling, led her in a different direction. In the early 1970s she worked at Maryland Psychiatric Research Center in the USA, where she selected the music used in conjunction with the experimental psychotherapeutic treatment of alcoholics and terminal cancer patients with hallucinatory drugs such as LSD. This work is described in a classical paper written in collaboration with Dr W. Pahnke (Bonny and Pahnke 1972). The use of LSD in research was prohibited in 1972, and Helen Bonny gradually developed a drug-free psychotherapeutic model: deep relaxation led to an altered state of consciousness and was followed by shorter selections of classical music, which were sequenced to assist deep psychotherapeutic work on different issues and problems. It is interesting to observe that Helen Bonny and Stanislav Grof, who had a common starting point in the LSD-based research at the Maryland Center, later found complementary ways in the music-based or assisted psychotherapeutic models: Grof went the 'ergothropic' way when he developed his holotropic breathwork (Grof 1988), while Bonny went the 'trophotropic' way with GIM (Bonny 1975, reprinted in *Nordic Journal of Music Therapy* 8, 2).

One of the problems in the LSD-based therapy was that clients could not remember much of their very strong experiences after the session, and GIM developed as a procedure utilizing the two non-drug components of the LSD therapy: the altered state of consciousness (facilitated by autogenic training (Schultz) or progressive relaxation (Jacobson)) and the dynamic evocative potentials of classical music. Gradually Bonny developed a session format in four phases and a series of music programs. The session format is described in detail below.

Today, more than 30 specific music programs are available, and new programs are added now and then (12 of these are so-called 'core programs'). In 1995–1996 Ken Bruscia developed a set of 10 CDs, *Music for the Imagination*, and he published a manual describing the complicated history of the GIM music programs, their later revisions by Helen Bonny and other GIM therapists, and their modifications in the new CD collection, based on Naxos recordings (Bruscia 1996). The music programs have a duration from 30 to 50 minutes and are composed of three to eight longer or shorter selected movements or single pieces from the classical music heritage, ranging historically from baroque to contemporary music, both instrumental and vocal. The music is sequenced in order to support, generate and deepen experiences related to various psychological (or physiological) needs, i.e. 'the experience of unconditioned support and a safe base', 'aggression support and stimulation', 'an invitation to delve into deep grief', 'creating a ritual of transition', or 'symbolic death and rebirth'. In the music travel the client has the opportunity to experience aspects of his/her life as imagery in many modalities. The images are (considered) metaphors of the client's problems and beliefs, strengths and weaknesses. GIM is an opportunity to tell and retell a life story in a symbolic medium, to reconfigure life episodes and the emotions connected with them. The music travel may assist the client in deconstructing old life scripts and stimulate him/her to 'tell a new tale'.

The session: procedures and techniques

The four phases of the GIM session are analogies to the sections of the sonata form: exposition – development – recapitulation – coda. The analogy or metaphor refers to the dynamic principle of both therapy and musical (sonata) form: it is a process where material is introduced, developed, transformed and integrated. However, in the following we will use the concepts normally used in GIM: prelude – induction – music travel – postlude. The interventions of the therapist are chosen and may be described within a spectrum of possible attitudes or orientations, and in the text this spectrum is made explicit. One end of the spectrum is more cognitive, the other more intuitive.

1. PRELUDE

The prelude (15 to 20 minutes) has, as a point of departure, the client's life world and conscious experience of his/her problems. During the prelude the therapist will gradually try to turn the client's attention from the outer to the inner world, and a focus point for the session must be identified. The transition from the conscious experience of the outer world to a more open awareness of the inner world is marked by the client's physical change of position – he/she lies down on a mat and closes his/her eyes. The therapist takes a position enabling physical comfort, full control over the audio system, overview of the full body of the client, and transcription of the dialogue (the therapist takes notes of dialogue and important reactions during the music travel).

2. INDUCTION, RELAXATION AND FOCUSING

This phase lasts from two to seven minutes, and within the spectrum of attitudes the therapist may choose Position A, to select elements of the client's conscious narrative, or Position B, listen carefully to identify a more emotional level, the level of the 'subtext'.

Example: The client gives a detailed report of her daily feelings of 'loneliness'.

From Position A, the therapist may chose to focus on a concrete situation that can be formed – like a 'Gestalt' – in the relaxation and in an induction image, e.g. 'Tense the muscles in part a … b … c … of your body as much as you can (without laying pressure on yourself) and … relax … Feel the difference …' (duration is approximately five minutes, without music). 'Now imagine yourself in a situation just before meeting X' (whom the client has described as playing an important role in his/her life). The music begins, and the therapist asks: 'How is the situation for you?'

From Position B, the therapist may choose a suitable metaphor or equivalent image, e.g. 'No-one is holding you'. The induction may sound like: 'Lift part a … b … c … of your body and feel how light or heavy it is.' The music begins and the therapist may say: 'Allow the music to help you hold part a … b … c … Can the music help you hold your body?'

The purpose of the induction is to facilitate a transition from ego-dominated to deeper levels of consciousness and to surrender to a more flexible experience of time and space. A focus, a limitation of the possible choices, is necessary in order to avoid insecurity or confusion in this exploratory timespace. The focus serves as 'a miner's lamp in the darkness'.

3. MUSIC TRAVEL

The therapist is the guide for the client, and the guiding may be quite directive in the first two phases. The choice of music is also the responsibility of the therapist. However, during the 'music travel' the therapist takes a non-directive attitude. He/she must be a trustworthy companion, who will follow the client anywhere the client chooses, and dares to go. Client and therapist share the imagery of the client, broadly understood as inner experiences in different modalities: visual, auditory, olfactory, gustatory, tactile. Memories and emotions are also included in the concept of imagery. The imagery of the client may be clear or diffuse, rapidly or slowly changing, personal or impersonal, disconnected or coherent. Every client has a specific 'style of travelling', and it normally takes a few sessions to develop optimum response to the imagery and the music. Again, the orientation of the therapist may be exemplified through the spectrum.

Example: from Position A the therapist understands the music as a stimulus evoking imagery. The music is a 'projection screen' on which the unconscious of the client may project its content. The therapist wants to know as much as possible about the image potentials of the music (pieces and programs).

From Position B the therapist considers the music as the core element of the experience. The imagery is a tool enabling a maximum outcome of the music experience. Some GIM therapists consider music an 'archetypal field of energy' where the mythical structures of the music operate and facilitate therapeutic change.

No matter what orientation the therapist may have, he/she will do his/her best to engage the client in music travel and the exploration of the imagery which may also lead to transpersonal experiences. The music travel lasts 30 to 50 minutes, depending on the program or improvised music choice of the therapist, and the client's actual imagery and process.

4. POSTLUDE

When the music comes to an end the client is guided slowly but surely back to a normal state of consciousness. As a standard element in this transition the client is encouraged to keep and concentrate his/her experience in a different modality – e.g. a drawing (*mandala*), a sculpture (clay work) or a poem. This may last 5 to 10 minutes. The last part of the postlude is a short dialogue (10 to 20 minutes) where the therapist helps the client to connect the experience to his/her daily life and the problem in focus.

Example: from Position A the therapist will guide the client into an interpretation of the imagery, aiming at new insight into the problem.

From Position B the therapist considers the music and imagery experience transforming in itself. He/she will probably stay in the metaphors of the imagery and encourage the client to explore the most important parts further.

Independent of attitude the therapist will acknowledge the client's own interpretation of the experience as authoritative.

Clinical applications of GIM

A classical GIM session is long, 90 to 120 minutes, and rather demanding. The client must have sufficient ego strength to trust and delve into the flow of images, and he/she must be able to distinguish between imagery and reality. Classical GIM is contraindicated for clients with reality (testing) problems, emotional instability and intellectual impairment. GIM has been used in a number of clinical settings and with many different client populations: self-development and transpersonal work of neuro-typical people, *music healing*, training therapy, drug addiction, abuse, neurotic disturbances, and, in the somatic field, clients suffering from cancer, and people living with HIV and other life-threatening diseases. The clinical field of applied GIM is broadening quite fast, mostly due to experiences with modifications of the classical format:

- sessions may be shorter (5 to 20 minutes of music)

- music and interventions may be supportive rather than exploratory and challenging

- including music other than classical

- guiding may be more directive, both with individuals and in groups.

Clinical projects and research indicate that modified GIM may be beneficial for psychiatric patients (Moe 2000), hospice patients (West 1994; Wylie 1986), patients with brain damage (Moe 1995) and autism (Clarkson 1998).

A well described and often used modification is *the guided group music travel*. This can also be applied to staff training, team building, music education and coursework in different fields. This is not a classical GIM technique, because the guide is quite directive during the music travel and because there is no dialogue during the travel, only a sharing afterwards. These 'fantasy travels with music' are useful for many purposes, and there are several published manuals and exercises (Bonny and Savary 1990; Bush 1996).

Documentation

The GIM literature covers clinical studies, clinical theory and research studies in both process and effect. A database of GIM literature has more than 300 entries from many countries. There are many case studies (single or multiple) based on the analysis of session transcripts of the therapeutic dialogue, the music selections and the mandalas (many of these are published in the *Journal of the Association for Music and Imagery* and in Bruscia 1991 and 1998a). In an extraordinary case study Ginger Clarkson (1998) has documented that GIM is an effective treatment modality for a man with autism – thus also demonstrating that autistics are not excluded from the world of imagery. Helen Bonny has bequeathed her papers, and other material, to Temple University, where a Bonny Archive will open in 2002 (together with a Mary Priestley Archive, see www.temple.edu/musictherapy).

GIM research is conducted both in quantitative and qualitative designs (see Bonde 1997). Effect studies have been conducted by Björn Wrangsjö and Dag Körlin (1995, 2001), and Torben Moe has studied the effect of modified GIM with schizotypical in-hospital clients (Moe 1998, 2000; Moe *et al.* 2000). There are several studies of the effect of GIM on cancer patients and people living with HIV (Bruscia 1991, 1998a; Bunt *et al.* 2000; Burns 2001). A very important qualitative research project was conducted by Denise Erdonmez Grocke (1999b), whose PhD dissertation 'The Music that Underpins Pivotal Moments in Guided Imagery and Music' also contains important information on the history of GIM. Grocke uses a phenomenological method of inquiry, where interviews with seven GIM clients are analysed with focus on pivotal experiences. The music underpinning these experiences is identified and analysed. Other researchers have studied transpersonal experiences and (music) transference in GIM.

Categorization

In Bruscia's systematic account of music therapy models (Bruscia 1998) GIM is placed at the intensive level as a transformative music psychotherapy, because in GIM 'the music experience is therapeutically transformative and complete in, of, and by itself, independent of any insights gained through verbal exchange' (1998, p.219).

3.2 Analytically Oriented Music Therapy – The Priestley Model

Analytically Oriented Music Therapy (AOM) is a further development of what was earlier called Analytical Music Therapy. Together with the tradition of Nordoff-Robbins music therapy, AOM is the most widely used active music therapy form in Denmark. In this music therapy modality the clients are actively involved in clinically organized musical activities and the most applied form of musical performance is improvisation. The improvisations can be tonal as well as atonal and it is the clients' way of expressing themselves in improvising music that influences the form and style of the improvisations. Composed music can also be used, or the activity of composing songs or instrumental music, as a part of the work. In all cases personal and/or functional development of the clients are in focus and not an evaluation of the aesthetic quality of the musical product.

Historical development of Analytical Music Therapy

Analytical Music Therapy (AM) was founded at the start of the 1970s by the English professional violinist Mary Priestley, who undertook her music therapy training at the Guildhall School of Music and Drama in London. As Mary Priestley simultaneously went through a personal psychoanalysis for many years, she began the development of a specific theory to combine music therapy and psychoanalysis. In her clinical work she tried to combine a psychoanalytical and psychotherapeutic understanding of the transference phenomena between the client and the therapist with the understanding of meaning and form of expressions in musical improvisations. Her books and articles mirror this deep interest and her important contribution to music therapy in developing Analytical Music Therapy (Priestley 1975, 1994).

No training programs in the 1970s had this combination. Priestley created a supplementary training module for qualified music therapists that mostly contained a comprehensive ETMT (experiential training of music therapists) module including individual music therapy and *intertherapy* with the students in the client role.

Priestley defines AM as follows:

> Analytical Music Therapy is the name that has prevailed for the analytically-informed symbolic use of improvised music by the music therapist and client. It is used as a creative tool with which to explore the client's inner life so as to provide the way forward for growth and greater self-knowledge. (Priestley 1994, p.3)

Clinical applications and applications in training

Mary Priestley primarily developed AM in work with psychiatric clients and in her counselling work with private clients. The application of the method today spreads over a whole range of clients where the symbolic use of improvised music (often combined with fairytales or other stories) in work with ego-weak children and adolescents can also create an indirect way of being better integrated or of helping to get a stronger and more clear self-picture and self-understanding. From being a supplementary training AM has been further developed and expanded to be the foundation and primary theoretical basis for some three- to five-year music therapy training programs. The idea of integrating ETMT into a MA program that is methodologically broad-based (as in Aalborg University) is to give the students basic tools to work psychotherapeutically, with music as the primary tool, with clients with complex psychological problems. The basic idea of ETMT training is to develop the students' sensitivity to a level so that they can better resonate with the problems of their clients.

In work with clients with complex psychological problems this training is important for building up alliances and trustful relationships in the music therapy work. In work with other populations (e.g. multiply disabled children) it is more an underlying source of information for the music therapist to get to know what to do, when to intervene and how to understand acts and interventions, as these clients cannot feed back verbally.

Analytically Oriented Music Therapy – a way of understanding and analysing the music

In Denmark and in Germany the term Analytical Music Therapy is no longer used. It has been replaced by the term Analytically Oriented Music Therapy (AOM) which indicates that the method is no longer solely based on psychoanalytical or analytical psychology theories. It is also based on communication theories, on developmental psychological theories and theories concerning the psychosocial components in developing one's personality. This development can be seen as a logical outcome, where AM is being incorporated as a basic modality in eclectic training programmes.

The understanding and analysis of the music can be examined from different ports of entry.

It is still a tradition that a joint analysis of all three components – the music therapist, the music and the client – is truly emphasized in understanding stages of development in AOM. As an example, Bruscia's Improvisational Assessment Profiles (IAPs) (1987) are often used to focus on certain aspects or stages of development in the musical improvisation most often recorded for the aim of being analysed. This includes using the same profile for both the client and the therapist. Another model for analysing uses Stern's terminology in describing mother/infant communication and can be applied to understand the improvisation (see Chapter 4.1).

As you can see it is important that the music is analysed as a unit that includes both the meaningful expressions of the client and how these expressions influence the simultaneous meaningful expressions of the music therapist. In other words a lot of emphasis is placed on the transference phenomena and the relationship between the therapist and the client.

The session: procedures and techniques

In individual work with AOM the therapist works alone. In group work there are usually two therapists working together adopting roles as primary therapist and co-therapist. In work with clients who are able to verbalize, a session typically starts with the therapist and client intuitively exploring verbally what is meaningful for the client here and now. From there they create a working topic formulated into a playing rule as an inspiration for a musical improvisation. During the music performance this working topic is non-verbally explored and the music therapist can be supportive or creative, improvising in connection with the client's music. He/she can also play a certain role that has been decided beforehand. The music can start tonally or atonally and develop in different directions. It often occurs that a slightly altered state of consciousness arises for the music therapist and client during the act of improvising music. This phenomenon can help in creating new ideas in playing/expressing oneself and in understanding the problem. The responsibility of the therapist is to let go of a full 'controlling' consciousness, while at the same time keeping an overview of the total act of interplaying. So the therapist is working in a condition of double awareness. Strong feelings expressed musically by the client must be supported or contained by the therapist. Finally, the client may want to play alone and to 'be listened to carefully' by the therapist. The client may also, on occasions, want the therapist to play some familiar classical music or 'caring' improvised music for him/her while he/she is listening and 'being nursed' by the music. A basic problem for psychiatric clients is to be motivated to stay engaged in an activity in order to give a chance for a process to be developed. Overall AOM is a caring method but the work can develop into a strong emotional confrontation for the client, when sufficient trust is present between the therapist and client.

It is important in AOM work that there is a verbal reflection after the playing activity in order to give the clients the possibility to make conscious the inner movements that were provoked in the musical improvisation. Normally a session ends with a final music improvisation where the material that was brought up in the session is digested as much as possible.

Philosophically AOM can de defined as music in therapy, as the music is used to symbolically express inner moods, emotions and associations. It often happens though, that the music 'takes over' and starts to live a life of its own during an improvisation, so that new and unexpected sounds, tones, rhythms and melodies turn the client and therapist away from the intentions they began with. Therefore one can say that AOM often becomes both *music in therapy* and *music as therapy* simultaneously. It is therefore important that the music therapist is flexible in his/her abilities of playing the piano, the drum-set and also other instruments.

PLAYING RULES

To find a focus or a topic for the musical improvisation is called: (creating) playing rules. Many different categories of playing rules can be created and used according to the type of problem. In the form of short-term AOM, there is often both an overall working topic for the course of treatment, and also playing rules created in each individual session. The task of the playing rules is to make the client connect with, and express, certain emotions, fantasies, dreams, body experiences, memories or situations through the music. The playing rule acts as an inspiration and a basis for the inner imagination and for the emotional and sensational experiences that emerge during music improvisation.

At the same time improvisations are unpredictable. Even if the players start with a clear awareness of what they want to express, the music in itself can surprise and transform what is being expressed so the transformation in itself becomes a part of the curing elements. Most often the client is prepared for the music performance through one or more centerring exercises.

Documentation

Priestley herself has written two books on techniques and theory creatively exemplified with a lot of clinical narratives (Priestley 1975, 1994) and she has also edited a range of articles on certain aspects of AOM. AOM today extends all over Europe and influences a number of training programs. Over the last 10 years interest in AM has been growing in the USA, where Scheiby today offers a supplementary training module based on Priestley's original AM model for trained music therapists. AOM is still identified by most music therapists primarily as a method for work with psychiatric clients and for counselling work. In Denmark two books in a series of books on music therapy in psychiatry (Lindvang 2000; Pedersen 1998) are based on AOM, and many chapters of international books (Bruscia 1998a; Wigram and De Backer 1999b) also are AOM oriented.

In AOM work with all kinds of client populations, the focus is on the client's self-healing forces and mental resources. In work with multiply disabled clients who cannot verbalize, AOM can be used to gain contact and to communicate at a very basic level. Understanding of stages of development has to be based on the condition of the clients and often has to be seen as tiny nuances.

AM practice has given much inspiration to qualitative research projects, where PhD projects by Langenberg (1988), Mahns (1997), Hannibal (2001) and Hadley (1998) should be mentioned. Bruscia (1998, p.219) places AM (here AOM) on the advanced level of treatment as this therapeutic modality aims at letting the client obtain deep insight, integration and transformation of complex psychological problems.

3.3 Creative Music Therapy – The Nordoff-Robbins Model

Paul Nordoff, an American composer and pianist, and Clive Robbins, a British trained special educator, collaborated together to pioneer one of the most famous improvisational models of music therapy developed over the last 50 years. This approach is now called Creative Music Therapy, and is known worldwide as the Nordoff-Robbins approach.

The history of Creative Music Therapy

Their method, developed between 1959 and 1976, has been taught in several countries, including Great Britain, Germany, USA, Australia, Japan, South Africa, Canada and Norway, and students of this method tend to continue using the approach in their clinical work. Most of the early development of Creative Music Therapy was aimed at children with learning disabilities, from the mild end of the spectrum to the severe, including Down's syndrome, emotionally and behaviourally disturbed, mentally and physically handicapped and children with autism. Paul Nordoff died in 1976, and Clive Robbins then further developed his work with Carol Robbins, his wife, introducing a new focus with hearing-impaired children, while maintaining the application of this model to mainly handicapped and emotionally disturbed children.

Philosophical orientation

In their early years of developing a music therapy method, Nordoff and Robbins were influenced by the ideas of Rudolf Steiner and the anthroposophic movement in humanistic psychology. Here they developed the idea that within every human being there is an innate responsiveness to music, and within every personality one can 'reach' a 'music child' or 'music person'. This idea was very important in their work with the handicapped population, where despite severe degrees of learning disability, and often severe physical disability, they believed in the potentially normal and natural responsiveness to music, and the power of music to enable self-expression and communication. Later, Robbins and Robbins related their therapeutic goals to the humanistic concepts of Abraham Maslow, including in their framework the aspiration towards self-actualization, peak experiences and developing special creative talents. Their relationship with the client is built on a warm, friendly approach, accepting the child as he/she is, recognizing, reflecting and respecting the child's feelings, allowing the child choice, and a non-directive approach to give the child autonomy, and the therapist the role of following and facilitating.

Method and approach in sessions

The Nordoff-Robbins style of work is unique and often easily recognizable. To begin with, it involves placing music at the centre of the experience, and musical responses provide the primary material for analysis and interpretation. They argue the need for highly skilled musicians and, as the use of a harmony instrument is central to their working style, they have predominantly trained therapists in the sophisticated use of piano (and in rare cases, guitar) in improvised music making. In individual therapy, the clients are typically offered a limited channel for their musical material, mainly the cymbal and drum, together with a strong encouragement to use their voice. In group work other instruments are involved – pitched percussion, reed horns, wind instruments and various string instruments.

In much of the individual work, and very much as a mark of their style of therapy, Nordoff-Robbins (where at all possible) work in pairs. One person establishes a musical relationship from the piano, while the other therapist facilitates the child's responses and engagement. This idea is based on the model of work employed with Paul Nordoff as the pianist/therapist, and Clive Robbins as the other therapist. Paul Nordoff's own music, mostly tonal in style, has also formed one of the foundations of the musical engagement, by which we mean that he developed a unique style of improvising that is evident in their two books of playsongs for children. Mostly, the therapists use creative improvisation, and create an engaging musical atmosphere from the moment the client enters the room to the moment he/she leaves.

The style of work, and their approach, comes within the conceptual framework of *Music as Therapy*, where the music provides the therapeutic catalyst through which change will take place. Music occurs almost throughout the session, and the therapeutic relationship is formed *in* the music. The therapists work through phases in their therapy:

> Meet the child musically...Evoke musical response...develop musical skills, expressive freedom, and interresponsiveness...(Bruscia 1987, p.45).

Clinical applications and process of therapy

Nordoff and Robbins offered a significant perspective on how music can be used in music therapy. The improvisational style must be free from musical conventions, and flexible. Intervals are important and represent different feelings, when used in melody. Triads and chords can be used in special ways – for example, the tonic triad to indicate stability, while inverted triads represent dynamic movement. Improvised music should also include musical archetypes, such as *organum*, exotic scales (Japanese, Middle Eastern), Spanish idioms and modal frameworks.

Music-making is the primary focus of therapy sessions, and from the early development of individual therapy, the experience of music was all-pervasive during the session. When working with children, clients are frequently brought into the therapy room while a welcoming music is being played by one therapist on the piano, and at the end of the session, they go out of the room to music. Music in the form of 'clinical improvisation' is used to establish a relationship with the client, provide a means of communication and self-expression, and effect change and the realization of potential. It is the belief in music itself as the medium of growth and development that is at the core of this approach, and the belief that in each person, regardless of disability, ill health, disturbance or trauma, there is a part which can be reached through music and called into responsiveness, thereby enabling healing and the subsequent generalization into the client's life (Etkin 1999).

The therapists often provide a musical frame, frequently establishing clear rhythm and pulse, and particularly, singing about what a patient is doing while they are doing it in order to bring into focus the experience that is occurring. Any musical expressions produced by the client, vocal or instrumental, are incorporated into a frame, and encouraged. The skill of the therapist is brought into play in providing an appropriate musical frame or context for the client's expressions, matching, mirroring or reflecting their musical material. The therapist pays close attention to responding musically to the quality, timbre, pitch, dynamics and inflection of the client's vocal, instrumental and body expression.

The clinical application of Creative Music Therapy has been introduced in a wide-ranging and diverse way. The graduates of the courses in the Nordoff-Robbins method, particularly in New York, London, Sydney, Pretoria and Witten/Herdecke in Germany, have diversified the approach to work with adult patients in the areas of neurology, psychiatry and terminal illness. The method has been tremendously developed through research and extension of applications (Aigen 1991, 1996, 1998; Ansdell 1995, 1996, 1997; Brown 1999b; Lee 1996, 2000; Pavlicevic 1995, 1997; Pavlicevic and Trevarthen 1994; Streeter 1999a; Neugebauer and Aldridge 1998).

Documentation

This model of music therapy has also developed methods of analysing what is going on and how the therapy is progressing. A number of scales have been generated including:

- thirteen categories of response
- child-therapist relationship

- musical communicativeness

- musical response scales: instrumental rhythmic responses, singing responses.

Case studies are the most typical way by which therapists working in the Nordoff-Robbins tradition document their work. The material is often presented as a 'story', a narrative description of the process and progress of therapy. Howat (1995) presented a lengthy and detailed account of individual work with a young 10-year-old girl with autism called Elizabeth, documenting more than 100 sessions over a five-year period. The narrative descriptions, sometimes brief and sometimes more detailed, mainly focused on her musical behaviour in the sessions, explaining how she played with many examples and interpretations of the emotional expression present in her playing. Life events were also included in order to make a context for the musical process in the therapy.

Etkin (1999) described a period of therapy with an emotionally, physically and socially abused and deprived child called Danu. She described the way that Danu played during the initial assessment session, and then set out the case study in the stages of therapy: early work – emergence of songs and stories – disclosure – endings. A method of improvisation called 'singspiel' or 'sprechgesang' featured strongly in the therapy sessions, and there was significantly more verbal material than is typical in other case studies from this tradition. From this example, it is clear that while the original conceptual model of Nordoff-Robbins provides the basis for a strong and grounded training, individual therapists develop methods and techniques out of their primary approach. Piano-based improvisation still forms the foundation, but guitar-based improvisation developed by Dan Gormley in the USA, jazz and blues improvisation styles more culturally effective with some populations in New York developed by Alan Turry, and Aesthetic Music Therapy recently defined by Colin Lee in Canada, amongst others, have emerged from the initial foundations of Creative Music Therapy.

Because Paul Nordoff and Clive Robbins lived in Denmark for a period of time, and also taught in Norway, there are therapists in both countries that follow their style of work, and others who incorporate their concepts at a more general level with certain clinical populations. Claus Bang, the Danish music therapist and audio-speech therapist, has translated the playsongs for use in Denmark.

Creative Music Therapy has lasted the test of time, and is a much practised model of music therapy, more now than ever before, as can be seen in the increasing number of case studies using this approach in the music therapy literature. It is relevant to look first at the writings of Paul Nordoff, and Clive and Carol Robbins (1971, 1977, 1980, 1998). Many other examples of case material can be found in the many anthologies and books, including amongst others *Clinical Applications of Music Therapy in Developmental Disability, Paediatrics and Neurology* (Wigram and De Backer 1999a), *Case Studies in Music Therapy* (Bruscia 1991), *Music for Life* (Ansdell 1995), *Music Therapy in Context* (Pavlicevic 1997) and *Being in Music: Foundations of Nordoff-Robbins Music Therapy* (Aigen 1996).

3.4 Free Improvisation Therapy – The Alvin Model

Juliette Alvin was a pioneer of music therapy and developed a foundation model for improvisational music therapy between 1950 and 1980. She was an internationally famous concert cellist, studying with Casals, and she strongly believed in the effect of music as a therapeutic medium. Her own definition of music therapy was:

> The controlled use of music in the treatment, rehabilitation, education and training of adults and children suffering from physical, mental or emotional disorders. (1975)

The History of Free Improvisation Therapy

In 1959, Alvin founded the British Society for Music Therapy, and subsequently founded the post-graduate course of music therapy at the Guildhall School of Music and Drama in London in 1968. During her extensive travels in Europe, the USA and Japan, she was invited to start a course in music therapy at university level, but she firmly believed in the importance of highly trained and experienced musicians as potential music therapists, so she chose to begin her course at a music conservatoire, where the emphasis was on musical training and skill, rather than academic knowledge. The programme at the Guildhall School of Music is still running (now in collaboration with the University of York, which validates it), and graduates from her courses, including Tony Wigram (Denmark), Leslie Bunt (United Kingdom) and Helen Odell-Miller (United Kingdom), have furthered her methods in other training courses. Mary Priestley (United Kingdom) also trained with Juliette Alvin, and went on to found Analytical Music Therapy. Many therapists and teachers of music therapy have been influenced by her methods, and her model of Free Improvisation Therapy is still taught and used in clinical practice (Alvin 1975, 1976, 1978).

CLINICAL AREA

Alvin worked in psychiatry, and also focused her work on children, including those who are autistic, mentally handicapped, maladjusted, and physically handicapped.

She argued that the analytical concepts of Freud underpin the development of music therapy, as music has the power to reveal aspects of the unconscious. While not requiring one to be 'Freudian' to believe in this important concept, Alvin's theory was built on the primary statement: *'Music is a creation of man, and therefore man can see himself in the music he creates.'* This idea was developed alongside Alvin's perception of music as a potential space for free expression. She cites Stravinsky as one of the single most important influences on music in the twentieth century, because his compositions broke the 'musical rules' in terms of harmony, melody, rhythm and form, and allowed us to make and experience a range of dissonant and atonal sounds that had previously been taboo. This opened the door for her development of free improvisation therapy, where clients and therapists can improvise without musical rules, and where the music can be an expression of the person's character and personality through which therapeutic issues can be addressed.

SESSION FORMAT

Alvin's method is musical:

- All the client's therapeutic work centres around listening to or making music.

- Every conceivable kind of musical activity can be used.

- Improvisation is used in a totally free way, using sounds or music that are not composed or written beforehand.

- By sounding the instruments in different ways, or by using unorganized vocal sounds, inventing musical themes allows great freedom.

- Free improvisation requires no musical ability or training, and is not evaluated according to musical criteria.

- The therapist imposes no musical rules, restrictions, directions or guidelines when improvising, unless requested by the client. The client is free to establish, or not establish, a pulse, metre, rhythmic pattern, scale, tonal centre, melodic theme or harmonic frame.

These were revolutionary concepts for music therapy in the 1960s, as the main schools in the USA used conventional, precomposed music in more behaviourally orientated therapy. Only Paul Nordoff and Clive Robbins' approach in Creative Music Therapy came close to this, although their music was more conventional and structured, and analytical theory was not inherent in their method.

Alvin taught about the importance of developing the client's relationship with music. In her work with people with autism and developmental disability in particular, she proposed that the client's relationship with the instrument was the primary and initial therapeutic relationship. The musical instrument, for Alvin, can be the container of the negative feelings projected by the client, and represents a 'safe intermediary object'. After this, clients become attracted to, and form relationships with, the instrument of the therapist, centring their feelings in the music created together. It is after going through this process that the development of a relationship directly between client and therapist occurs. So her concepts relating to the objectives of the therapy, the process of the therapy and the successful outcome of the therapy start and develop in the musical relationship. This was a seminal and unique contribution to the theory and understanding of music therapy from a psychotherapeutic point of reference in the 1950s and 1960s and was picked up and developed by leading figures in music therapy all over the world.

From a psychotherapeutic and theoretical point of view, Alvin worked within the concept of an 'equal term relationship' where the therapist and client share musical experiences at the same level, and have equal control over the musical situation. This is very significant as a concept, and explains much about the remarkable effect of her therapeutic approach, and her success in drawing out the potentials and strengths of clients with whom she worked. Autistic, maladjusted and physically handicapped children responded eagerly to her approach, when she would offer them an empathic and sensitive musical frame.

Clinical applications: approach and method

Alvin proposed the potential to use different approaches in different situations, and this 'eclectic model' has caused some controversy. She mainly worked from a humanistic and developmental point of view, often describing in her many cases, changes in the client's behaviour that represented underlying changes in their capacities. When working in the field of psychiatry, she approached clients from a more analytical perspective.

Alvin believed the therapist's instrument was his/her primary means of communication and interaction. She herself used a method of 'empathic improvisation' when she used her cello. This involved gaining an insight and understanding about a client's way of being, mood and personality, and then reflecting it back through improvised playing on her cello. This was 'playing for the client' and therefore receptive in style. The therapists can also, through this method, introduce themselves to the client in a safe and non-threatening way, adjusting their playing to the listening responses of the client.

Documentation

Alvin wrote extensively about her concepts and ideas of music therapy in her main books and many clinical articles. Her books were:

- *Music Therapy* (1975)
- *Music Therapy for the Handicapped Child* (1976)
- *Music Therapy for the Autistic Child* (1978).

Probably the most useful overview of Alvin's theory, method, clinical approach and methods of assessment and evaluation can be found in Unit 3 (Chapter 3) of Bruscia's *Improvisational Models of Music Therapy* (1987). As well as what we know and understand about the psychotherapeutic functions of music in music therapy, Alvin placed emphasis on the importance of understanding the physiological effects. She said one needs to link the psychological effect of music with the physical effect, and used the examples of shamans and witch doctors from primitive cultures to illustrate this idea. Music therapists need to understand human physiology and the way the body reacts to music and sound to fully understand the influence of music within music therapy. Alvin has defined some important concepts for our understanding of music therapy within Free Improvisation Therapy:

- analytical concepts of music
- psychological functions of music
- physiological functions of music
- functions of music in group music therapy.

She formulated a descriptive approach to evaluating the effects of music and music therapy, including evaluating listening responses, instrumental responses and vocal responses.

Alvin's method, and her concept of the role of the music therapist, places the level of therapy at either augmentative or primary. In her own clinical work, Alvin worked as part of multidisciplinary teams in hospitals and units, but also with individual clients in private practice – as a primary therapist.

Alvin died in 1982, as music therapy in Great Britain was becoming a regulated profession within the health and social system. Her contribution both at a theoretical and clinical level was foundational in promoting the value of music therapy, and in beginning a course in the United Kingdom that placed music skill and competence at the centre of music therapy training and clinical practice. Alvin holds a place in history as one of the earliest and perhaps most eclectic and inspirational pioneers.

3.5 Behavioural Music Therapy

Behavioural Music Therapy (BMT) was mainly developed in the USA and still forms a primary method of intervention. It is a method that is defined as follows:

> ... the use of music as a contingent reinforcement or stimulus cue to increase or modify adaptive behaviours and extinguish maladaptive behaviours. (Bruscia 1998)

Dr Clifford Madsen, together with Dr Vance Cutter, published an article in 1966 describing BMT. It is a form of cognitive behaviour modification, and involves applied behaviour analysis. The main concepts are that music is used in treatment in the following ways:

- as a cue

- as a time structure and body movement structure

- as a focus of attention

- as a reward.

As in behaviour therapy, the focus of the treatment is towards the modification of behaviour – conditioning behaviour – which can be measured by applied behaviour analysis. Whether one is working with an autistic child or a depressed adult, the process involves the concept of stimulus-response, and music is used to change behaviour, and reduce symptoms of a pathology, rather than an attempt to explore the cause of behaviour. Research has been undertaken in the USA, and many of the studies have used recorded music in order that the studies can be replicated. Rigorous scientific standards are applied to ensure that the effects of BMT are accepted and recognized in the scientific community. The term behaviour is understood as an all-inclusive concept. Therefore the object of the therapy is the control and manipulation of many different types of behaviour including:

- physiological behaviour

- motor behaviour

- psychological behaviour

- emotional behaviour

- cognitive behaviour

- perceptual behaviour

- autonomic behaviour.

In practice, music in any form is used in conjunction with a behaviour modification program. An example of this would be a program to encourage a person with learning disability to increase their attention span in a group. If the person sustains their attention on a task, or on the therapist, they will receive music (perhaps in the form of songs or a played piece). If their behaviour deteriorates, music is withdrawn. Based on the assumption that the person wants music experiences, the program is designed to increase his/her attention because of his/her motivation to get musical experiences.

Another example is the research and clinical work from Professor Jayne Standley of Florida State University who measured the effect of music in reinforcing sucking behaviours in premature infants. When the babies sucked, they received musical stimulation, and when they stopped sucking, the music was withdrawn. The results of Standley's research showed that the introduction of the musical stimuli resulted in increased sucking, and improvements in weight gain and health leading to earlier discharge from the intensive care unit. Standley also investigated the music that was effective as a stimulus (Standley 1991b, 1995, 1998).

Participation in musical activities is also used in BMT. Whether one is working with geriatric patients, psychiatric patients or adolescents with developmental disability, the structuring and implementation of musical activities such as singing, music and movement, playing and dancing are used to encourage non-musical goals and objectives such as:

- social engagement

- physical activity

- communication

- cognitive processes

- attention and concentration

- enjoyment

- reduction and elimination of antisocial behaviour

- independence skills.

Research and documentation

The music that is used in BMT varies widely, and some research has been done to define what type of music will promote the achievement of therapeutic and treatment objectives. For example, pulsed, rhythmical music is used with patients with Parkinson's disease to promote good walking patterns (Thaut 1985). Old songs, familiar melodies and hymns are used with geriatric patients to promote attention, engagement and memory. Also, music with slower tempos such as largo, adagio and andante are used when attempting movement or dancing with older adults. With patients with senile dementia, short songs and pieces are recommended to cope with short attention span.

Applied behaviour analysis in BMT allows the therapist to measure over time the effect of music therapy intervention. If a child is acting out in school, the introduction of guitar-based music therapy sessions may give the child motivation and stronger self-esteem. Applied behaviour analysis can measure the number of defined, asocial behaviours that are targeted during periods when the child receives music therapy, and also when music therapy is withdrawn for a period. Using reversal designs and multiple baselines, the therapist and researcher can evaluate the actual efficacy of music therapy intervention over time, by comparing the number of behavioural incidents that occur during the different periods of intervention with periods of non-intervention.

BMT is a good example of music *in* therapy, as the role of music is to act as a stimulus and reinforcer of non-musical behaviour. Although the therapist may be interested in the patient's way of making music, and their expression and communication through music, the main focus for therapy and evaluation is to achieve changes in the client's general behaviour.

Bruscia (1998, p.184) places BMT at the augmentative level, because this therapeutic direction works with limits and goals that specifically address symptoms, and, to a lesser degree, with the client's personality or general development.

3.6 Physiological Responses to Music

'If music be the food of love, play on' – a well-known line from Shakespeare tells us of the place music holds in the emotional lives of people, particularly in its subtle and powerful psychological effect. We can also see in music therapy the frame music provides for reaching to a deep psychological level. However, Juliette Alvin, one of the foremost pioneers of music therapy, once said that we should never ignore the physical effect of music. She felt it was necessary to study physiology, to understand how music can affect the body, and that this aspect was often ignored because it was not 'romantic', and did not seem to relate to the more important psychological and psychotherapeutic processes in music therapy. Yet one cannot have the emotional effect of music without a corresponding physical effect, and all physical effects of sound inevitably provoke a psychological reaction. From the romantic point of view, John Sloboda, a leading music psychologist in Great Britain, referred to the 'DTPOTA' effect ('Darling, They're Playing Our Tune Again') in provoking physical 'goose-bump' responses through association, and the effect of music to recall memories and associations is very powerful.

Generally, the study of how music affects us physiologically has fascinated psychologists and physicians more than it has music therapists, resulting in some extensive investigations and quite detailed studies. More recently, the doctors, therapists and nurses associated with the International Society for Music in Medicine have looked carefully at how the brain perceives and processes music, as well as the potential for music to be used in medical and dental procedures. Whether it is psychologists, music therapists or doctors looking at the physical effect of music and sound, interesting results from the research studies have included the way music influences:

- heart rate

- blood pressure

- respiration

- skin temperature

- electrodermal activity (arousal levels)

- brain waves (electroencephalograph).

Stimulating music tends to enhance body energy, induces bodily action, increases heart rate and blood pressure, while sedative or relaxing music can reduce heart rate and blood pressure, reduce arousal levels and generally calm individuals. Some researchers have tried to establish links between heart rate, blood pressure and anxiety, but there are many reasons why heart rate and blood pressure will change, and individual differences make it difficult to establish that any specific piece of music will universally reduce or increase these parameters, even if the change may be linked to raising or decreasing anxiety. An example is the study by Landreth and Landreth (1974), who recorded changes in heart rate in 22 members of a college-level music appreciation society while listening to the first movement of Beethoven's Fifth Symphony. Taking measurements over a six-week period, before, during and after the experiments with listening to this music, they found significant changes (tachycardia and bradycardia) in different parts of the music. However, there was not a consistently reliable effect on listeners' heart rates.

Individual likes and dislikes in music mean that the effect will vary. For example, when using biofeedback methods to develop a music-based individualized relaxation training (MBIRT), Saperston (1989) found that a patient who identified with the hippy subculture of the 1960s was more likely to relax to rock music, whereas another patient relaxed to Indian sitar music.

In considering the physical effects of music, it is therefore more important to look at the elements in the music that might affect stimulation or relaxation. Wigram defined the parameters that influence whether a piece of music has such effects in terms of predictability within the music. If the musical elements are stable and predictable, then subjects will tend to relax, whereas if the elements in the music vary significantly over time, and are subject to sudden and unpredictable change, then the subject will maintain a higher level of arousal and stimulation.

Potential elements in stimulating music:

- unpredictable changes in tempo
- unpredictable or sudden changes in:
  - volume
  - rhythm
  - timbre
  - pitch
  - harmony
- wide variations in texture in the music
- unexpected dissonance
- unexpected accents
- harsh timbres
- lack of structure and form in the music
- sudden accelerandos, ritardandos, crescendos and diminuendos
- unexpected breaks in the music.

Potential elements in relaxing music:

- stable tempo
- stability or only gradual changes in:

- volume
- rhythm
- timbre
- pitch
- harmony
- consistent texture
- predictable harmonic modulation
- appropriate cadences
- predictable melodic lines
- repetition of material
- structure and form
- gentle timbre
- few accents.

In developing musical skills to use in clinical improvisation, music therapy students and qualified practitioners learn how the balance and effective use of these elements can be made in a very sensitive and subtle way to engage and help patients. Some clients *need* the stability and safety of predictable music, for example people with psychotic disturbance, whose world is chaotic and disconnected. Others, for example patients with autism, learning disability or anxiety neuroses, *need* to develop abilities to cope with an unpredictable world, and this can begin in developing adaptability to unpredictable musical experiences. So these elements of music that can determine the effect in receptive music therapy also play an important role in active music making with clients.

Vibroacoustic and vibrotactile therapy

One of the areas where music has been used specifically as a physical treatment is the 'vibroacoustic' form of therapy. Music is played through speakers built into a chair, mattress or bed on which the patient is lying. Therefore the patient experiences directly the vibrations created by the music. This is a receptive form of music therapy, which nevertheless still involves a client/therapist relationship. In Europe, the main pioneers of vibroacoustic therapy were Olav Skille in Norway, Petri Lehikoinen in Finland, and Tony Wigram in Denmark and England. Many vibroacoustic and vibrotactile devices have been developed in the USA and Japan. However, in England, the treatment has involved the use of pulsed, sinusoidal low frequency tones between 30 Hz and 70 Hz combined with appropriate and relaxing music. (Lehikonen 1988, 1989, 1993a, 1993b; Skille 1982a, 1982b, 1989a, 1989b, 1992; Skille and Wigram 1995; Skille, Wigram and Weekes 1989; Wigram 1991b, 1992a, 1993b, 1996b, 1997b, 1997e, 1997f, 1997g, 1997h.)

Anecdotal results accrued over many years of experimentation and treatment sessions can be looked at as helpful and guiding rather than statistically significant. There has been a certain amount of objective research into vibroacoustic therapy, including two doctoral dissertations (Chesky 1992; Wigram 1996b) although very few studies undertaken have been replicated. However, there has been a wide clinical application of this 'treatment,' and many results have been positive.

Collated reports fall into five main clinical/pathological areas: 1. pain disorders, 2. muscular conditions, 3. pulmonary disorders, 4. general physical ailments and 5. psychological disorders.

PAIN DISORDERS

There have been reports of the effective use of vibroacoustic therapy with colic pains, bowel problems, fibromyalgia, migraine and headache, low back pain, menstrual pain, dysmenorrhoea, premenstrual tension, Bechterew's disease, neck and shoulder pains, polyarthritis and rheumatism. Some of the treatments undertaken with these conditions have been successful. The use of frequencies recommended can vary considerably. For example, for polyarthritis, Skille recommended the use of frequencies between 40 Hz and 60 Hz, whereas for migraine and headaches, he recommended the use of frequencies between 70 Hz and 90 Hz. Low back pain should be treated with frequencies between 50 Hz and 55 Hz. The evidence for the specific use of certain frequencies as opposed to other frequencies is again purely anecdotal and not based on any research results. Over 50 reports collected by Skille have shown that over 50 per cent of patients treated for fibromyalgia have been successfully helped with a reduction in pain symptoms.

A detailed analysis of the effect of music vibration on the sensory and mechanoreceptors was undertaken by Chesky and Michel (1991) and Chesky (1992) in studies on pain. Their studies have found significant effects from the stimulation when compared to music alone or a placebo treatment on pain reduction using a specific frequency range (60–600 Hz) on pain receptors with the Music Vibration Table (MVT™). They have also drawn attention to the lack of specificity regarding the stimulus used in other studies, in particular the nature of the music used. Michel and

Chesky (1993) used equipment which was adjusted to generate greater activity in the frequency ranges known to produce pain relief (approximately 100–250 Hz).

Further studies documented the effect of vibroacoustic treatment on reducing pain with knee replacements (Burke and Thomas 1997), and the management of post-operative gynaecological patients (Burke 1997).

MUSCULAR CONDITIONS

Vibroacoustic therapy has been used to aid muscular problems, particularly when those problems can cause painful conditions. Cerebral palsy has received a lot of attention from researchers looking at the effect of vibroacoustic therapy in reducing muscle tone (Wigram 1991, 1991b, 1992a, 1992, 1996, 1996b, 1997a, 1997c, 1997d; Wigram and Weekes 1992). When treating cerebral palsy, the condition reacts with spasms to overexcitement, high stimulation or sudden stimulation. Therefore, relaxing music using low frequencies in the 60 Hz range has been important. Some of the treatments that have taken place with vibroacoustic therapy have also involved doing active physiotherapy during or immediately after the session.

Other muscular conditions that have been helped include: multiple sclerosis, Rett syndrome, spasticity, and muscular overuse syndrome.

Research in the clinic for children and adults with Rett syndrome at Harper House Children Service in Hertfordshire, England, has already indicated positive responses from clients to vibroacoustic therapy. Specifically, increased levels of relaxation, reduced anxiety, reduced hand plucking and reduced hyperventilation amongst clients have been noted (Wigram and Cass 1995).

Anecdotal reports regarding vibroacoustic therapy with people who suffer from muscular pain are interesting. One striking observation is that during treatment for pain in a specific muscle group, the patients have experienced that, as they are relaxing, the pain focuses on the particular muscle group where the damage has occurred. The effect of vibration has been to relax all other muscle groups or muscle fibres around this area. In this way, the treatment has pinpointed very clearly and located the primary source of pain and discomfort.

PULMONARY DISORDERS

Further anecdotal results have shown some effect on certain pulmonary disorders, including: asthma, cystic fibrosis, pulmonary emphysema and metachromatic leucodystrophy. Both metachromatic leucodystrophy and cystic fibrosis have similarities in that patients must cough up lung secretion to keep the lungs clear. Vibroacoustic therapy helps to do this by generating a vibration into the lungs and shifting mucus on the bed of the lungs causing a cough reflex to occur. Skille has reported that up to the end of 1994, four children with this specific disorder in Norway were having vibroacoustic therapy on a daily basis.

Asthmatic problems have been eased by vibroacoustic therapy, through the facilitation of easier breathing, reduced wheezing and decreased viscosity of the expectorations of the lungs. Because severe asthmatic conditions sometimes cause bronchial spasms, the spasmiolytic effect of vibroacoustic therapy has been helpful in reducing the severity of asthma attacks. Again, only anecdotal reports exist to support this.

GENERAL PHYSICAL AILMENTS

Clinical problems in this category might include the following: decubitus ulcers, reduced blood circulation, post-operative convalescence, and stress.

There is a body of thought that has found vibroacoustic therapy effective in reducing blood pressure, heart rate and improving blood circulation. Anecdotal reports of legs that have become purple through poor circulation turning to a more healthy pink or red colour have emerged. These studies provide conflicting data. Vibroacoustic therapy has been attempted in neurosurgical units on clients in coma. There is no recorded evidence that it has had a successful effect. Other areas in which good effects have been recorded are with post-operative cardiac surgery patients (Butler and Butler 1997), with idiopathic parkinson's disease (Del Campo san Vicente, de Manchola and Torres Serna 1997), in general medicine (Raudsik 1997) and with hospitalized children (Jones 1997).

PSYCHOLOGICAL DISORDERS

Vibroacoustic treatment can have an effect on psychological states which may or may not contribute to a physiological condition. In this group of problems, vibroacoustic therapy has been used in the treatment of insomnia, anxiety disorders (Hooper and Lindsey 1997), self-injurious behaviour (Wigram 1993b), challenging behaviour, autism (Persoons and De Backer 1997; Wigram, McNaught and Cain 1997), depression and stress.

Autism is an organic condition, and therefore should not, strictly speaking, be included in this group. However, there is no apparent physical disorder in the individual who has autism in terms of an illness. The main claims to effective vibroacoustic therapy in autism is that it relaxes clients, reduces their resistance to contact, and makes them more open to interaction. It is a tactile experience, so it can also stimulate a feeling of physical pleasure (Persoons and De Backer 1997).

Insomnia has been treated, and the reports have indicated that clients fall asleep more readily, and that they sleep for a longer period than is usual. Clients with depression have been treated with vibroacoustic therapy, and there is now significant evidence that changes have taken place in their condition.

Summary

The literature on this particular area of intervention, using vibroacoustic or vibrotactile stimuli, is extensive. Some of this is collected together in a volume of contributed papers (Wigram and Dileo 1997), while the rest is spread throughout the literature. While this chapter has gone into some detail regarding these forms of intervention, the general area of MusicMedicine, Music in Medicine, and Music Therapy in Medicine also accounts for a substantial range of research studies and clinical reports. These will be discussed in the next chapter, and range from the highest level of front-line technological medicine where magnetic resonance imaging (MRI) and PET scans have looked at the way the brain processes music, to clinical reports on the effects of instrumental study and performance on the physical health of musicians (Pratt and Grocke 1999; Pratt and Spintge 1996; Spintge and Droh 1992).

3.7 Music in Medicine

The application of music in the field of medicine has become more defined and precise in recent years. There is an International Society of Music in Medicine that includes mainly medical practitioners, but also nurses, psychologists and music therapists. The medical area includes all applications of music and music therapy which are aimed at the prevention, treatment, or recovery from medical conditions. In *Defining Music Therapy* (1998a), Bruscia defines Music in Medicine as:

> ... the use of music to influence the patient's physical, mental, or emotional states before, during or after medical treatment.

Maranto offers the following categorization of the place of music therapy in the field of medicine:

> Music therapy may relate to the medical treatment of the patient in a variety of ways:
>
> (A) Supportive to medical treatment (e.g. the use of music listening during kidney dialysis)

(B) As an equal partner to medical treatment (e.g. the use of singing in conjunction with medication as a treatment for respiratory disorders)

(C) As a primary intervention for a medical condition (e.g. the use of music listening to directly suppress pain). (Dileo-Maranto 1993a)

Medical and dental practitioners use music as a background relaxant, for example in waiting rooms, but this must be clearly differentiated from the specific application of music in a treatment process. This is important when considering the use of recorded music in a variety of situations where it may or may not have a therapeutic purpose.

Additionally, it may or may not have a therapeutic effect, something that the institution or unit using music in this way may or may not have intended, and of which they may or may not be aware. It has become common practice for surgeons to have background music in the operating theatre during operations. The music is to provide a relaxing and conducive atmosphere for the operating team, and is not intended for the anaesthetized patient. However, there is some research on the use of music in surgical procedures, particularly in operations where the patient is conscious and under spinal anaesthesia (Spintge 1982, 1988, 1993; Spintge and Droh 1982). Spintge (1993) describes the use of 'anxioalgolytic music' in medical and surgical procedures to reduce the distress, anxiety and pain suffered by patients. From a psychological point of view, Spintge's studies reported significantly reduced anxiety and improved *compliance*, particularly during the preparation phase before a surgical procedure. From physiological measurements, he reported a significantly reduced need for medication during surgery, especially during procedures where the mode of anaesthesia was other than a general anaesthetic.

Table 3.1: Musical parameters of relaxing music compared with anxioalgolytic music

Music element	Relaxing music	Anxioalgolytic music
Frequency	600 Hz–900 Hz	20 Hz–10,000 Hz
Dynamics	little change	little change
Melody	in dynamics	in dynamics
Tempo	60–80 beats/min	50–70 beats/min
Rhythm	constant: little contrast	floating: no contrast

(Spintge 1993)

Spintge looked at the musical elements he was using, in order to define differences in music he would describe as 'relaxing music' and the elements in the music he would describe as 'anxioalgolytic music'. In order to select appropriate music that he expected would have the effect of reducing anxiety, Spintge suggested some specific parameters for 'anxioalgolytic music' that differentiated it from relaxing music:

Looking at the role of music in pacification/stimulation of premature infants of low birth weights, Standley (1991b, 1998) found that music is an optimal early intervention stimulus for infants and parents with medical, social or psychological problems. She commented that music is 'heard' and 'learned' by the foetus; therefore it may affect development prior to birth. 'After birth, music in the neo-natal intensive care unit can mask the aversive sound level of the isolette, thereby facilitating *homeostasis* which increases the infant's neurological development. Music is a singular stimulus which can both pacify and stimulate in socially beneficial ways, with implications for future preference and interaction' (Standley 1991b, 1995).

Standley (1995) has conducted a meta-analysis of the variety of applications where music is used as a therapeutic intervention in medical and dental treatment. These analyses provide evidence from studies of a wide variety of medical or dental interventions, including objective studies on pain, cardiac conditions, pre-operative anxiety, childbirth pain and neonate weight gain, which support the use of music as an effective element in treatment.

Further studies have looked more specifically at the use of music in the control of human pain (Brown *et al.* 1991; Chesky and Michel 1991; Spintge 1993) and the effect of music on premature babies (Standley 1991b). Brown's study was mainly concerned with evaluating the attributes of music for pain control and considered that the music had two specific qualities which could be used in developing effective pain-coping skills: an attention-distraction dimension and an affect dimension. In terms of the attention-distraction dimension, music had the potential to hold one's attention, challenge the intellect and modify the emotional state regardless of personal preference or knowledge of the music and it required the individual to commit himself or herself to the experience moment by moment. Therefore, music has the potential to alter one's perception of time, and a sensation of pain may not necessarily be diminished, but the suffering involved would be greatly reduced. As far as affect is concerned, music can be mood-evoking and can arouse emotional experiences that can provide a heightened meaning to a situation, stir up past memories or allow self-catharsis.

The effect of recorded music on pain relief was investigated by Curtis (1986). Here, personal preferences in music were an important consideration and the researchers prepared 15-minute studies based on the patient's stated preference and perception of the calmness of musical excerpts presented from a master tape. The music selections were drawn on the basis of procedures defined by Curtis (1982). This study pointed to the efficacy of music as an intervention tool with terminally ill people, although the sample group in the study was small and a recommendation was made for replication of the study using a larger patient group.

The field of Music in Medicine is more focused than that of music therapy, and tends to be orientated around specific clinical and pathological disorders. Professionals contributing to this field have mainly been music therapists and medical practitioners. The field is very well documented (Dileo 1999; Dileo-Maranto 1991a, 1991b, 1993a; Spintge 1982, 1988; Spintge and Droh 1982; Standley 1995).

A comprehensive analysis of some of the Music in Medicine studies was also undertaken by Dileo-Maranto (1994a, 1994b) who reviewed studies evaluating the effect of music in neonatal intensive care, coronary and intensive care, pulmonology, surgery, specific medical procedures, radiology and oncology. The majority of the 77 studies reviewed by Maranto in her paper employed recorded music in the experimental condition as the method of therapeutic intervention.

Some studies record reductions in blood pressure (Bonny and McCarron 1984). Maranto points out that there have been inconsistencies in physiological results from some trials that have been undertaken, and that 'knowledge of the physiological and psychological effects of music is far from complete, and recent research has been addressing the specific influences of musical elements such as rhythm, tempo, harmony, timbre, etc. on these parameters' (Dileo-Maranto 1994a, 1994b). Hodges (1980) has also referred to the conflicting evidence of the effects of music on heart or pulse rate. For example, some studies indicate that, in general, stimulating music will increase heart rate whilst sedative music will cause a decrease in heart rate (Darner 1966; De Jong et al. 1973; Ellis and Brighouse 1952). Other studies have found that there are quite unpredictable results or that music has no effect on heart rate (Barger 1979; Bierbaum 1958; Coutts 1965). There are equally contradictory findings from studies on the effect of music listening on blood pressure. Hodges also comments on the difficulties in summarizing and collating the literature studying the effects of music on muscular and motion responses. He points to certain conclusions, which influence issues discussed in this study:

- There is no significant difference in muscular activity during stimulative and sedative music in listening situations. (Lord 1968)

- Consistent neuro-muscular responses were detected through Electro-Myography (EMG) as individuals saw and heard music. (Holdsworth 1974)

Music has been proposed as a therapeutic intervention for stress and stress-related disorders (Dileo 1999). This field has become a focus of interest for music therapists and doctors, as disorders which have no clear organic origin present may be affected by stressful life situations or significant events. Aldridge and Brandt (1991) studied the value of music therapy for inflammatory bowel disease on the basis that this disorder could have an immunological basis influenced by chronic stress. This research focused on the value of music therapy as a process that stimulated positive emotions, enhanced coping mechanisms and enabled recovery. In their study, Aldridge and Brandt sought correlations between the behaviour of patients with inflammatory bowel disease and elements of their musical improvisation. For example, a lack of gut motility is evident musically in a lack of rhythmic flexibility, and an unresponsiveness to tempo changes. This study is important in scientifically evaluating evidence of a pathological condition through improvisational music therapy.

Therefore, whereas in passive approaches, and in the principles of Music in Medicine generally, music can influence physical behaviour including autonomic activity, it can also be found that music affects and elicits psychological response, by influencing mood and affective responses in individuals. In addition, these studies demonstrate how the pathological behaviour or state of a patient may influence, and be evident in, music-making. This has also been found to be useful in the use of music therapy as a medium for diagnostic assessment (Wigram 1992b, 1995a, 1999a, 1999b, 1999e, 2000a, 2000b). In the field of Music in Medicine, there are more detailed and scientific experimental studies with quantitative methodology and design due to the influence of a medical milieu, and due to the requirement for objective data indicating physical changes in the patients as a result of the application or intervention of music. Music therapists working within a psychotherapeutic framework, as found in Europe, would not consider the use of Music in Medicine to be a form of music therapy, as it does not involve a developing musical relationship with the patient. However, it is nevertheless a therapeutic use of music, used by both music therapists and practitioners in other disciplines, and Music in Medicine offers a lot of relevant information also for music therapists, e.g. in connection with pain management (Bonde 2001b).

3.8 Music and Healing

Man has used music for healing purposes since the dawn of civilization. There is a direct line from classical Greek music philosophy (see Chapter 1.2) to many current healing practices based on sound vibration, or music healing. The crucial difference between music healing and music therapy is ontological. It becomes obvious when answering the question: where does the healing power of music come from? What is it that promotes (healing) change?

In the different models and methods of music therapy described earlier in this chapter therapeutic change is promoted by the dynamic 'triad': client–therapist–music (experience). In healing practices the changing agent is 'the universal forms of energy in music, and their elements – sounds and vibrations' (Bruscia 1998, p.202). For the same reason music healing is often connected with an inclination towards spiritual practices, rituals or procedures with a background in religion or nature worship. The basic idea is that everything in the universe is vibration. Some vibrations can be felt in the body, some can be seen or heard, while others can only be perceived in altered states of consciousness. The vibrations of a living body can be in or out of harmonic balance, and with sound and music the disturbed inner balance of a human being (or the balance between the individual and the universal) can be restored.

Bruscia makes a distinction between *sound healing* (which is considered a form of music therapy, when music plays an important role) and *music healing*. He writes: '*Sound healing* is the use of vibrational frequencies or sound forms combined with music or the elements of music (e.g. rhythm, melody, harmony) to promote healing. (The use of sound alone, without music, is called *vibration healing*, ed.) *Music healing* is the use of music experiences and the inherent universal energy forms in music to heal body, mind and spirit' (p.204ff). In other words, the difference is a matter of the understanding of the aesthetic dimension of music and of music as a means of interpersonal communication.

It is obvious that it is difficult to distinguish clearly between physiological methods like vibroacoustic and vibrotactile therapy (Chapter 3.6) and sound healing on one side, and between music healing and music therapy for self-development and spiritual purposes, like Guided Imagery and Music (Chapters 3.1 and 4.7), on the other. The common denominator of the traditions is that music is used *as* therapy or as an agent of healing. The differences lie mainly in the understanding of man and music, in the understanding of the potentials of the therapeutic relationship (client–therapist–music), and above all in the understanding of the healing potentials of the music experience: whether it is the work of the individual client (the potential of self-healing) and the therapeutic relation – or the work of universal, collective, possibly divine powers that are externally channelled into therapy.

There are many different procedures, variations and techniques within vibration, sound and music healing (see Campbell 1991, 1997; Gardner-Gordon 1993; Halpern 1985; Hamel 1979; McClellan 1988; an overview is given in Bruscia 1998, Chapter 20). We shall only mention a few practices that are common in Europe (after Bruscia

1998, Chapter 20). For a critical discussion of music healing theory and practice, as found in the 'New Age' literature, see Summer (1996).

Procedures within sound healing

Body and voice work. The use of breathing, body and voice exercises and techniques to set the voice of the individual client free, in a process aimed at the elimination of muscle tensions, energy blocks and limitations in body, mind and spirit. Examples: the voice-building principles of the Roy Hart Theatre, and the 'therapeutic voicework' of the British therapist Paul Newham (Newham 1993, 1998).

Healing with sound bowls, gongs and/or overtones. The use of the voice and/or ancient Eastern 'instruments', their fundamentals, vibrations and rich spectra of overtones to promote resonance and balance in the listener. The ancient instruments are often used in combinations with meditation, Gregorian chant and/or overtone chanting. Examples: Michael Vetter, David Hykes and the Harmonic Choir, Igor Reznikoff (see also Moreno 1988).

Toning. A technique utilizing the conscious sustaining of sounds and tones produced by the voice of the client(s) and/or the therapist, directed inwards, to the body, or outwards. It may be a question of finding, sustaining and exploring a specific tone (frequency and sound quality) by using, for example, different vocals, consonants, rhythms or mouth positions, but without text or melody. The purpose may be that the client finds his/her own 'personal tone' or 'fundamental', cell changes in body tissues, pain reduction or the activation of energy centres or chakras. In group work toning can be a powerful technique to achieve attunement of group dynamics and energies (see Gardner-Gordon 1993; Garfield 1987; Myskja 1999).

Crowe and Scovel (1996, in a special issue of *Music Therapy Perspectives*) divide the field of sound healing into six areas:

1. self-generated sound (toning, overtone chant, chakra sounds)

2. projection of sounds into the body (Cymatic therapy, radionics, tuning forks)

3. sounding the body (the 'Sirene technique', projection of overtones, resonant kinesiology, bioacoustic systems, low frequency sounds)

4. listening technologies (for the improvement of hearing and sound perception, e.g. the Tomatis model)

5. healing compositions (healing songs, instrumental pieces and special ethnic music; 'therapeutic voice work' (Newham); music in Pythagorean tuning;

'drumming' (Flatischler 1992; Hart 1990); 'entrainment' (Rider 1997, 1999; Saperston 1995); HemiSync; special instruments, e.g. singing bowls and gongs; specially composed healing music, e.g. Halpern, Kay Gardner)

6.   sound environments/vibrotactile apparatus ('ambient music', 'sound environment', the Somatron, many types of vibrotactile equipment (Chesky and Michel 1991; Standley 1991a; Wigram and Dileo 1997)).

Crowe and Scovel suggest that music therapy and sound healing are considered two poles of a continuum covering all forms of healing with sound and music.

Techniques within music healing

Music rituals. The use of music rituals belonging to a given community (religious, social, cultural) for healing purposes. The ritual(s) may already exist – or they can be created and developed for the specific group purpose (Kenny 1982).

Shamanistic music travels. This ancient healing tradition has survived in remote parts of all continents, and it has seen a contemporary revival, modified to meet the needs and problems of people living in modern Western cultures (Harner 1990). The shaman (the 'music therapist') uses drums and rattles, songs and hymns to bring himself and the client into an altered state of consciousness, enabling access to healing powers and spirits. The relationship between shamanism and music therapy has been studied by several music therapists (Cissoko 1995; Kenny 1982; Kovach 1985).

Many music therapists have a solid anthropological knowledge of the use of music for healing in ancient cultures, and they know the potentials of ritual for the modern man, whose life is poor in rituals. This knowledge of the potentials of shamanism and rituals is used consciously when the music therapist creates and develops the therapeutic field of play and interaction (Kenny 1982, 1987; Moreno 1988; Winn and Crowe 1989; Winn, Crowe and Moreno 1989).

Many of the books on music and self-development are based on or refer to especially Eastern traditions of music healing, and often the chakra system (a vibrational system uniting man's body and mind) is used as a basis for the classification of different types of music and exercises (Gardner-Gordon 1993; Hamel 1978; Kjærulff 2001). Also Western spiritual influences on the understanding of the transforming potential of music and sound can be found (Pontvik 1996; Steiner 1983; Tame 1984).

CHAPTER 4

Music Therapy in Clinical Practice

Introduction: Referral Criteria and Clinical Practice in Music Therapy

It is still typical in many countries that professionals from other disciplines may not know why they should refer someone for music therapy. If you have a language disorder or delay, it is obvious to refer to speech and language therapy, and if you have cerebral palsy or some other physical handicap or disability, physiotherapy is clearly indicated. If you have suffered from a major trauma, psychotherapy or psychological counselling can be prescribed, and if you have a mental condition such as schizophrenia or depression, you will be referred to a psychiatrist and may be treated with medication. But some people may still think they are referring someone to music therapy for musical activities, development of musical skills or just to make them happy. Referral criteria for music therapy are frequently formulated in an appropriate way within different clinical areas, and then clarified with the rest of the multidisciplinary team or school department. There are differences in the ways people understand how and when to refer patients to music therapy, depending on whether they are working in health, educational or social situations. The criteria in the health field, for example, may originate more typically from identified problems or therapeutic needs that need to be addressed based on diagnostic criteria as one finds in ICD10 and DSM IV. However, in the field of education, and particularly special education, referral criteria may be more closely identified with educational and developmental goals.

In clinical practice, it is important, therefore, whether working in health, education, social services or more specialized areas, for music therapy to have defined criteria of areas of need for which it can offer helpful and potentially successful interventions, and be able to make recommendations regarding the expected length of intervention.

An example: in the case of autistic spectrum disorder, referral criteria will relate specifically to the disorder. They are closely connected to pathological indicators, and contain all aspects of autism, which form the working goals of music therapy.

Criteria for referral and needs that will be met by music therapy:

- difficulties with social interaction at verbal and non-verbal level
- lack of understanding or motivation for communication
- rigid and repetitive patterns of activity and play
- poor relationships
- hypersensitivity to sounds
- lack of ability or interest in sharing experiences
- significant difficulties in coping with change
- apparent lack of ability to learn from experiences
- lack of emotional reciprocity and empathy
- poor sense of self.

Expected length of intervention

The second criteria involves trying to define the expected length of therapy. It is difficult to predict the amount of therapy needed to achieve progress and development and to meet the above needs. But health and education systems cannot write a blank cheque for an indefinite period of treatment. Music therapists offer a framework for assessment, treatment and evaluation over time in order to start and then continue therapy. This can be supported by the results documented in the literature for assessment, short-term therapy and long-term therapy.

An initial baseline assessment of two to four sessions is a critical period when you can see both the potential of the child and the potential of music therapy treatment. The need for this is supported by people who have described assessment work (Grant 1995; Oldfield 2000; Schumacher and Calvert-Kruppa 1999; Wigram 1999c). This assessment gives the criteria for the first period of therapy, which should be 10 to 12 sessions. This is supported by the results gained by Edgerton (1994) in her study. There should be a mid-therapy assessment to report on the progress and process of therapy, which will provide evidence for the need of a longer period of therapy. Beneficial effects of therapy can emerge quite rapidly, but it can, in some cases, take months to see substantial and lasting results.

The second period of therapy could be a further 20 or more sessions. There are many case studies in the literature (Alvin and Warwick 1991; Brown 1999b; Bruscia 1991; Clarkson 1998; Di Franco 1999; Etkin 1999; Robarts 1998; Warwick 1995) showing effects over an extended period of time. Howat (1995) documented a case study of an autistic girl who had music therapy for more than five years – that was a continual process of development. Finally, an end-therapy assessment with a report on the outcome is very important to summarize a period of therapy. A final report will detail the results and will be related closely to the referral criteria, the needs of the client and the expectations of the therapy.

Overview of the assessment, treatment and evaluation period in a music therapy referral:

1.   Initial assessment 2 to 4 sessions

2.   First period of therapy 10 to 12 sessions

3.   Analysis, evaluation and recommendations for further therapy

4.   Second period of therapy 15 to 20 sessions

5.   Second (and final) analysis, evaluation and conclusion.

4.1 Music Therapy with Psychiatric Clients

Introduction: pioneers of music therapy in psychiatry

In Europe, music therapy as a psychoanalytically based psychiatric treatment (see Chapter 2.3) started in England in the beginning of the 1970s, when Priestley was employed at several hospitals in London. Further pioneers include Lecourt (1993, 1994), who was developing work in France from a psychoanalytic perspective, Di Franco in Italy (1993), Odell-Miller (1999), and Streeter (1999a). Many have been inspired by Priestley's model and approach, and have further developed this (De Backer and Van Camp 1999; Langenberg 1996; Pedersen 1998; Scheiby 1998).

However, the roots of Priestley's professional work go back to Juliette Alvin, who established the first actual training program for music therapists (a one-year post-graduate diploma at the Guildhall School of Music and Drama, see Chapter 3.4). This program started in 1968. One of the main disciplines was the study of musical techniques, where improvisation was seen as the key element in establishing musical contact between therapist and patient. Alvin's clinical practice was primarily based on work with children in psychiatry – especially autistic children – but she also worked within the field of hospital psychiatry (see Chapter 3.4).

Priestley further developed elements of Alvin's improvisational methods. At the same time, her work was based on a psychoanalytical background and understanding of psychological symptoms. She felt that these symptoms were rooted in traumatic experiences of early childhood. Priestley comprehensively developed Alvin's ideas about a psychoanalytic approach and formulated psychoanalytic and psychodynamic theories for her music therapy practice in the 1970s (see also Chapter 2.3).

Priestley's methods and techniques were developed through her work with adult psychiatric patients. A characteristic procedure for Priestley is the use of 'playing rules' or 'titles' to stimulate improvisations. The playing rule is defined before the start of the improvisation, either by the therapist himself/herself or with the help of the patient. Another characteristic of the Priestley model is that the therapy session alternates between improvisational parts and verbal, reflective parts. During the musical improvisation the therapist uses disciplined subjectivity, described in classical psychoanalysis as techniques developed through work with regressive patients: 'containment', 'holding environment', 'empathic affirmation' or 'professional empathy'. During verbal reflection the therapist also uses clarification and interpretation, including interpretation of transference phenomena, as described in classical psychoanalysis. These techniques are primarily used with neurotic patients.

Priestley emphasizes that professional empathy and involvement in the patient's situation are the therapist's most important ways of relating. At the same time, she uses the classical technical rules of interpreting and seeking insight together with the patient. She does not see the principle of neutrality as central to the therapist's way of being present in therapy. In this way, her theory differs from that of classical psychoanalysis (see Chapter 2.3). The patient's experience of continuity and his/her possible insight are the primary goals for the therapy. Priestley emphasizes the therapist's sense of timing in interpretation (intervening at the right moment) as an important factor, if the interpretation is to have a healing and integrating effect.

Analytical(ly) (Oriented) Music Therapy in Psychiatry

In order to practise Analytical Music Therapy (as developed by Priestley), a therapist must, in addition to his/her music therapy education, complete a psychotherapy training module with music as the therapeutic agent. In Denmark, this training module is an integrated part of the five-year Master's program at Aalborg University (see Chapter 6.5). After completion of this module, a music therapist can call himself/herself an Analytical Music Therapist, according to Priestley. The psycho-therapy training module creates a basis for understanding that is very suitable for work with psychiatric patients, and it can also be applied to other clinical areas, such as special education and medicine.

The training module is based on theories from classical psychoanalysis, ego psy-chology, object relations theories and self-psychology, as well as transpersonal psy-chology (see Chapter 2.3)

As mentioned earlier, Priestley worked in psychiatry for many years. She believed that uncovering and re-experiencing early childhood traumas were the healing factors in the therapeutic process. Music plays an important role in this process, by stimulating memories and by generating emotions and fantasies in the moment – and thereby actualizing and making audible early traumas, both in actual relationships and in transference relationships between the patient and the therapist. Priestley developed the use of musical improvisation as a 'stage' for the re-enacting of early relationship experiences – as a specific psychotherapeutic method.

From her clinical experiences, she developed a differentiated definition of empathy and countertransference. Priestley was a pioneer, in that she never used interpretation of transference alone – she was very conscious of the need for a warm alliance and a deep and authentic involvement in the patient and his/her conflicts.

As early as 1975, Priestley developed her differentiated definition of countertransference from a psychoanalytic frame of reference, primarily through her work with psychiatric patients (Priestley 1975). She distinguishes between empathic countertransference (E-countertransference) and complementary identifi-cation or countertransference (C-countertransference). (See definition in Chapter 2.3.)

The influence of classical psychoanalytic therapy

As mentioned above, music therapy in psychiatry (Analytically Oriented Music Therapy) focuses to a great extent on transference relationships between the therapist and the patient, and on the music therapist's way of being present in the therapist/patient relationship.

Seen from a classic psychoanalytical point of view, the music therapist relates to a wide variety of patients, including neurotic patients, in the same way that a classical analyst would relate to patients with *regressive symptoms*. This means that the patient can develop and strengthen the self – by continually being seen and heard through the therapist's empathic affirmations and through the musical duets, where the therapist identifies with the client's psychological reality.

For the music therapist, it is often less relevant to act as a neutral 'projection surface'. It is more important to create a setting where the patient feels secure enough to interact with the therapist here and now – through the music and with the resources he/she possesses. Music therapists are, however, trained to use neutrality as it is described and developed in classical psychoanalysis, when the clinical situation demands this. This can be in situations where the therapist is in danger of becoming 'trapped' into the patient's re-enactment of compulsive relationship patterns. But neutrality is one of many possible techniques that can be used in music therapy – it is not a characteristic of a specific method.

At the same time, interpretation of transference is often very relevant for the therapy process. The clinical concepts of resistance and repetition compulsion are used in interpretation, but with a focus on the fact that they represent the best possible solutions the patient could choose, in order to survive earlier anxiety-producing situations. The aim is not to break the resistance, but to regulate it, by developing new patterns of behaviour. This often weakens the repetition compulsion.

One of the distinctive features of music therapy is that improvisation is described as an (inter)active process. Experience shows that patients with severe relationship dysfunctions and weak egos in particular can benefit from music therapy. These patients' tendencies to interrupt dialogue can be 'played out' with great effect in musical improvisations. The setting created by the music can make it possible for the patient to oscillate between *primary and secondary processes.* The therapist follows these processes empathically, but at the same time he/she must – with a disciplined presence – listen from 'outside' this state. In this 'floating' state, the patient can re-experience early relationship patterns that he/she repeats in life. The *split-off* or 'locked-in' affective world can be re-experienced and transformed.

For patients who are stuck in this fantasy state, music represents the possibility of meeting and relating to another person in the music – without the demand of having to leave the fantasy world first. A playing rule for a musical duet could be: 'We play what comes to us, and we let the music grow out of that which is inside of us, that which wants to be expressed.'

Music therapy in psychiatry doesn't look exclusively to psychoanalytical models in order to understand the emerging phenomena in therapy. But a psychoanalytical orientation creates the basis for establishing a therapeutic space, where subconscious fantasies and interactional patterns can be made audible, and where embodied, perceptual experiences are a part of the whole, within the mutual dialogue.

The transference relationship in music therapy – regardless of theoretical basis – has a particular quality, by virtue of the sensory experience: the direct resonance of the music is perceived physically. This sensory aspect vitalizes the 'meeting' between the therapist and the client, which is a crucial part of the relationship process.

Although active music therapy – primarily improvisation, but also performance and composition – is the most widely used method in psychiatry today, receptive music therapy is being developed as a systematic treatment modality and as a tool for improving quality of life. In receptive music therapy, the patient and the therapist listen to selected pieces of music and reflect on their experiences afterwards. Here GIM (Guided Imagery and Music, see Chapter 3.1) is most prevalent, often conducted in a modified form for use with patients with weak egos. After finding a psychological issue as a focus for the session, the patient listens to specially selected music and verbalizes his/her experiences during music listening. The GIM therapist accompanies the patient empathically, by affirming and exploring the patient's experiences. During the music listening phase, he/she writes a log of the patient's experiences/images and helps to integrate the preconscious images into the patient's self-identity.

Music therapy in hospital psychiatry in Denmark

Music therapy as psychiatric *treatment* is relatively new in Danish hospital psychiatry. Music has been used as a *recreational activity* in psychiatry for many years, in the form of music groups playing mainly pop, rock and jazz. Musical arrangements and levels of difficulty are adapted to the skills and strengths of the individual group. A well-established example of this is the *Chok Rock* project at the Psychiatric Hospital in Risskov (Århus). Music groups are a service offered to patients in several psychiatric hospitals in Denmark.

The purpose of music groups is to create a setting where the patients can express themselves musically and where they can maintain or develop the musical skills they already possess. A prerequisite for joining the group is either having played music earlier (and feeling 'at home' on an instrument) or having the desire and courage to participate in a simple arrangement of a song or piece of music. The individual patient becomes an equal and valuable participant in the group social activity of music-making. Each participant plays an equally important role in making the music 'work'. A safe and secure atmosphere is important for these activities.

During the last 10 to 15 years, the use of music as a therapy in psychiatric treatment has become more common in hospitals in Denmark, so that music therapy is now one of the services offered in their total treatment plans. At this point in time there are music therapists employed in nine psychiatric hospitals in Denmark. Several of them are alone in representing music therapy at their hospital. The music therapist can act as a centrally placed treatment 'unit', offering services to all patients in the hospital, depending on resources available. The music therapist can also be associated with one particular ward in the hospital, and at the same time offer treatment to patients from other wards. The music therapist works as a part of a 'treatment team' together with psychiatrists and psychologists. Some hospital music therapists' salaries are funded through both the budgets of the ward staff (nurses and other care-givers) and of the 'treatment team'. This can cause some confusion as to where music therapists 'belong' and under which conditions they should work. In most hospitals, music therapy is now understood as a potential substitute for verbal psychotherapy. This means that the patient cannot receive other types of psychotherapy while participating in music therapy. However, the patient can receive medication and psychosocial activities/treatments along with music therapy.

The music therapist can also offer group activities of a more supportive nature on closed wards, often open group activities such as active music-making with simple improvisations, singing familiar songs or listening to the patients' own preferred music.

Patients who begin in individual music therapy or more insight-oriented music therapy groups are referred by a psychiatrist. Often the psychiatrist has discussed this with the music therapist prior to the referral. If the referral is deemed relevant, the music therapist and the patient have a preliminary conversation. After this, if the patient is motivated, the music therapy begins with a trial period of three to six sessions. When the trial period is over, it is determined whether or not short-term or long-term music therapy is relevant for the patient.

During the trial period, the music therapist presents different playing rules and 'givens' that structure the improvisations. These 'givens' are chosen so that the patient can try a variety of musical instruments and playing techniques. In addition, they help to uncover the patient's potential for relating to the therapist musically. The focus is on the patient's relationship to music and musical instruments – his/her involvement in the music and ability to experiment. Additionally, there is a focus on the patient's ability to relate or listen to the music therapist in the music, and on the relationship between non-verbal and verbal expression and interaction.

The music therapist participates in the trial period, and tries out different music therapy techniques, such as matching the patient's personal musical expression and supporting the patient's music. He/she also uses more confronting techniques in relating to the patient and his/her music. Some music therapists make it a rule that the patient's doctor or *contact person* is an observer during the trial period (Jensen 1999). Musical improvisations are recorded on audiotape or video, to the extent that the patient allows it. This makes it possible for the patient to hear the music later, and is also useful for the therapist's analysis (De Backer 2001).

Music therapists regularly receive professional *supervision/consultation* from psychiatrists or psychologists, where transference and resistance issues can be addressed, based on the cases presented. During *supervision*, the therapist can also identify which of the patient's issues are suitable for music therapy work.

Issues in treatment and criteria for treatment

Important themes for music therapy sessions in psychiatry are: intimacy/distance, aggression/non-aggression, dependence/independence, acting out/emptiness, being present/disappearing, moving from one position to another, and creating boundaries/breaking or testing boundaries. Although music therapists work with the patient's whole personality, there are certain symptoms that seem to be common for patients who benefit particularly from music therapy. Some of these are intellectualizing, severe communication disturbances, weak emotional contact, obsessive-compulsive symptoms and productive psychotic symptoms.

If the patient is to benefit from music therapy, these basic requirements must be met:

- The patient must be able to attend therapy regularly.

- The patient must be able to reflect verbally or musically.

- The patient must be able to articulate goals for the therapy or to have an opinion regarding the music therapist's suggested goals.

- The patient must be able to enter into a therapeutic alliance (see Chapter 2.3) or wish to work with his/her problems in entering into such an alliance.

- There should be careful awareness of any risk of psychotic relapse.

Previous experience has shown that it is often easier to establish a positive working alliance in music therapy than in traditional psychotherapy, among non-productive psychotic patients with communication disturbances, intellectualization, obsessive-compulsive symptoms and difficulties in expressing emotions. A positive working alliance in this case is defined as the motivation to co-operate within the structure of the music therapy session and with its goals.

Among productive psychotic patients it has been especially beneficial to use music therapy to establish a working alliance with patients who have dominating autistic traits, megalomania and/or self-devaluating thoughts. Common themes for these patients in therapy are establishing an alliance, moving in and out of contact, etc. In quite a few cases, this has helped to motivate the patient to move forward in a treatment plan, with or without music therapy.

Music therapy in child psychiatry has been developed in Denmark in the form of a two-year project, funded by private grants. In this project, the music therapist worked with music therapy assessment and individual sessions with preschool children (Irgens-Møller 1998a, 1998b). Goals for the individual sessions varied – from working through emotional issues, to development of communication skills, impulse regulation or increasing self-esteem. For half of the children, a visible development in relation to the child's important problems was seen, and in half of the cases, observations from music therapy sessions contributed to new information about the child.

In addition to music therapy practice, the music therapists regularly attend case conferences and referral meetings, when relevant, as well as meeting with the individual patient's psychiatrist and *contact person*. Music therapists also teach other psychiatric colleagues, through workshops and lectures, about music therapy and its uses. An important part of the music therapist's job in psychiatry is communicating about, and documenting, their work.

The Music Therapy Clinic at Aalborg Psychiatric Hospital (Centre for Treatment and Research) publishes the annual *Musikterapi i psykiatrien (Music therapy in psychiatry)* with case study presentations and theoretical articles on aspects of music therapy, written by music therapists in Denmark. This group of music therapists has also formed the group Music Therapists in Hospital Psychiatry (MIHP), in Denmark that meets four times a year to exchange ideas, experiences and methods for assessment and research.

CASE STUDY EXAMPLE AND PATIENT NARRATIVE

A male patient (41 years old) was referred to psychotherapy at a psychiatric hospital. During the referral meeting it was decided that he should be offered music therapy. He was referred with the diagnosis 'personality disorder/disturbance of personality structure', which was the conclusion after an evaluation using the following tests: WAIS, Luria's 10-word test and the Rorschach test.

Characteristic traits were intellectualizing, obsessive-compulsive behaviour, and very little contact with his emotional life. The patient attended hour-long music therapy sessions as an outpatient once a week for two years. The aim of the therapy was defined as follows: to work towards the patient establishing better contact with himself and with others – primarily women. Partial aims were working with boundaries and autonomy, and supporting the patient in clarifying future employment possibilities. In the following, excerpts from the case are described, illustrated through music examples 3 to 8 on the enclosed CD.

CD example 3: The therapist and patient both improvise on the piano (separate pianos)

The excerpt is from the first music therapy session. The patient has been asked to choose an instrument (he chooses one of the two pianos in the music therapy room). He is asked to play a note, listen to it carefully and let the note lead him to the next note. In other words, he is asked to try to direct his attention to the sound of the note, instead of focusing on his preconceived idea of how it is supposed to sound. The patient plays alternately in the high and deep register, avoiding the middle register. He seems to become gradually more absorbed in listening – to immerse himself in the sound.

The music therapist plays a simple repeated note as an accompaniment during the whole improvisation (one note in the middle register of the piano). The notes of the therapist and the patient join together and create harmonies that invite them to focus inwards and listen. The patient's body language shows intense concentration in the improvisation. The music therapist hears quite a lot of intentional contact between the patient and the therapist in the music.

In the conversation after the improvisation, and after hearing the tape of the music, the patient states that he barely heard the therapist's music. However, he had a sense of a musical centre somewhere that he felt drawn to. He knew he needed this centre, in order to allow himself to be aware and present in his own music. In this case, the patient gave his permission for the examples to be used for analysis and research. When he was invited to the clinic four years later and listened to this example, he was asked to focus on the contact between the patient and the therapist. He was asked to score his interpretation of the contact on a scale of 1 to 10, where 1 meant no contact and 10 meant very close contact. The music in this example was scored at 9. This shows that the patient's perception had changed significantly through the treatment.

CD example 4: The therapist plays a metallophone; the patient plays the piano

This example is from session 14. The patient himself now asks the therapist to act as a focus point in the music – or in this case, to be a lifeline, while the patient challenges boundaries, allows himself to take up more space and allows more aggressive energy in the music.

CD example 5: Both the therapist and the patient improvise vocally

This example is from session 32. The patient has started to dream very intensely, after not having had dream activity for many years. The patient often starts music therapy sessions by relating a recent dream. He also paints watercolours between sessions. He brings these with him and says a few words about them in the sessions. Finally, he writes a journal, which he gives to the therapist (his own idea) so that she can read it between sessions. Comments on the watercolours and the journal notes come primarily from the patient himself.

In this session, the patient relates a dream. In the dream he is running around, looking for something. He comes to a barbed-wire fence and climbs over it. On the other side there is a frozen lake. In the middle of the lake there is a patch of ice so thin that the patient can see a petrified sea urchin through it. He says that the sea urchin is a part of him that needs to come alive. We decide to try to use our voices to express the sea urchin. This is the first time that the patient improvises with his voice. The therapist attempts to match the patient's pitch and expression. There is a movement from very little vibrato to much more vibrato in the vocal sound towards the end of the improvisation. This can be understood as 'something that is frozen, beginning to thaw'. The therapist matches empathically and supports the patient in his expression.

CD example 6: Both the therapist and the patient improvise vocally

This example is from session 42. The patient is now much more familiar with vocal improvisation. The night before the session he has dreamt of a black panther, and this is the symbol that we attempt to express together through our voices. This makes the patient use a much deeper voice, and he experiences this as an expression of something masculine. He also finds that it is much easier for him to make himself heard and 'stand alone' with his voice when using the deeper pitch. This gives him the confidence to express himself as intensely and 'primitively' as he does in this case. The therapist matches his expression and, through her sounds, she tries to encourage the patient to explore his own boundaries in the vocal improvisation.

CD example 7: The patient improvises alone vocally

This example is from session 44. The patient uses in this case an integrated vocal sound, which contains both 'light' and 'dark' (high and deep) sounds. The patient feels surer of expressing himself and can do so independently. He feels that his feminine and masculine sides are more alive and present and that they are more integrated.

CD example 8: The therapist and the patient both improvise with voice and piano

This example is from the last session – number 57. The therapist and the patient play freely in the 'flow' of the music. Both of them contribute to the music with new ideas and let themselves be immersed in the music of the moment. There are no defined roles. The therapist feels free to express herself and play her own ideas, inspired by the joint improvisation and without thinking of supporting, amplifying or accompanying the patient in another way. The music sums up many of the elements that have been expressed in earlier sessions. This is the first time that both the therapist and the patient have improvised vocally and played the piano at the same time.

The patient made his own decision of when to end music therapy. He felt that he now was ready to go out into the world and try out his strength – using his experiences from music therapy. The same patient wrote, by request, the following patient narrative, three years after the music therapy ended. (Patient narratives are not very common in music therapy literature. A good anthology is Hibben (1999).) As seen in the following narrative, the music helped the patient to achieve a more 'spacious' self-identity and greater personal freedom. Regarding the aims defined at the start of the therapy, the patient developed more flexible, yet clear boundaries and a greater degree of autonomy, in this way improving his contact with himself and others – including women. The patient was fully rehabilitated shortly after the termination of music therapy.

We have included seven of the patient's watercolours, with his permission, as an illustration of some of the inner processes he went through during the course of music therapy. The seven paintings are selected out of a collection of 63 watercolours that the patient brought with him to therapy sessions.

See the seven watercolours on the following pages.

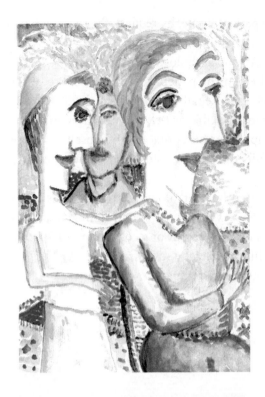

1. A little boy reaches out to a mother figure, who is distant. The green man in the background, who is an observer of reality, is the most important figure here.

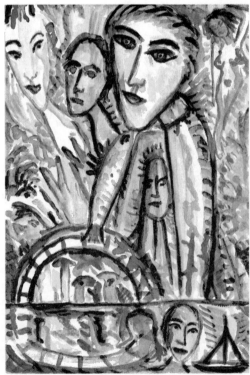

2. The petrified sea urchin that appeared under the ice in a dream has become a face here. It is still under the surface of the water.

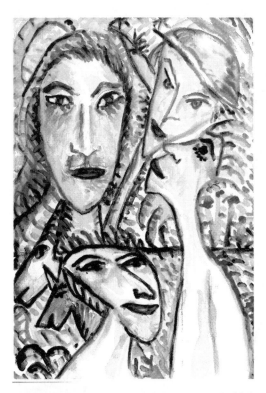

3. *The face has now come up above the surface of the water – this creates insecurity in relation to other people.*

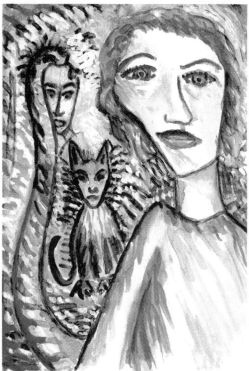

4. *An indescribable anxiety has broken loose and is manifested in dreams and fantasies of devils and snakes.*

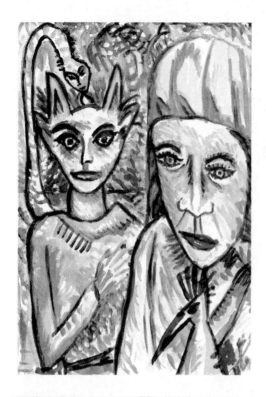

5. The devil is growing. It can be experienced now both as dangerous and as an important, not acknowledged source of energy.

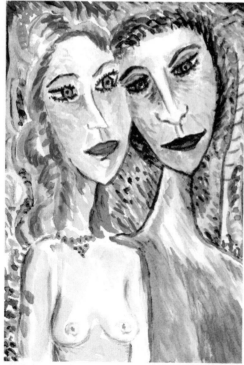

6. I now experience a better balance between the feminine and masculine sides.

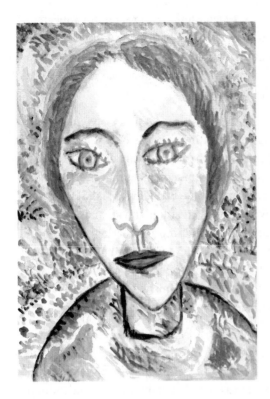

7. I feel much younger now, but much more integrated.

Figures 4.1–4.7: Art pictures from a patient in therapy

Patient narrative

The background for my participation in music therapy was a very long period of illness and absence from my job as a preschool teacher; a job that got on my nerves more and more, where I became more and more stressed, nervous and confused from having to relate to so many people and new impressions. Finally, I completely lost perspective, and as a result I constantly forgot what I was in the process of doing. A thorough psychological test confirmed that this job wasn't the right one for me. Based on this, it was suggested (and I accepted) that I start psychotherapy in the form of individual music therapy once a week.

I was nervous when I went to the first session. I wasn't sure of what music therapy was, had never heard of it before. I had also grown up in a very unmusical family, and my experiences in school were limited to getting hit on the head for not singing or for singing out of tune. It took some time, about a half-year, before I started feeling like I could find my own space in the music. Early on, it was the piano that I was drawn to; the piano with its many keys ranging from the very deep to the very high. In the beginning I was most drawn to the dark, sorrowful, melancholy sounds; later lighter, higher notes appeared. First they were opposed to each other; later they began to relate to each other, to play together and dance in and out and around each other. I experienced more and more that there was a space in the music; at the same time my daily life seemed more and more sad and full of anxiety.

After a good while, in the course of the therapy, I started using my voice as an instrument; this I especially felt was a breakthrough – something that was difficult but that also gave me direct contact with/access to my deepest feelings. Shortly after this, dreams poured forth, long dream sequences that I wrote down as they came – among others, dreams from the time when I was on LSD, dreams of persecution, dreams where there were strange creatures and animals like crocodiles, panthers, snakes, etc … A lot happened during this period; I felt like a child again, 'Palle Alone in the World', in a good, new and exciting way. I started being more aware of where I was and what I wanted. Three or four months later I made the decision to end therapy, felt that it was finished; now the time had come to go out into the world again and test my strength.

About three years have gone by since the music ended. Quite a lot has happened since then. I feel that I have changed quite a bit, in some ways I'm still the same person, but at the same time I have a feeling of being able to 'fill myself out' much more today. Earlier I felt like I was a sad, lonely and misunderstood 'steppenwolf', sitting in a waiting room, and when I was with other people, I often felt like the spy who came in from the cold. I'm still a 'steppenwolf', but now a much freer, more spontaneous, active and cheerful one – instead of a silent and speculating wolf, I'm now a wolf who joins in, barking with pleasure. I've become much better at being aware of my own needs, and the fear of hurting others has moved into the background. The morning crises I used to have, crises that could last all day, and where I felt that catastrophe was lurking right around the corner, have more or less disappeared. Although music therapy officially has ended, I feel that it is still going on. All the experiments, notes and themes that I played out in the music, I now use in different encounters with other people, and it gives me a great feeling of freedom; freedom understood in the way that I have many different keys to play in – many different ways to tackle situations. I still do voice exercises to become aware of how I feel right now, deep inside. This is a good tool for me to relax knots and tensions that are forming.

4.2 Music Therapy with Physically and/or Developmentally Delayed Clients

Music therapy for children and adults with developmental disability is sometimes misunderstood to be a form of 'music teaching'. The degree by which the therapeutic direction can veer towards developmental goals, functional goals or psychotherapeutic goals varies from country to country, and also between training and working approaches within countries. However, as a general principle, music therapists formulate and implement non-musical goals in their treatment of this population, whether they are working in schools, hospitals, community units or private practice. The primary therapeutic goals in many European countries involve working with contact, communication and sensory stimulation. Music and musicality as a tool can evoke the expression of feelings and emotions in people with physical and developmental disability.

In the European literature of music therapy, one can find well-documented evidence that music therapy is both a suitable and an effective form of intervention for this population. Perhaps the most important rationale behind this argument is that these clients often have significant limitations in their use of formal language and their potential for normal development, particularly in the area of communication development. With the multi-handicapped clients there is often a total lack of verbal language, and therefore they need other media of communication for self-expression and to interact with their surroundings. Music is a good tool for this as it has often been described as a 'language' in itself.

In an article for the *Nordic Journal of Music Therapy*, Muff (1994) described the relevance of music therapy for this population in the following way:

> The ability and the possibility to establish contact and communication with others is the most important basis for human development. A characteristic of the developmentally disabled is precisely a reduced level of language development, both in reference to spoken and body language. A language is fundamental for contact, and the music therapist's strategy is to improve this by initiating fundamental and systematic work with language and expression. This can be expressed as follows:

> A single note, a phrase of notes, sounded on an instrument, a vocal sound, a clap on the leg or hand, to sing, hum, whistle, dance, march etc. is to express through music. When one expresses musically, playing together with another, one is communicating and 'talking together' in music. The music therapist can, as such, have a very wide musical understanding, that also includes the developmentally disabled person's non-verbal symbolic and body language. Based on this foundation of language and expression, the music therapist operates at the

level of and with reference to the weaker intellectual and motor abilities of the client. The developmental process can start where the client's language and expression is improving thanks to possibilities for emotional expression. This strategy is a primary objective in the therapeutic work with people with developmental disability. (Muff 1994)

Music therapists working with people with developmental disability are very conscious of the power of music-making, and its value in evoking pleasure, motivation, stimulation and joy. People with Down's syndrome are often reported in the literature as being particularly responsive to music, to be able to play in tempo, rhythmically skilled, and demonstrating potential for being part of group music-making. This concept of music being 'enjoyable' and 'fun' has been both an advantage and a disadvantage in the serious perception of music therapy as a treatment. For example, if a client is referred to music therapy, the question that needs to be addressed is, 'Why does he/she need music therapy?' The answer has often been, 'Because he/she loves music – is very responsive to music.' For the music therapist, this is useful to know, and encouraging, but not a clear rationale for treatment. To find a better rationale we need to explore the client's psychosocial, emotional, physical and psychological needs (Smeijsters 1999; also Chapter 4.3). Educational and remedial goals have also been included in the objectives of therapy because many pioneers in music therapy worked with school-age children.

In Denmark, England, Norway, Holland, Germany and many other countries in Europe, therapists working in the field of developmental disabilities have combined a psychotherapeutic approach with a more developmental orientation to meeting clients' needs. Juliette Alvin, Paul Nordoff and Clive Robbins all worked with methods to help people with these disabilities to benefit from creative experiences and achieve their potential.

This population need creative experiences through which they can enjoy relative success and through which they can develop.

Areas of need and potential development

Music therapy focuses on specific areas of need including perceptual awareness, physical and psychological stimulation, communicative abilities, emotional expression, cognitive ability, social behaviour and the development of individual resources and capacities.

Perceptual awareness: music is used to stimulate and enhance awareness of their body, of the potentials of hearing, seeing and touching, of the therapist, of the environment, and of the relationship between the creation of sound, and the sound they hear. Awareness of vibration is a first step, especially for more severely handicapped patients, and music/sound is created through vibration. To use the vibration of the instruments as a form of 'deep sensory experience' is, especially in the work with the multiply handicapped clients, a means to direct their attention to the self and to the sound. The client must be able to 'feel' the music to understand cause and effect and the production of sound. For example, a stereo or TV producing complex sound through a speaker in a box is not as effective in capturing attention and developing awareness as a guitar or drum pressed against the body, where one can both feel and hear the sound produced. The sounds and music must be at the level of their awareness and understanding or it ceases to be therapeutically effective.

Physical/psychological stimulation: music is physically stimulating, motivating and can be exciting. Conversely, it can be calming and relaxing. To promote engagement and contact, music therapists create stimulation and excitement in music with variations in tempo and dynamics, and the music becomes 'psychologically interesting' through the context of harmony and melody, texture and phrasing. When clients with developmental disability both experience stimulation and learn how to initiate and motivate themselves through the stimulation of music-making, their potentials increase and they develop greater engagement with the external world and the people in it.

Communicative ability: The use of music in a therapeutic way to encourage contact and communication is a primary function of music therapy with the developmentally disabled. Taking turns, sharing, reciprocal interaction, intersubjectivity and vocal/verbal expressions emerge in music-making. The earliest patterns of communication, found in mother–baby interaction, where timing is an essential ingredient in the development of meaningful, pre-verbal communication, are found in music therapy interaction through shared music-making. Music provides a raw form of non-verbal communication, where the therapist uses the elements of music with this population to create communicative intentionality – shared meanings, by the development of a shared repertoire of events that have meaning and context for therapist and client.

Emotional expression: Music is a language, with the inflections, nuances and emotions of speech and, in the use of a simple musical instrument, sounds can represent happiness, sadness, anger, frustration or joy. While the perception of fellow professionals, and the public, might be that music therapy is a medium for making people with developmental disabilities 'happy' and 'content' (and this is undoubtedly one of its functions), the skilled music therapist can also enable the handicapped client to externalize other necessary emotions, such as anger, sadness and melancholy. A very high percentage of people with developmental disability also suffer from psychiatric disorders such as anxiety and depression, so the potential of music therapy is also to allow negative emotions and conflicts to emerge. Music, both improvised and precomposed, can contain and facilitate many emotional characteristics.

Cognitive abilities: for developmental, educational and remedial objectives with the developmentally disabled, music can be used in a therapeutic way to promote attention, concentration, organizational skills, memory, sequential and simultaneous processing skills, and problem solving. This is perhaps the more functional use of music in therapy, and is where the use of music in therapy aims to achieve developmental goals. Many case study examples illustrate where attention and concentration is improved, short-term and long-term memory is stimulated, and people develop capacities to organize sounds into patterns and phrases, and connect experiences together through associations.

Social behaviour: While individual work is sometimes more specifically and intensively focused on the client–therapist relationship, there are some examples in the literature of the power and value of music-making in group music therapy to promote and develop social engagement and interaction between clients, as well as between clients and therapist. Improvisational music therapy is live, active and innately social – and for people with developmental disabilities, for a variety of reasons, this is a critical area of need. Some clients are very limited in their awareness and contact with their environment because of their extensive mental and physical handicaps. Others have difficult and challenging behaviour, with obsessive, ritualistic or antisocial patterns of behaviour. Confrontation with aspects of the outside world that they have difficulty understanding often provokes reactions of anxiety and fear. Music-making can be a non-threatening, safe and interesting way to develop social engagement – a natural development from acquired alternative methods of communication.

Individual resources and capacities: people with developmental disabilities tend to be perceived as quite dependent, and are often underestimated. The subtle and skilful development of the clients' ability to play within musical interaction leads to choice-making, initiative, spontaneity, musical independence, confidence, improved self-esteem and creativity. Music therapy offers a creative medium for developing potentials, particularly because music-making is such an incredibly motivating experience.

Music as a medium for basic contact

For some clients with severe developmental disability, their abilities to achieve a basic level of communicative contact with others (either reacting to stimuli or taking the initiative) is very poorly developed. It is therefore quite difficult for the music therapist to see whether the client can sense an attempt at contact made by the music therapist. Anne Steen-Møller, who has been working with multiply handicapped children for many years, has developed a model of understanding levels of contact in her work with this population (Steen-Møller 1996). She has defined five levels of contact.

LEVEL 1: 'THE THERAPIST FEELS THE CONTACT WITH THE CLIENT'

- At this level there is very little contact, and it is almost unnoticeable and inaudible.

- *Goal*: the music therapist aims to communicate with the client, and to give the client a possibility to want to – to dare to – direct his/her attention outwards towards the therapist and the environment. The client needs to feel secure and accepted and the therapist must be totally aware and open without any expectations in the interaction. The music used here can be seen as a 'mother–baby' form of contact. The mode of expression must be familiar and shared by both: the therapist glides into the client's form of expression – sounds, movements, rate of breathing – in order to create an atmosphere of security and pleasure which is the prerequisite for meeting the client.

LEVEL 2: 'THE THERAPIST HEARS AND SEES THE CONTACT'

- At this level the awareness of the outside world is established and can be widened through the use of music. There are obvious reactions to the therapist's approach in sound and music – often expressed in the pauses between the stanzas that the therapist plays. These reactions are not yet conscious communication, but a reaction to the impressions from the outside world which the client is now able to perceive as something separate from himself. Self-awareness is not yet clearly established.

- *Goal*: the goal is to develop the self-awareness of the client – hearing the musical reactions of the therapist gradually makes the client conscious of his/her own expressions. A development can be observed in the following three areas. Time: reactions become faster, pauses shorter. Quality: more marked but not necessarily new reactions; greater attention. Recognition of sounds and music: this shows that clients at this level actually remember and learn from experience.

LEVEL 3: 'THE CLIENT NOW CONTROLS THE CONTACT'

- At this level the client is aware of himself/herself and of his/her ability to make sounds to call for the attention of the surroundings. These expressions are goal-oriented and the interaction is now based on the initiative of the client.

- *Goal*: the goal is to increase the client's awareness of communication and motivate him/her to experiencing being in control. The role of the music is now increasingly a reaction to the client's active participation. The length of time and the quality of the participation of the client are still important issues in the perspective of development. The way of playing the different instruments becomes more relevant and new patterns of movement are incorporated.

LEVEL 4: 'OUR CONTACT TAKES THE FORM OF DIALOGUE'

- The client is now conscious of our interaction. We can take turns at producing sound and listening and he/she can direct his/her attention on me and on himself/herself in our interaction. That is to say that the interaction now takes the form of a dialogue.

- *Goal*: The goal is to create two-way communication in which the client experiences that his/her mode of expressing himself/herself becomes the starting point of a dialogue. Music is here used as reciprocal communication. It offers the client the possibility to enter into a dialogue and his/her awareness of communication thus materializes through the music. At this level the client is able to play the basic beat and may learn small rhythmical patterns.

LEVEL 5: 'WE CONTACT EACH OTHER THROUGH FREE, IMPROVISED MUSIC'

- At this level the client has a clear understanding of himself/herself interacting with the surroundings. There are the beginnings of a verbal communication but it is very limited.

- *Goal*: The goal is to support and prolong the client's experience of being part of an on-going exchange. Music provides a non-confronting space for the client to experience independence and autonomy. The music is free from demands and expectations which these clients are very sensitive to. In the musical interaction he/she may further develop communicative skills such as sensitivity, flexibility, creativity, listening and responding to what you hear etc.

The model can be seen as a tool through which one can establish a developmental perspective of the music therapist's work within this field. It is a tool for elucidation of a client, for developing music therapeutic methods and for the documentation of our work.

Conclusion

For this population, music breaks down barriers of disability, rigidity and age. Therapists may use classical, pop or folk music, and while improvised music provides the best medium for creative development, songs and pieces from the repertoire also allow the expression of emotion and communicative participation in a musical experience. An elderly person with profound disability responds just as positively and emotionally to a child's nursery song, or a simple folk song, as a six-year-old boy. Monotonous pulsed playing can evolve into creative rhythms and syncopation, and range, inflection and accents can develop from monotonal singing. The development of a musical and therapeutic relationship has been demonstrated in many articles and case studies where the therapeutic process involves both musical and non-musical goals.

4.3 Music Therapy with Paediatric Clients

Music therapy with children with a variety of different diagnoses is a comparatively large area of work to review in a limited overview, and it has been an area of development for music therapy pursued by music therapists in many different countries. Perhaps this was a popular and immediately valued area of work because of children's positive and enjoyable experience of music. Another reason is that the evidence today suggests that early intervention pays, economically, and for humanitarian reasons. As well as children with significantly late, undeveloped or disordered language, as are referred to in Chapter 4.4, one can also find music therapy used as an intervention with children with the following illnesses and/or disabilities:

- children with chromosomal or inborn metabolic disorders (Down's syndrome, Williams syndrome, Speilmeyer syndrome, Vogt's syndrome, Rett syndrome, Asperger's syndrome, fragile X syndrome etc.)

- children with childhood autism (or whose disabilities can be diagnosed as an autistic spectrum disorder)

- children with global developmental delay and mental retardation
- children with early emotional damage (adopted children/children from dysfunctional families
- children born with drug or alcohol dependency
- children with specific learning disorders
- children with Deficits in Attention, Motor Control and Perception (DAMP)
- children with Attention Deficit Hyperactivity Disorder
- children with weak left brain function
- children with brain damage (cerebral palsy, spasticity and athetoid disability)
- children with hearing impairment
- children with tuberous sclerosis
- undiagnosed children (with behaviour, communication, social or attentional problems)
- children who are hospitalized for surgical procedures or serious illness.

The goals and objectives in working with children are always adjusted to an individual child's presenting strengths and weaknesses, and with attention to his/her unique individual personality. The music therapist must create a foundation for supporting an individual child's developmental potential. The intervention often starts with a period of observation and evaluation, where the therapist both observes and enters into the individual child's specific way of communication with and relationship to the world outside.

The music therapist's aims, as a rule, are always a part of the general aims in a multidisciplinary approach with other professionals involved (speech therapist, physiotherapist, teachers in special education and educational psychologists). The main focus of the work of music therapists with handicapped children is often to draw out the potentials and resources of a child, developing a therapeutic relationship with the child as a frame for eliciting engagement and contact. It is not unusual that in music therapy hidden resources and responses are 'discovered' in the child, sometimes resources that have not been seen by others, but that can reveal another side of a child (see for example the case study 'Joel' in Chapter 5.3)

General goals are:

- to strengthen a child's potential for responding to and initiating contact and communication (with consideration to personal expression and expression within a dialogue)

- to develop the child's understanding and contact with their emotions and feelings

- to improve their quality of life through experiences of sharing, giving and receiving

- to improve their awareness of situations, a feeling of identity and ability to concentrate

- to develop social skills. (Alvin 1975; Bean 1995; Bruscia 1987, 1991; Flower 1999; Grant 1995; Wigram 1999a; Wigram and De Backer 1999a; Wigram and Weekes 1985)

As well as this, music therapists often focus on quite specific objectives:

- to strengthen the child's use of their voice (Di Franco 2001; Etkin 1999)

- to stimulate language development

- to stimulate motor co-ordination skills (Bean 1995; Voigt 1999; Wigram and Weekes 1985)

- to develop 'turn-taking' skills when playing together (for example, dialogues) (Edgerton 1994; Holck 2002a, 2002b; see Chapter 4.4)

- to develop body awareness and identity (Strange 1999)

- to develop a use of fantasy in thought and play (Brown 1999b)

- to make a framework where the child can experience and express different emotions. (Flower 1999)

Music is an ideal medium to work with the many different problems of handicapped children, because children have always incorporated and integrated music as a part of their everyday life. They sing while they play, singing and 'calling' to each other. As children grow up, music becomes more externalized – for example, something one can listen to on a radio or CD, or something at which one can be skilled. Everyone can express themselves through the use of the basic elements of musical communication: intonation, rhythm, timing and tone-colour. We have all used these elements in our earliest communication with the external world.

The majority of the clinical populations listed above will typically include a degree of developmental disability or learning disability to a greater or lesser degree of severity in their profile. However, some populations, such as those with early emotional damage, hearing impairment, unclear diagnoses, those with drug or alcohol dependency, and children who are hospitalized for treatment, may have no learning disability, and for them a treatment with music therapy, either as an intensive or as an augmentative treatment, will have some different objectives.

Music therapy for hospitalized children was not reported in the Danish publication of this text because there is a much smaller prevalence of this specialized area in Europe when compared with the USA or Australia. A leading music therapist from Australia, Jane Edwards, has recently completed a fine doctoral thesis in this area of work (Edwards 2000). She demonstrates clearly the role music therapy has in meeting the needs of children in coping with painful and difficult procedures as a result, for example, of severe burns (Edwards 1995, 1998, 1999). There are also evident advantages when addressing psychosocial needs for comfort, support and self-expression (Chetta 1981; Cowan 1991; Dun 1993; Edwards 1995; Robb 1996), alleviating anxiety and offering opportunities to express feelings (Dun 1993; Froehlich 1984; Gfeller 1992), management of pain in coping with serious illness and injury, and cancer (Kennelly and Edwards 1997; Standley and Hanser 1995; Turry 1999), and in improving recovery and growth (Nöcker-Ribaupierre 1999; Shoemark 1999; Standley and Moore 1995).

The function of music

Music can be used by the music therapist in many different ways, and what follows are some explanations of these different applications when working with these very different populations.

FREELY IMPROVISED MUSIC

Here, music is used as a sort of bridge between the inner and outer world of a child, and is developed as a common language between therapist and child. Musical dialogue develops through rhythmic, vocal or other types of exchange. The music therapist can support, stimulate and challenge the client. Improvisations can be made with voice, body or instruments and can be very free, or the music therapist (or clients) can create some 'playing rules' (for example, 'Let's play a beat each on the drum'). Sometimes the repertoire of improvisations can be at a simple level, but may nevertheless be almost insuperably difficult for the most severely handicapped child to deal with. In some cases a very simple musical expression is needed to enable the child to develop their first sensation of communication and contact with others – and for them to experience being seen and heard.

MUSIC WITH A GIVEN STRUCTURE AND FRAMEWORK

Here one can use well-known melodies, which can create structure in a social situation, or use well-known songs at the point in a session to establish a routine that is stable. Familiar 'Hello/Goodbye' songs are a typical example of this. Songs provide a good framework for recognition, security and the possibility of relating to past experiences. They can express feelings, moods or themes that otherwise can be difficult to draw out.

As a part of this structure the music therapist and the child can compose or improvise a song together, or the music therapist can do so alone, that can sum up the quality and value of the relationship that has developed in this individual session. For example, the music therapist can create a frame and a structure around the child's expression by singing to the child what he/she is doing. This may help the child to focus, and to extend and augment their playing, relating to developed attention and expression. Play songs can be structuring when working in social problems, and it is very helpful to use this type of song to help children experience working together with a music therapist, and also with other children.

MUSIC AND SONGS AS A MEDIUM FOR TRAINING

Musical activities can be organized so that a child can come in with a decisive 'hit' on an instrument at a certain moment as part of a whole piece. This can act as training for better co-ordination, concentration, precision of movement and hearing abilities. In addition, motor co-ordination, body movement, tempo and other motor skills can be included as a training through music and dance.

RECORDING AND PLAYING BACK MUSIC

One technique that is employed is the recording of an improvisation, song or musical activity to play back to the child so that they can actually hear their own musical production. From this, the child may gain some insight about themselves, while listening to their own expressive musical sounds. Then the issues or problems that the child is working with, or their fantasies, might be included in a new improvisation.

THE MUSIC THERAPIST'S ROLE WHEN WORKING WITH CHILDREN WITH DIFFERENT DISORDERS

The music therapist often seems to have many roles – both in the team around the child, and in the progress made during the individual sessions. Seen from outside, the music therapist might be perceived as some sort of music teacher in one situation, voice therapist in another, and a containing, caring mother or a playmate. There are many possible roles. The music therapist must be flexible and adaptable in fulfilling his/her role so that the child's needs, identified in the objectives of the work, can be met.

DOCUMENTATION OF THE STAGES OF DEVELOPMENT

There are many written results of music therapy work with this client group. There are also examples of systematic research in this area in international publications. Literature in this particular clinical area describes developments in the following areas:

- increased concentration and learning
- better use of language
- maturing of social play (children make more and different forms of expression, move more to music, and become more independent – taking the initiative)
- greater variation of expressive abilities (voice, body and musical expressiveness)
- greater degree of extroversion (the child is more communicative, and engages for longer periods in music-making)
- greater degree of emotional balance
- greater self-confidence
- improved rhythmic sense and body experience
- improved social understanding
- better contact with themselves and with others.

The music therapist often has contact with the child's parents, and a part of the work lies in developing a good relationship with the parents and informing them about often small, but nonetheless important, developments experienced in working with the child. The music therapists will write assessment reports and reports on the periods of treatment giving information about specific music therapy goals. Reports can also form a part of a multidisciplinary team report together with physiotherapist, speech therapist, teaching consultant etc.

Conclusion

It can be hard work to communicate the specific possibilities of music therapy for the individual child to the caseworker of the community or to other authorities who can give licence for music therapy treatment, if these authorities don't know the profession.

Gradually, the fact that music therapy can offer another contact form than the one offered through verbal language is becoming better known and accepted. There is also generally more knowledge that music therapy can be a necessary contribution in work with relationship and communication abilities in children who are not able to use, or have difficulties in using, verbal language.

Music therapy with children focuses on resources more than problems. In the treatment the children most often have nice and positive experiences of themselves and of the resources they have. Music therapy offers a frame for these children, where they can express themselves on their own premises and thus can be seen, heard and valued through something they create themselves from inside, and not only from something they perform and imitate by learning from outer structures and schemas. Most children react spontaneously and with interest to music – also including children who are difficult to contact otherwise.

Case study examples

CD EXAMPLE 1

In the following we describe two short case study extracts from music therapy work with a five-year-old boy. The extracts are illustrated through the music examples 1 and 2 on the music CD in this book.

In the first example you can hear the first meeting, through sound and music, between the music therapist and the boy. The boy had suffered from meningitis when he was nine months old, which caused a stop in his speech development at that time. Even now, at five years old, he makes use of an infant's sounds like 'gigi' and 'gaga'. At the same time he is very communicative within the narrow span of different sounds he uses. As he has shown no sign of being able to imitate sounds from other people or surroundings, the speech therapist has given up on him for now. In co-operation with her and other pedagogues in the special kindergarten he is visiting on a daily basis, it has been decided to give the boy an offer of music therapy treatment.

The aim of music therapy is defined as: trying to expand his repertoire of sounds and raise his communication ability. The music therapist doesn't demand of the boy that he shall imitate or say specific sounds or words in the beginning. The music therapist makes use of the sound repertoire of the boy and puts these sounds into musical frames such as rhythms and melodies, and communicates with the boy from there. The short melody, which is created during expressions of the infant sounds at the end of the first example, is so simple that it can be remembered by the boy and can be repeated in the next sessions. Some kind of form gradually arises and becomes a part of the joint communication. The boy is ready to take part in creating other small rhythm and melody patterns as long as it does not implicate that he has to change his infant sounds.

CD EXAMPLE 2

After some months have passed, where the two have been playing around with repetition of sound patterns and small melodies as well as with instrumental improvisations on piano and drums, the boy has become more clear and eager in communication with other people, although he is still keeping his own repertoire of sounds. The music therapist matches the energy level of the boy in the music and sometimes even tries to overtake him. In one case it develops into a game with melody, dynamics and putting different voice sounds together (still sounds from the sound repertoire of the boy). During the game the therapist is playing a melody from a children's song at the piano and, in an energetic way of playing together, the therapist keeps the melody and the dynamics, but suddenly replaces the voice sounds from the boy's sound repertoire with voice sounds the boy normally doesn't use. The therapist sings 'vov vov vov' instead of 'gaga' and 'gigi'. In the quick tempo the boy is seduced and he does not notice that he very clearly and loudly imitates the therapist's sounds. Immediately afterwards, the boy stops singing and he looks very surprised. After a short break he is willing to repeat it.

It was the first step for the boy to very gradually start to imitate sounds from other people and thus a first step towards an opening of his closed universe. After six months of music therapy the boy could start again at the speech therapist and there gradually have his repertoire of sounds and words expanded.

Here, the music therapy was, as in some other cases, the first step in a developmental process – the step which breaks the isolation or a necessary obsessive pattern of habits. In these examples it is obvious that the techniques are based on seduction by the help of musical elements such as melody, crescendo and dynamics. It is only possible to use such techniques when a basic trust is created between the music therapist and the child.

4.4 Music Therapy for Children with Communication Disorders (Ulla Holck)

This chapter is about music therapy for children with severely delayed, disordered or absent language development. Some of these children may have developed a few functional words or signs, but they have no language (in the real sense of the word) that enables them to express themselves or be a part of a community of language. For communicative development to take place, a child must have the desire, ability and possibility to influence the environment and be influenced by it. In this area of communication, music therapy particularly has potential to help these children. It would also be useful to consider that while this chapter is concerned with children, concepts within it can also apply to music therapy for adults with disordered language development, but not to those with late brain damage or others who have lost earlier language skill.

Based on the latest infant research, two perspectives from which to understand music therapy for children in a pre-verbal stage of development will be presented. The first is a *developmental theory perspective* that shows a clear connection between early musical ability in the infant and pre-verbal development. The second is an *interactional theory perspective* that points to relational interactions as the basis for all development.

A developmental theory perspective

In pre-verbal development, infants and parents communicate by means of sounds and movements in interplay, consisting of mutual imitation, turn-taking and, especially, affective attunement. When infancy researchers such as Daniel Stern (1985, 1989) and Colwyn Trevarthen (1999) describe sound dialogues between mothers and infants, they employ 'musical' terms. When describing *tonal qualities* they use the terms pitch, timbre and tonal movement, and when describing *temporal qualities* they speak of pulse, tempo, rhythm and, especially, timing.

At a very early age, the infant possesses the ability to perceive sound qualities and sound patterns (Trehub, Trainor and Unyk 1993), and, importantly, is able to use these abilities to participate in communicative interplay. From this perspective, acquiring language is merely the natural development of a communicative process that started much earlier. Based on his acoustic analyses of sound dialogues between mothers and infants, musician Stephen Malloch speaks of *communicative musicality* as fundamental to all human communication:

> … it is our contention that the ability to act musically underlies and supports human companionship; that the elements of *communicative musicality* are

necessary for joint human expressiveness to arise, and lie beneath, to a greater or lesser degree, all human communication. (Malloch 1999, p.47, my italics)

The early dialogue is of course not music, in the sense of a *formed cultural expression*, but on the other hand, music is made up of the same elements that form the communicative bond between parents and infants. It is no wonder that all cultures have music as a common human phenomenon!

When a music therapist works with a child (or an adult) with no language skills, he/she can work on communicative levels that developmentally precede language, while at the same time taking *the child's chronological age* into consideration. A ten-year-old boy, whose language skills and mental ability are that of a one-year-old, can express himself and be 'met' on both levels through the music.

'COMMUSICAL' INTERPLAY

There are some important and inherent processes involved within shared music-making that contribute significantly to the communicative part of musical engagement. The word 'commusical' actually came into being by a slip of the tongue. It was a spontaneous, but not completely random, contraction of the words 'communicative' and 'musical'. However, the expression is quite precise, for which reason it will be maintained and elaborated here.

Sound is appealing. An important precondition for interplay is, naturally, attention, and music has an obvious appeal – both the musical sounds as such and the act of playing musical instruments. Also, music moves through time. It is this link between sound and time that catches and holds the attention – and therefore makes concentration possible for shorter or longer periods of time. I will come back to this later, after a more specific description of commusical interplay.

Response-evoking techniques

Music therapy uses a number of *response-evoking* techniques. These techniques are similar in *character* and *function* to the way that parents elicit responses from infants, but with *music* as a means, the effect is increased strikingly. This is especially necessary with children who do not respond to usual invitations to interplay.

Imitation. Imitating a child's expression, whether vocal sounds or beats on a drum, often results in a positive response from the child. Normally-developing infants respond at a very early age to being imitated. Comparative studies show that developmentally disabled and autistic children also respond with increased interest upon seeing or hearing others imitate them. Musical parameters such as pitch, tempo, rhythm, etc., are easy to vary slightly from one moment to another. This makes it possible for the music therapist to imitate the child's initiatives at a general level, and at the same time vary them at a more detailed level. Besides imitating the music itself, the music therapist can imitate the way in which the child is playing, with small responses, or more exaggerated movements.

Turn-taking. Turn-taking refers to interactions where partners take turns making vocal or instrumental sounds. These interactions usually consist of sequences of imitation and variation. In the beginning there are fixed roles, but later the child and the therapist 'exchange roles' and take turns being the initiator and the imitator. Exchanging roles is a particularly important element in *mutual* communicative interplay. This mutuality is only possible if the child has the ability to direct attention outwards – ability communication-disordered children reveal significant limitations when starting music therapy. In some cases explaining the structure to the child, 'now you follow me, now I follow you', can be helpful, but often changes in turn-taking happen gradually, and it can be difficult to see who is following who.

Pausing or 'freezing'. Another frequently used response-evoking technique is the unexpected break in the middle of a melodic phrase. The break has an even greater effect if the child is moving to the music, e.g. rocking, swinging or jumping. At the same time the therapist can make his/her intention clear to the child by gesture and facial expressions, for example by looking surprised and 'freezing' his/her body movements. Other response-evoking techniques are, for example, unexpected melodic leaps, discordant sounds, sudden changes in tempo, or beats played 'across' the pulse (syncopes).

Expectation. Response-evoking techniques presuppose the fact that the child recognizes the 'surprise' element; that is, that the child has developed a musical expectation within a musical structure. Most (but not all!) children will spontaneously respond to simple musical surprises such as sudden breaks in the music, while other more advanced musical surprises demand more experience. This matter was described in detail by the Norwegian music therapist researcher Even Ruud (1990). A musical expectation can be built up in a very simple manner. For instance, a series of beats on a drum, in a steady tempo (pulse), will very quickly create an expectation of when the next beat will come. As soon as this expectation has been built up, the therapist can surprise by hesitating with a beat or by playing a little faster. Musical humour is closely linked to expectations; for example, when an expectation within a musical structure is not fulfilled, this is a type of musical 'surprise'.

Variations on a theme. Another way of building up a child's musical expectations is by creating small, recognizable themes together with the child. This is done by starting at the child's level of ability and, through repetition and variation, developing small structures or 'themes', to which child and therapist can return from session to session. This can consist of a few familiar lines or accompaniment from a children's song. A theme can be a small rhythmic motive, which the child is able to play, or a certain vocal sound that is characteristic of the child. The crucial element is that the child is able to participate actively, and that the therapist – with music as the means – can start with what the child is able to express and can create a setting that invites the child to further interplay.

By using a common 'theme' with small variations, a balance between the familiar and the unknown can be maintained, so that both partners can return to the familiar if the unknown causes too much insecurity. Variations can consist of changes in melody or temporal shifts – as in the above example, where the steady pulse of the drum is suddenly changed.

Movement through time. An important aspect of actions, feelings and experiences is that they move through time. Without time, there is no course of action. Music is also experienced through time. By structuring and directing sounds in a period of time, a common human field of experience can be created. This is why music is seen as a temporal art.

Small musical-drama sequences. In the music, it is possible to create shorter or longer sequences with a child, depending on the child's ability to perceive impressions as meaningful units and integrate them. The sequences can be very simple dynamic sequences where both partners spontaneously play faster, slower, louder or softer. They can also be sequences where the therapist uses various musical techniques to create musical tension that attracts the child's attention, leading to a climax. As described above, this type of interaction can have a humorous character in the form of a musical surprise: the therapist 'cheats' the child of his/her expectation, after which the child looks up wondering, catches sight of the smiling face of the therapist, understands the intention and begins to smile. Similarly most therapists have experienced 'golden moments' where the child attempts to surprise the therapist musically, for example by playing faster, in order to see if the therapist can keep up.

Both Stern and Trevarthen focus on such narrative sequences between infants and parents as being crucial to the child's *emotional attachment and development.* In describing these musical and pre-verbal interactions, they come very close to descriptions of music therapy practice. This has given rise to mutual inspiration (see for instance Colwyn Trevarthen interviewed by Brynjulf Stige, 1997).

An interactional theory perspective

The relationship between the child and the music therapist is typically very asymmetrical, and often it can be difficult to 'read' the actions of the child as meaningful. This particularly applies to children with severe attention disorders (Irgens-Møller 1998a, 1998b), children within the autistic spectrum (Schumacher 1999; Wigram

1999c), children with limited physical and mental abilities (Møller 1995; Plahl 2000), or children who, in addition to other disabilities, are born deaf or deaf-blind (Bang 1979/1998; Hauge and Tønsberg 1998). The question is, then, how the music therapist can structure the interplay with the child, in a way that *gives meaning* for both parties.

Interactional theory emphasizes that *all human development takes place in relationships with others*, regardless of disability (Sameroff and Emde 1989). What is important in this context is the fact that relationships always have a *history* that creates continuity and forms *the expectations* each part has to the other. Stern describes this in the following way:

> Relationships are the cumulative constructed history of interactions, a history that bears on the present in the form of expectations actualized during an ongoing interaction, and on the future in the form of expectations (conscious or not) about upcoming interactions. (Stern 1989, pp.54–55)

In this way, repeated actions over time create a common history of expectations, which gives the actions meaning. If the music therapist stops at a surprising place in the music, this only makes sense to the child if he/she has expectations of where the music is going. Only because of earlier experiences can the therapist know that the child is playing in a certain way, because he/she expects to be imitated. Through a jointly constructed relationship or musical history, it is possible for the child and the music therapist to 'read' each other's actions as meaningful and intentional. This actually applies to all relationships, but because of our ability to accumulate experiences from one relationship to another, we rarely focus on this fact when relating to children who function well.

Predictability and meaning are thus closely linked. Predictability can become a part of the interplay by means of the 'outer' structures with which the therapist creates the setting. But rather more interesting are the 'inner' structures that are created *between* the child and the therapist in the form of themes repeated from one session to another, as described above.

How much progress can be made in music therapy depends on the child's capacities and limitations, but also on the music therapist's experience in bringing out the communicative potential in this group of children, as well as his/her co-operation with parents and/or the interdisciplinary team.

The background for this chapter/section is a PhD research project (Holck 2002).

4.5 Music Therapy with Older Adults (Hanne Mette Ochsner Ridder)

Working with older adults in music therapy means working with a very non-homogeneous group. At one end of the spectrum of differences there is the group of wise, serene elderly, representing big resources for younger generations. At the opposite end of the spectrum are the weak and dependent, needing 100 per cent help and care, with severe memory, communication and functional deficits. This group includes amongst others, older adults suffering from dementia.

Elderly persons who are no longer able to take care of themselves will have the possibility to enter an old people's home, where they are offered the care they need. They are in a situation where they may be coping with a progressively degenerative brain disease, and at the same time they face significant upheaval and change in their lives, as well as unfamiliar and difficult situations with which they must cope. In summary, they face many of the following problems:

- relating to new surroundings

- a changed everyday life

- new routines

- many new faces

- other residents that might have disturbing behaviour

- staff that might invade personal space in care situations

- staff that don't always have enough time when the person needs it.

For these reasons many people suffering from dementia are in a situation where they are in further need of support and empathy and have a special need to express inner feelings and to feel understood. There are various ways to use music therapy with an elderly population, and the following two case study examples show different approaches based on the different needs of the participants, who in these examples are both suffering from dementia. This chapter will place clinical examples at the beginning to highlight the importance of the individual person and his/her everyday needs. Following these two important examples, a more general view, firstly at an international level and subsequently at a national level, will place the therapeutic value of music therapy with older adults in a broader context.

Case study vignette 1 – Mrs F

Mrs F was athletic and straight, with a short haircut. She was 72 years old and a new resident on the unit. The colour of her face indicated an active outdoor life, and she was still an active woman. She walked up and down the corridors grabbing every door handle she passed. She seemed restless and seemed to be searching for somebody or something. Newer laws in Denmark require all doors in residential homes to be accessible and unlocked, even in special care units, and one staff member was ready to walk outside with Mrs F – and later guide her back – if she left the house.

Mrs F suffered from dementia (Pick's disease). She needed help to get dressed, often put her shoes on the wrong way round, would put on three sweaters even when it was warm, or walk out wearing no coat when it was raining. Her family informed the unit she used to be very tidy, but now she was not able to lay the table, and tableware was spread in random piles. She lost her parents when she was a child, lost her husband when she was middle-aged, didn't raise children, and seemed to like her job as an office worker very much. She still liked to write, but what started as a sentence on the paper ended up in big squiggles. When Mrs F talked, a few favourite words were repeated in endless variations, sometimes with joy and laughter, other times angrily, in a threatening attitude. Time and time again the police had picked her up from places very far away from where she was living, which was one of the reasons for her move into a residential home. Even when staff went with her for long walks every day, she was still restless and constantly active. If she felt watched over, she would become angry and hit out. The same would happen if a fellow resident was in her way or seemed threatening to her.

Mrs F was in a chaotic situation. She had lost her language and her identity and didn't understand what was going on around her. Staff kept an eye on her all the time. Sometimes she enjoyed contact with a staff member; sometimes she tried to escape the supervision, even though the staff tried to make it appear and feel as natural as possible.

Mrs F was invited to join a group singalong activity. For more than one hour she sat relaxed in a chair. She nodded her head to some of the songs and smiled to some of the other participants. The singalong was an open group activity. People joined in no matter if, or how, they sang. Well-known songs, ballads, folk songs, hymns, sea shanties, cradle songs, patriotic songs, love songs, historical songs etc. were sung. A music therapist accompanied the songs on the piano and entertained with quiet, easy-listening music in a coffee break halfway through. The family informed the unit that Mrs F was not engaged in music in her former life. She did not play an instrument, go to concerts or even listen to music on the radio. But she joined the singalong sessions every week, and over time she was successfully integrated in more and more activities including music. She enjoyed the folk-dancing where the group did simple, well-known dances, the music and movement activity where the group sang, played ball and did simple exercises sitting on chairs, and finally the

'Friday coffee singing' where residents, staff and relatives listened to music in a calm and warm atmosphere, and sang, chatted and drank coffee.

Mrs F was unable to find rest, but for periods of time she calmed down when she was in a group of people singing together. Even if she did not join in the singing, she was still a member of the group. Most of the songs were part of her cultural background and therefore part of her identity.

She seemed to recognize the songs. Recognizing a song in her circumstances, where chaos was reigning, was like recognizing a bit of her self. She was attentive to the environment and she was part of what was going on 'here and now'. In the process of recognizing, the 'now' is connected with former 'nows', as on a string of pearls. This meant she was a person with a past and a present – and therefore also a future. Thus there was a structuring perspective forwards and backwards, and at the same time a perspective reaching out from the present – out towards those people sitting around her. She showed attention towards the other participants and often made eye contact – a calm, watchful eye contact not containing the often-seen aggression and desperation.

Mrs F did not like social gatherings where people talk, chat, laugh, and certainly not where a serious discussion was taking place. She did not understand what was going on and felt left out. It made her feel insecure and very often angry and aggressive. Reports indicate that music gave her a frame where she could handle being together with other people. Mrs F was one example of a person to whom the 'being together with others' in a musical situation was essential to her quality of life.

Case study vignette 2 – Mr G

In contrast to Mrs F, Mr G liked socializing and talking. Mr G suffered from dementia (Alzheimer's disease) and was 77 years old at the time of music therapy. He was clear about why he was staying in a residential home, and that his wife was not able to take care of him any longer. He was eloquent (even if he often had problems remembering the nouns) and liked to talk about his childhood and youth.

Mr G was very bitter:

- towards his wife for having placed him in the home

- towards his daughters for not visiting him

- towards staff never giving him another cigar when the one he was smoking was soon finished

- about the coffee being cold

- about the food being miserable

- about staff treating him like a spoiled child.

Thus, apart from the enjoyable moment with Mr G as the entertainer in the centre, he was angry and scolding.

Mr G was offered two, weekly individual music therapy sessions taking place in his living room. In the beginning he preferred talking about events from his youth, but soon the songs came to the fore. Mr G did not want to play any instruments, but he liked to sing with the music therapist. Every session he asked the therapist to sing the well-known Danish song 'Altid frejdig, når du går' (by Chr. Richardt, 1868), originally sung by a knight in the drama of the fairytale *Sleeping Beauty*. He tried to join in the first lines, but every time he burst into tears, and cried while the therapist sang the song. He was not able to put into words what was going on in the music therapy. However, the fact that he, in this period, was searching for a way to express some very strong feelings can be construed as his way of handling essential conflict-ridden themes without being badly affected by it. To many people in Mr G's generation, the song 'Altid frejdig ...' is associated with funerals, sorrow, leave-taking – or with associations to the Second World War where young people, maybe friends, died too young, associations to the Danish resistance movement, to good fighting evil, or to more archetypical themes in this direction.

To be overtaken by a progressing, incurable brain disease meant, to Mr G, that he was leaving his home, his well-known surroundings and his everyday life, together with his wife. These conditions caused him to have to face many losses. In individual music therapy he found a way to express and contain intense feelings through the songs, and to share those feelings with another person. After the therapy sessions he seemed relieved and started to share some pleasure when his wife came on her daily visits.

To understand some of the processes that are going on in this type of therapy work with older adults, it is useful to look at some of the literature at a national and international level to see the direction and objectives of music therapy with this population.

International perspectives

A literature review of studies, journal articles and books in the English, German and Danish languages dealing with the subjects of music and dementia reveals a large number of different approaches (Ridder 2001a). First of all music as a medium is used in quite different ways and is implemented in activities or in therapy by, for example, activity personnel, staff and therapists. Music is used in group or individual sessions in general with one or more of the following foci:

- relaxation
- physical stimulation
- social stimulation
- cognitive stimulation
- behaviour management
- communication or interaction.

The results of a systematic review of 73 studies examining the use of music with a population suffering from dementia show that:

- The number of studies has increased steadily since 1980 and shows a growing interest in the field.
- A majority describe the use of active techniques and a third describe receptive techniques.
- In Europe there is a higher tendency to document individual sessions.
- In Europe there is a tendency to report longer periods of therapy.
- In the USA there is a tendency to describe short-term interventions.
- Only a few studies indicate a precise specification of stage of dementia.
- A majority of the studies use controlled designs (control/experimental groups, AB-designs where the participant serves as his/her own control, or pre/post designs).
- A third of the studies use case study descriptions.
- In 73% of the American studies the function of music as a stimulus is examined.
- 43% of European studies examine interaction in music therapy.

Many different interventions are described in the literature and show what a richly faceted job a music therapist can expect, either implementing the different interventions or supervising staff members. The following music interventions are described and studied in the literature:

1. Music therapy employing:

    - *improvisation* (G. Aldridge 2000; Ansdell 1995; Eeg 2001; Gaertner 1999; Munk-Madsen 2001; Odell-Miller 1996; Simpson 2000; Wellendorf 1991)

    - *singing* well-known songs (Fitzgerald-Cloutier 1993; Ridder 2001; Tomaino 2000)

    - *vibroacoustic* therapy (Clair and Bernstein 1993)

    - *stress-reduction* techniques (Hanser and Clair 1995)

2. Music therapy/music interventions, often in teams:

    - *music and movement* (Baumgartner 1997; Groene *et al* 1998; Newman and Ward 1993; Smith-Marchese 1994)

    - *folk dancing/*social dancing (Clair and Ebberts 1997; Götell 2000; Newman and Ward 1993; Palo-Bengtsson *et al* 1998; Pollack and Namazi 1992)

    - *vibrotactile* stimulation (Clair and Bernstein 1990b)

    - *singalong* (Carruth 1997; Clair 1996a; Olderog-Millard and Smith 1989; Prickett and Moore 1991)

    - *music reminiscence* (Ashida 2000; Brotons and Koger 2000)

    - *music stimulation* (Brotons 1996; Brotons and Prickett-Cooper 1994; Christie 1992, 1995; Clair 1991; Clair and Bernstein 1990a; Clair *et al* 1995; Clair and Ebberts 1997; Gardiner 2000; Groene 1993; Götell 2000; Hanson 1996; Korb 1997; Pollack and Namazi 1992; Riegler 1980)

    - songwriting (Silber 1995)

3. Interventions mostly implemented by staff members, maybe under supervision from a music therapist:

    - *background music* (Clair and Bernstein 1994; Denney 1997; Goddaer and Abraham 1994; Ragneskog 1996; Sambandham and Shirm 1995)

    - *music listening* – individual listening to music (Casby and Holm 1994; Clark *et al* 1998; Foster 1998; Gerdner and Swanson 1993; Glynn 1992; Johnson *et al* 1998; Korb 1997; Lipe 1991; Norberg *et al* 1986; Tabloski *et al* 1995; Thomas *et al* 1997)

- *play along* – open groups using instruments to accompany taped music (Lord and Garner 1993)

4.   *Music therapeutic care giving*: interventions where staff members use live singing in the personal caregiving of, for example, agitated persons (Brown *et al* 2001)

Working as a music therapist at day care centres or in special care units demands flex-ibility and an all-round knowledge about the many different ways of using music to focus and maintain attention, regulate arousal level, and involve a client in dialogue. A recent publication (D. Aldridge 2000) contains a rich resource of literature in the field of music therapy in the care of people with dementia.

Working with music therapy and the elderly in Denmark

For the moment in Denmark, in gerontological music therapy there is a focus on music therapy in dementia care. Out of a population of around five million, 77,000 older adults are living in residential homes (Ridder 2001a).

   Working as a music therapist in gerontology is an all-round job. You will often see the music therapist function as a piano entertainer, leading very different groups where music is integrated in some way, as well as carrying out individual music therapy sessions. The elderly generation has a strong song tradition in Denmark and this has an influence on many activities.

   In Denmark there are only a few full-time positions for music therapists in homes, units or institutions for older adults. On the other hand, there are a number of part-time positions and a large number of people are paid by the hour to play music and lead activities at residential homes, nursing homes, hospitals and day care centres. Musicians are mostly employed in these hourly-paid jobs, working for a few hours a week, thus having a peripheral status concerning the daily life of the institu-tion. A few trained music therapists work like this as well, maintaining individual sessions, group activities or supervision. This large number of music interventions going on in the care of older adults indicates a need to involve music in activities in daily life and in therapies, and the focus on dementia in recent years has made more residential homes increase the number of people employed. More music therapy positions have been offered, and music projects have been initiated and economi-cally supported (Eeg 2001; Munk-Madsen 2001). At the doctoral programme in Aalborg one research project deals with music therapy in dementia care (Ridder, see Chapter 5.2).

   Apparently music therapy is expanding in the care of older adults, building on the work of the pioneers who started up the work several years ago. Synnøve Friis started to work using music with older adults in the beginning of the 1960s. She, Bojsen-Møller, Thorup and Varsted have written the Danish book *Musik i ældreplejen* (Friis 1987), where music is described as a means to contact people. They give concrete suggestions of how to carry out different activities. Friis is a qualified music teacher and trained further in music therapy in Germany, Switzerland and the UK. Her work is inspired by the Australian music therapist Ruth Bright (1997). Friis taught occupational and physiotherapy students and different groups of staff throughout Scandinavia before she retired. Thus she has influenced the tradition of music therapy in many residential homes and institutions, and often points out that to carry out music therapy you need to be a trained music therapist, whereas the different activities described in her book are meant to involve and inspire staff in general working with a population of older adults.

There is only one music therapy course in Denmark, a five-year study at the University of Aalborg, but over time, when more and more students qualify, it is hoped that all those sporadic temporary jobs will be replaced by permanent positions, where the music therapist works in the milieu of the patient/client and as a member of a team. The elderly individual will benefit from co-ordinated activities and therapeutic interventions where a trained professional is able to set up a safe structure that enables the participant to enter a dialogue. The weakest group amongst the elderly have often sustained several losses caused by dementia. They might have lost the ability to communicate with words. Here, other approaches are needed for the elderly to express their identity and inner feelings. This means a need for therapists who are able to work with a population with difficulties in communication and with difficulties in understanding and being understood (Sundin 2001) – a need for trained music therapists with theoretical knowledge and human, musical and therapeutic experience.

Conclusion

In spite of all the deficits in functions in the weakest group of the elderly, music in particular can draw out important resources. Some musical abilities might be preserved, e.g. the ability to hum, or to recognize a melody or a rhythm. The ability to be involved in some musical activity might trigger response, behaviour, memory, consciousness and the ability to enter a dialogue. Where memory for everyday events has become inconsistent and, in some cases, almost completely absent, the long-term memory in music for songs and pieces, and the associations and memories provoked by that music, will enable recall of a life history, people and a nostalgic reminiscence of the past.

Recognizing a melody is a gift when everything else in the environment – even the face of a loved one – is strange and incomprehensible. This gift can be linked to feelings of happiness, longing, sorrow, etc., and thus serves as a key to express oneself in situations where words are failing, and a key to experience company and coherence.

4.6 Music Therapy as Milieu Therapy, Social Treatment and Self-Management

Some music therapists work in therapy teams in social services or community psychiatry. Music therapists can also be employed in educational programs, or in municipal rehabilitation projects (for example, psychiatric halfway houses).

Institutional systems

A *community psychiatry home* is often a patient's first place to be after being discharged from a psychiatric hospital, and outpatient institutions often become homes for formerly hospitalized patients. Here the patients/residents can continue the treatment that was planned for them during hospitalization, often in the form of medication, and they can receive personal and social support to begin rehabilitation.

A patient receiving music therapy during hospitalization often continues treatment as an outpatient, while enrolled in a community psychiatry program. Ideally there is a close connection between hospital psychiatry and community psychiatry, and it often happens that a patient is readmitted to the hospital while participating in an outpatient treatment program. The aims of music therapy in hospital psychiatry are directed in part towards relationships and qualitative encounters with patients, and in part towards the patient's psychological development in a deep sense – often at the same time reducing anxiety and strengthening identity. Therefore, in most cases, it is natural for music therapy to continue after hospitalization, which is focused on diagnosis and clarifying treatment modalities, especially in order to prevent readmission.

Music therapy in hospital psychiatry focuses on the individual and the individual's self-healing potential, as this is manifested in interactions with others. The goal is to improve quality of life and coping skills, privately as well as socially (see Chapter 4.1). In community psychiatry and even more in rehabilitation programs, the focus for treatment, education and group activities is directed outwards – towards social conditions and experiences, and social functions. However, the contact between the patient and the staff member is still the most important tool in this work. At this point in time psychiatric services, as a whole, are undergoing structural changes in many European countries, and the model from this book that will be referenced in connection with this is Denmark. The objective of these changes is to increase coherence in treatment and rehabilitation for the individual patient and to decrease problems caused by the fact that some programs are financed by regions and others by local municipalities. There is a focus on strengthening social psychiatry.

Social psychiatry is defined today as:

> The work done to support individuals who, because of a psychiatric illness, cannot get their social rights and needs fulfilled through ordinary social services. The central element is, thus, that patients'/clients' social rights are fulfilled and that they have a cohesive and reasonable daily life despite the illness and the problems it brings. (internal memorandum, Aalborg Psychiatric Hospital, 2000)

Common to clients using social psychiatry is that they have a psychiatric illness that makes it difficult for them to provide for having their own rights guaranteed – rights that they are entitled to as human beings and citizens. They have problems coping with life, both personally and socially. Some have difficulties recognizing that they have unfulfilled needs. The psychiatric illness can result in a daily life characterized by lack of initiative, communication difficulties and isolation. Often these are people without a network, who find it hard to participate in the reality surrounding them, or to create structure in their daily lives. They can suffer from insecurity and anxiety, as they often have difficulties controlling their own behaviour. The primary goals in social psychiatry can be seen as the sum of goals defined by the various municipal institutions working within the social sphere. It appears that this will potentially become an important area of employment for music therapists in the future.

MUSIC THERAPY IN VARIOUS INSTITUTIONS

Below is a summary of experiences made by music therapists working in community institutions in Denmark, on a continuum that ranges from social services based therapy in hospital psychiatry to rehabilitation centres (including halfway houses) and adult education. The last two mentioned institutions focus on social treatment, general education and specialized education.

In *social services*, the aims of music therapy are, for example:

- to create a milieu/space where the patient/client or resident can unfold and express himself/herself through social activities with others (living/learning situations)

- to adapt the activity to the patient's actual skills, interests and needs (use an open listening attitude and be available to the patient)

- that the activity takes place in accordance with milieu therapeutic principles, where values and attitudes are emphasized more than expectations for a specific result (the basic principle here is that the patient is the expert in his/her own life).

Here, music contributes with a spiritual dimension, as musical activities are experienced as something that gives nourishment to the soul, where the patient can be mirrored in a positive way and discover his/her own potential.

Generally music is used as:

- a means of contact and communication, to motivate and create an atmosphere that breaks isolation

- a 'co-therapist' that, together with the milieu therapist, influences the patient

- a means of strengthening identity – through the patient's relating of his/her own experiences, in group music-listening or in individual contact with the therapist

- a means of bodily expression through dance, song and musical performance

- a means for the patient to tell of his/her own life, by writing songs and melodies

- a *transitional object* – an object for positive and negative emotions; a space where the patient can experience that emotions can be expressed, amplified (made audible) and contained in a musical form

- a social activity in the form of group singing, musical ensemble or listening groups

- out-of-house activities such as concerts or music festivals.

The music therapist must first and foremost provide an atmosphere where the patient can be 'met' and supported in expressing himself/herself through creative/musical activities. Because the music therapist in social services concentrates less on 'products' and more on the patient's whole personality (including symptoms and inner resources), he/she is often process-/development-/value- and attitude-oriented. The music therapist has the important, but difficult to measure, task of creating a setting where the patient can experience being present and aware, and being seen and heard – without high achievement demands. Typical colleagues of the music therapist in a social services team are nurses, psychiatric caretakers, nurse assistants and occupational therapists.

In *municipal rehabilitation centres*, music therapy shares common goals with the other services offered as a part of the social treatment plan. These goals can be differentiated in three levels: a societal level, an organizational level and an individual/group level. The main goal is a greater degree of self-management for the individual client/resident, so that he/she can achieve greater self-determination and freedom of educational and vocational choice, and in this way a better quality of life.

- On the *societal level* the goal is a greater degree of self-management regarding employment, education, financial situation and social conditions.

- On the *organizational level* the focus is on the quality of the milieu therapy team's work, both in relation to the main goals and to the wellbeing of clients and staff.

- On the *individual level* the focal point is the client's learning. From a humanist/existentialist educational basis, the emphasis is on the client achieving a more conscious relationship to himself/herself, learning to be more responsible for himself/herself, and learning to be more aware of personal needs as well as getting them fulfilled. Finally, there is a focus on the client's being able to enter into social relationships and develop their social skills.

Music plays an important role in the daily life of these institutions. Recorded music is often played, either brought by the clients/residents themselves, or by a staff member (often the music therapist) who talks about the music and encourages clients to join the discussion. In addition, the music therapist often accompanies singing groups during special events, and the music therapist initiates projects with clients, where songwriting and composition are central components. The importance of these musical 'products' should not be underestimated: for clients with low self-esteem, there can be great value in holding in their hand a cassette tape or CD of music created by themselves – or in performing music in a concert for other clients or at an open-house event. (Music examples 20 and 21 on the CD are examples of this type of work. They will be described later.)

In this case, music is used as a tool in learning processes that have to do with training stability/attendance, concentration, developing mutual respect between participants, finding strategies for solving conflicts, learning to master an instrument, developing staying power and experience in working with a process – and possibly also making a creative product – over a long period of time.

When these goals are reached, the individual's self-esteem is usually strength-
ened – at least for a time. Music activities in day centres or community centres are
often much sought after. Therefore they are a good means of motivation, as they
often are a part of a 'package deal' of activities, where the client must commit to the
whole 'package' in order to participate in music activities. The music therapist in a
rehabilitation centre often plays several different roles in the course of a
workday/week. They can range from having responsibility for practical details to
development of educational ideas, to directing projects or acting as *contact person* for
a few clients.

The music therapist is employed under the same conditions as other team staff
and is expected to perform similar tasks. However, the music therapist is also
expected to bring music into the work in the way most suitable to the situation.
Typical colleagues are occupational therapists, social workers and community-based
teachers. Day centres in Denmark are supported financially by the state and city in
combination, and they actually function as a part of general education, which is
characterized by:

- being open to everyone

- being voluntary

- being free of exams

- being based on the spoken word

- having a personal aim, but at the same time presupposing community.

The courses aim to strengthen the individual's personal development and improve
his/her educational and vocational possibilities. Typical goals are: to improve
quality of life, develop self-esteem and self-worth, improve social skills and gain
knowledge and practical experience within the subject that is being taught. Last but
not least, the goal is to break old patterns that the clients/participants subconsciously internalized earlier in their lives – patterns that now prevent them from
actively fulfilling their needs.

Music therapy in the Danish day centres is typically part of a module (for
example, two days a week for six weeks), as an experiential creative/musical activity
with an emphasis on group dynamics. Activities involved can be improvisation, psychodrama with music, voice training, *psychodynamic movement*, guided fantasy with
music (inspired by GIM), simple choral arrangements, drum exercises, group
singing, sound healing, dance and movement, stretching exercises and
bioenergetics.

Partial aims for music therapy in these centres can be for the participant to:

- improve his/her non-verbal communication
- be able to listen and to express inner feelings
- be able to give and receive
- develop his/her creativity, imagination, ability to find new solutions, ability to improvise
- develop empathy and co-operation
- become more conscious of his/her private space and that of others – i.e. practise limit-setting
- be able to open himself/herself to, and close off from, contact with others
- become more aware of body and emotions and be able to verbalize experiences and needs
- be able to release tension and experience being present – through listening to music
- become open to and understand his/her own symbolization (in dreams, fantasies and creative expression)
- develop his/her voice and increase its power and variation
- learn to use the voice as a means for nurturing self and others
- have the courage to exceed boundaries and expand his/her 'playspace'
- have the confidence to use new sides of himself/herself
- practise new social and personal skills in a musical/dramatic form
- learn about the music of other cultures.

A course lasts three to four months and the participants react differently to the various activities offered. Some choose not to participate in improvisation, while others participate with great enthusiasm and integrate their experiences into their daily lives. Some students/clients choose to continue instrumental training after the course has ended. Typical colleagues are bodywork therapists and relaxation therapists. It is a constant challenge for the music therapist employed at a day centre to keep transference issues and regressive reactions within the frame of experiential education – instead of therapy.

Case study examples

VIGNETTE 1 (FROM A DAY CENTRE)

In a series of improvisations the participants are told to play instruments by following their inner impulse, with the aim of becoming more aware of their own needs and wishes, and being able to act on them:

> M, a 42-year-old woman, goes to the big drum and plays with slow heavy beats. She says afterwards that she felt it was a 'survival pattern' that she played the drum at all. Inwardly, she tries to convince herself that it is better for her to play than to sink passively into the chair. Neither of these two extremes feels right, but for M there have only been these two possibilities: passive despair or willed action. Gradually she becomes aware of an aversion to doing what the teacher tells her to; she wants to leave. She discovers that she has been too adaptive, and that she has blindly done what authority figures have told her to, and has made this her own truth. Maybe there is an alternative, a middle ground? Through this insight her improvisations change: she starts giving herself permission to move around the room and play instruments when she feels like it. She communicates with the rest of the group, teasing, searching, with new-found pleasure. Parallel to this there is a development of her inner symbolic world. In the beginning she sees herself being cast about in the waves – she sees herself as a victim of greater powers. But later she herself is sailing on the water – she starts to feel that she can influence her own life and do something. M starts to take initiative regarding future vocational possibilities.

VIGNETTE 2 (FROM A DAY CENTRE)

The participants are also given voice lessons and trained in awareness of their own vocal sound – both within the body and as sound projected outwards. The aim of this is for them to become conscious of inner resources and of possibilities for clearer communication and expression.

> K, a 55-year-old woman, is working on improving her self-esteem. When she hears the sound of her own voice inside her head, she is frightened by its loudness. She comes into contact with childhood memories, where she feels like kicking and screaming over the things she experienced. When she was a young girl, she wanted to be a singer, but was denied this chance by her family. During the course, K becomes more and more confident vocally, although she can still become frightened after using her voice. It takes time before she gives herself permission to experience her own strength and to speak out, and there are many things in her life that she needs to 'settle accounts with'. Towards the end of the course she sees an inner image of herself on a big stage, where she is singing

with Julio Iglesias. Inspired by this, she sings alone for the group, and makes plans for a small performance after the end of the course.

Examples of remarks made by participants after completing a course are:

- I am more grounded, more robust, and can contain more intense emotions.
- I've learned to be aware of my feelings.
- I have changed – I'm less prejudiced and my thoughts aren't as chaotic.
- I've become stronger, can stand up for myself, don't let people exploit me anymore.
- I've been helped to open my mouth and get in touch with my strength.
- I like myself a little better, am better at getting angry.
- I'm going back to my old job with renewed energy.

Songs from the Heart

The CD *Songs from the Heart* is the final result of a music therapy project in the City of Aalborg Youth Centre that took place in the autumn of 1996 in connection with the youth centre's 25th anniversary. The CD's nine cuts are studio versions of the songs that were written during the project. The songwriting project was a part of the psychosocial treatment of a small group of youths at the training schools in Aalborg. The only requirement for participation was that the individual have the desire to write a song (with the necessary help) – a song that would be performed with a band at the anniversary celebration. There were seven participants in the project. All of them wrote a song, and all of them got on stage, more or less nervous and shaky, and sang their song. On the CD there are two additional songs, written by two girls who were 'infected' by the atmosphere of the project and wished very much to participate in the studio recording of the songs. The two songs chosen for this book's example CD are written by two participants in the project, both of whom used the songs to verbalize their life situations.

CD EXAMPLE 20

In the song 'Ludwig', a 21-year-old songwriter tells of his loneliness, and how he experiences his contact with his surroundings. The song is written in a rock style, which acts as a socially acceptable channel for this man's aggressive and frustrated emotional energy. The song has, in this way, become a container for the man's sadness and loneliness and, at the same time, a means to express emotional chaos.

CD EXAMPLE 21

The second song, 'I Want Out', is written by a woman in her early twenties, who, because of long-term illness throughout childhood and youth, has periods of hope-lessness and despair in regards to creating a good life for herself. This song has a brighter tone that supports the message of hope in the lyrics and the need to break out of the chains of loneliness and feel joy in living.

Common to both songwriters is the fact that singing has always been very difficult for them, but also the fact that songwriting and singing in this project was one of the best experiences they ever had.

Summary

Music is used in the various institutions of community psychiatry and social services in an active form (group singing, ensemble, improvisation, dance, drama, movement activities), in a receptive form (music listening groups, guided fantasy) and as a creative media (songwriting, musical composition) that can result in own produc-tions. In all of these types of institutions, music contributes specific and significant perspectives in the total treatment plans.

4.7 Music Therapy for Self-Development

Introduction

It is possible to use both active and receptive music therapy in work with personal growth processes with non-clinical clients (people without a diagnosis of any kind). The application of music therapy can be:

1.   focused developmental work with anxiety, inhibitions, grief, crises, and other natural existential life problems which can influence the subjective, experienced feelings of self-confidence by the one who asks for music therapy

2.   as a tool to explore and integrate new areas of the conscious mind – and thus it can also be an opportunity for people seeking therapy who want help and guidance to the processes of being able to open up for more spiritual dimensions of life experiences.

The models of music therapy which will be in focus in this chapter are Analytically Oriented Music Therapy (AOM, see Chapter 3.2) and Guided Imagery and Music (GIM, see Chapter 3.1) as both these models are suitable for work with these two aims of self-developmental work.

Methods of music therapy in Self-Developmental work

1. EXISTENTIAL NEEDS

The Experiential Training in Music Therapy (ETMT) also includes music therapy as self-development. These elements of any training course focus on the perspective of understanding self-development as a tool for the 'student client' to become a future professional music therapist (see Chapter 6.5). Music therapy as self-development is mostly asked for by clients who, on a voluntary basis (and most often with a very positive motivation), wish to explore a change in or an expansion of potential for action and ways of being present and clear in their experiences in everyday life. In this respect it can be relevant to look at which qualities in the medium of music make it suitable as a tool for this kind of work.

Specific qualities of the music which make music therapy applicable as self-development

Here we emphasize the following qualities (see also Chapter 3.9):

Music is ambiguous (it does not have one, and only one, clear meaning)

There is no consensus made up in society that music has one, and only one, meaning and thus the therapist neither can nor should interpret the client's musical expressions in an unambiguous way. This aspect can be positive for clients who are afraid of being evaluated and of being misunderstood. In everyday life they may often resist expressing themselves verbally because their anxiety of being evaluated is bigger than their need of expressing themselves. At the same time they do have a need for expression – and this creates physical and psychological tensions. The music can offer those people a channel for ambiguous expression.

At the same time they can experience a 'way of being together' in playing (expressing themselves) with one or more other people. It can help to break the isolation, which is caused from all kinds of inhibitions in self-expression. Often, the clients engage in a new experience by this form of self-expression: the experience of being heard and met in their own personal style of expression.

From practical experiences there are many stories of clients who have developed a greater trust in their own ability of expression through music – in a way that gives them possibilities of transferring these experiences to other life situations, where verbal spoken language is the tool of communication. One can also say that through music therapy they have negotiated and have found a better balance with their own superego function.

The language of music is comparable with the language of emotions

This statement was first written by Langer (1942). Langer did not mean that specific pieces of music express specific emotions – rather she argued that the form of emotions and the form of music are very alike. Music is a language expressed in a very dynamic way which is similar to the way emotions arise, are expressed and die out.

From a therapeutic perspective this argument is a very good theoretical explanation of why music generally promotes emotional experiences and can 'modulate' these in a specific direction (e.g. towards melancholy or something amusing). Music can reinforce the client's connection with some emotions which are hidden just under the surface of consciousness, and music can also break through barriers which prohibit a person from getting in contact with a certain emotion. An example would be: a person is paralysed by sorrow and mourning, but he is not able to express these emotions either in words, in crying or in other ways. The person is also not able to submit himself to the emotion. In such a case the music can be the channel which opens the connection with one's emotional life and makes this life more rich. In some cases the music can even reinforce and develop the life of emotions.

Both active music playing and music listening can be facilitators in such a process. In therapeutic work with the aim of integrating childish and adult parts of the same person, the method of letting the childish parts express themselves through voice improvisation can lead to shouting and crying outbursts. These outbursts can facilitate a process where childish parts are no longer only childish but grow into a real, deep, grown-up feeling of oneself as being able to better contain being hurt and being sad. The expressions can become a part of a person's grown-up way of understanding himself/herself and thus expanding his/her self-perception.

Active work with 'an inner child' (childish ways of sensing, experiencing, expressing and acting) of a person can be very intense and very releasing. It is a suitable method for people who suffer from disturbing feelings of having been rejected as a child or who have had experiences of any form of abuse. The term 'the inner child' comes from the contemporary theory of psychoanalysis and is to be understood on the basis of the grown-up person's subjective memories of the historical childhood which is still influencing contemporary ways of experiencing, relating and acting.

For example, a grown-up person might not be able to imagine that he can be accepted in a social community unless he always gives something to the community, and unless he himself is, all the time, aware of the needs of others and tries to fulfil those needs (an irrational belief). In the musical interplay he will most often repeat this pattern and play music that is very close in style to the music of the others, or he will be creating his music from the expectations he thinks the others have of the music as a whole. Thus he will never be able to demonstrate confidence in his own musical expression. It is a huge challenge for such a person to be given the role of being a soloist in a musical interplay and it is also a further challenge for him to let himself try playing exactly what he likes to play, irrespective of the music of the others.

In receptive music therapy it is a great challenge for such a person to be allowed to listen in a slightly altered state of consciousness to music (mostly in a lying position) and to get to know that he need not be active in doing something during listening – but just receive the music. Here the music can take over the role of being a positive, caring, grown-up person who gives something to the listener just because of who he is, and not because of what he performs or produces. In an active music therapy modality he can get an experience of being a subjective, creating human being, who can be recognized, respected and affirmed for his own expressions, and not for expressions which are more like appendages to other people's expressions, and thus formed to meet other people's expectations.

Music is unfolded in time and space

Music is a form of art which is unfolded and experienced in time – in contrast to the art form of pictures, which are created over time but the product is presented in the space as a concentrated result of the process. Music is also an art form which is created and experienced as space, where sounds and noises can be experienced as close by or far away, as high placed or low placed. The picture of the sound can be tight and compact or it can be scattered and diffuse. In this context, Christensen refers to music as: 'Music is a virtual timespace' (Christensen 1996). Both the dimension of time and of space are used in music therapy. In a musical improvisation the whole process can be heard from the first tiny notion to the phase of working through until the last sound fades out. This means that both important ideas – their sources, the way they are built up (what comes before) and the digestion or the working through them (what follows) – and also the transitions between them are audible in the product which comes out of the process. Such a musical product is often saved in the form of a recording, which can be re-experienced in the space and can be further developed – verbally or musically.

Some clients have a compact and stressful everyday life situation, where phases for transitions and digestion are of a low priority, or are not even recognized by the person. Such clients can learn through the improvised musical interplay to slow down (by being present in a very aware way in the musical process as it unfolds itself) and to increase their consciousness about variations in intensity in everyday experiences.

Clients who, on the other hand, have a more empty and emotionally flat way of coping with reality – where nothing seems to happen – can learn to build up tensions actively in the music and to submit to the changing levels of energy in the music. Thus they can increase the consciousness of shifts of intensity in everyday life experiences.

The music therapist can also empathically follow the client in total and complex emotional phases of experiences from their early growth until they eventually release their emotions into a climax – and then fade out. The music therapist could also play an accompaniment which functions as a sounding musical 'carpet' during the solo performance of the client on their scenario of experience in the therapeutic situation.

Time is a relative phenomenon in music therapy. Clients can have the experience that an improvisation which lasts half an hour or more can be experienced as a moment, or vice versa. At the same time the factor of time is important in the experience of the level of tension or the elasticity of tension of the improvisation. It is not unusual that a group of clients, in a situation where they play together and where they receive an instruction that they themselves shall subjectively listen to and be aware of when the end of the musical improvisation is, shall often have different sensations and listen differently to a subjectively experienced moment of ending. Sometimes a group stop exactly at the same moment except for one person who continues and who might not even notice that the other participants have already stopped. In such work the focus is very much on the participants' consciousness in being present during active and listening activities with musical interplay. (Do I listen to the others, listen to myself, listen to the music as sounding material; or am I sitting and dreaming, or thinking of something totally different out of the situation I am in, and just playing more or less mechanically in my musical part?)

Music has the effect of being like a lullaby

Most people know the feeling of sitting down and putting some quiet classical music on the stereo (e.g. classical chamber music with a string or a wind instrument in the foreground) when one can feel like one is almost being stroked on the skin and the body by the music. Typically it can calm one down and renew one's energy in a stressful everyday life. In active music therapy it can be relevant for the therapist to play this type of music to a client who, for some reason, is not able to be active in the situation. Playing this music again becomes the function of being nourishing and affirming for the client, and thus gives the client a possibility to receive something from outside without giving anything back. This technique is mostly not an aim of the work as it will create an inexpedient dependency on the music therapist by the client. As a client once said: 'What does it matter that in here, in the music therapy room, I receive care, and experience being in "paradise", if everything is just the same when I am on the street again?'

The aim of using this quality of the music is to connect it with work for personal integration where, as the first step, the client gradually risks accepting himself/herself, and his/her own helplessness and feeling of being very small and meaningless as a person. Then this step can be followed by further steps of integrating these accepted feelings and helping them go into dialogues with other parts of the client's personality. It can be easier for a client to submit to affirmation from another person through music than through words or through touching.

Music doubles the self

Most people have experienced walking along a dark road when they start whistling or humming a melody because they are afraid of the darkness and nothingness. In music therapy a basic therapeutic curing tool is a phenomenon of experiencing oneself as bigger, filling oneself out more, or as one who can feel oneself through the help of active music playing.

The phenomenon is especially noticeable during improvisational music performances, because the player himself/herself creates the frame of his/her doubling of the self in the music: he/she creates his/her experience of being bigger, and totally present in his/her expression. An example from practice is where some clients easily experience that they have lost contact with their body, or they have lost their feeling of being grounded, or they have lost their orientation in time and space. These people can often use a little melody or part of a melody as an 'anchor function' in such moments. They identify with the melody and the melody gives the security of not having totally disappeared from the world (or totally 'lost' awareness). The melody is repeated and repeated and functions as a lifeline for the consciousness, which can gradually dissolve the condition of the client from being what is in diagnostic terms called 'dissociated'. The melody creates both a sensory connection to the body, and to a sounding landscape around you, and simultaneously it offers a structure the client can hold on to.

In other examples from practice, where the topic is not the client's experience of disappearing from the world but where focus is more on expanding one's ability of being able to experience at all, melodic material can facilitate an expanding of one's experience of the self. Therefore it can be experienced as if the self is melting together with something bigger than one's self. This is very often in the form of a spiritual experience. Thus the client can, at the same time, feel as one with the cosmos and also feel enriched from an enormous power. The client can gain enough self-confidence to realize how small and insignificant one is compared to something much bigger. It is not only melodies which are active here but often complex classical compositions with an inner 'drive' of harmonic, dynamic, melodic and sounding elements which 'carry the self' out of the well-known level and into a bigger context.

Specific active music therapy methods in work with self-development

In Analytically Oriented (active) Music Therapy, methods are used which can create frames for the client where the client can:

- act out an inner child part
- work on difficulties with boundaries
- act out, balance and enrich his/her emotional life.

Some prototype exercises are developed, such as letting the clients work together in couples, with closed eyes, sitting back-to-back on a mat on the floor. From this point of reference a variety of issues can be worked on:

- Both clients express their imagined quality of an inner, caring part through voice improvisation while at the same time they keep in contact with each other through their back-to-back contact and sensed breathing patterns.

- One of the clients expresses an inner child without judging what comes out and the partner simultaneously gives attention to the child's sounds through voice expressions from his/her inner, caring part, still keeping a close and warm contact through the lower part of their backs.

The position of sitting back-to-back for some people gives the association of having a mother figure close by (back support) and at the same time allows the possibility of expressing oneself in one's own private space (the space in front of me) without being observed by others. Like a little child who explores and notices the world and feels safe by having a mother in 'the back', the warm and intense contact through the back can help in melting feelings of resistance connected to expressions of childish emotions and voice sounds.

For many people the use of the voice for free improvisation is almost stepping over the bounds of propriety, and it quite often produces very authentic experiences. The voice can be experienced as an almost 'naked' instrument which expresses something from very deep inside oneself. The expression comes directly from inside

– it is not passing through the hands, or through sticks or a bow. The voice is the most basic and original instrument.

It is very important in such kinds of work that the clients explore and become familiar with their own caring resources. These can be more conscious through being expressed and concretely heard by the owner himself/herself. In situations where a grown-up person is almost overwhelmed by a childish voice, sound or a 'violent crying', the person has to learn not to hold back, but also to be able to have trust that he/she can contain what comes up. Without a success in this learning process it is very difficult to really accept these expressions or to understand that they can be positive steps in the process of growth.

Case study examples

CD Example 9

A man in his thirties asks for music therapy and relates that he is experiencing much anxiety and also that he experiences himself as being split into two equally strong, quite different parts in his personality – half of him being a nice little boy and the other half being a demon. The split-off in his self-experience creates some quite psychosomatic dislikes such as loss of energy, and strong pain from physical tensions.

The music therapy work starts by identifying how these two different parts of the client sound in the music, which can be heard in example 9 on the CD. The 'nice boy' plays scales up and down the piano, while the 'demon' plays in a more violent, dynamic and atonal way. The music therapist supports both parts and tries to encourage the client to fully accept both parts as being fundamentally parts of himself.

CD example 10

This procedure is repeated over and over again and one day the music therapist suggests that the client not only plays the two different parts of his personality, but to go on after this just playing: 'I allow myself to be abnormal in my playing.' It is clear to the therapist that being split-off is experienced as being normal by the client, as this is what he knows and identifies with.

The client starts, as usual, by expressing the two separate parts of his personality, but he continues the improvisation on other instruments as he remembers the instruction of allowing himself to be abnormal. He continues on metal instruments (as can be heard in example 10), on a gong, a metallophone. Then he suddenly gets hold of a hand-drum on which he plays a steady, repeated rhythm which is sha-man-like in its character and sound. This way of playing makes him use his voice in a primitive form with much energy and full sound – a form of voice expression which is unknown for him. He 'submits' to this voice expression for a while and after the improvisation he says that he feels his body and himself both physically and psychologically in a different and new way. He reflects further verbally that it seems like the two parts of his personality individuated in the improvisation.

He continues using his voice and the hand-drum in this way for the next sessions and gradually gains a better feeling of integration and self-value at the same time as he experiences less anxiety and less loss of energy. The function of the music therapist here was mostly to be supportive and facilitating.

Specific methods of receptive music therapy in self-developmental work

Therapeutic music listening is a procedure well suited for personal growth work, and the GIM concept (Chapter 3.1) can be regarded as a prototype for receptive self-developmental work.

Music is used to stimulate imagery as a means either to facilitate emotional expression or to explore the images as metaphors or symbols of qualities that may give the client new experiences and insight. The therapist – and music, the 'co-therapist' – supports the client in his/her process of accepting, exploring and integrating the images and emotions emerging during the session. Existential needs (referring to Wilber's fulcrums between levels 4 and 5, and levels 5 and 6; see Chapter 2.3) can be explored through metaphoric imagery, and this can be used by the client to understand and eventually reject old 'life scripts', roles and strategies, and to experiment with new 'scripts' or attitudes in the imagery. Gradually the client will be able to experience and tell his/her life story in a more constructive way. Within the framework of narrative theory this is called a 'reconfiguration of the metaphors to a new narrative' (Bonde 2000).

No matter whether client and therapist follow active or receptive procedures, it is important that the client's experiences (facilitated through improvisation or music listening) are made conscious and reflected by the adult part of the client's personality. The goal is to integrate child and adult personality parts and make them more flexible and more easily accessible in the client's inner world (self-image), so that they are available also when the client needs them in the outer world (interpersonal exchange).

Methods of music therapy in self-developmental work

2. SPIRITUAL NEEDS

As mentioned earlier, GIM is an advanced psychotherapeutic model, well suited for therapeutic work with both existential and spiritual needs. From the early years GIM has been connected with client experiences transcending the normal borders of ego consciousness, and with the needs mentioned above. From the very beginning this has demanded a broader theory of consciousness than Freud's and even Jung's and Grof's. In the 1970s Helen Bonny designed the so-called 'Cut Log' diagram (Bonny 1999, see Fig. 2.5, p.81), visualizing the layers of consciousness as 'year rings' in a trunk. The outermost rings or layers are the transpersonal, where the client in his/her music experience transcends the personal history and taps into something numinous. In the 1970s Bonny related GIM to Assagioli's psychosynthesis (Assagioli 1965; Bonny and Savary 1973/1990 Appendix 2). Today GIM refers to Ken Wilber's 'Integral psychology' (Wilber 2000, see Chapter 2.3).

It is not easy, if at all possible, to describe transpersonal experiences, as they connect man with the realm of the spirit, which is beyond words, language and concepts. In verbal exchange the transpersonal can only be formulated in metaphors, paradoxes, enigmas or metaphysical statements. Transpersonal experiences are not a prerogative of special clients with certain preconditions or extensive therapeutic experiences, and they are not related or limited to special music selections. A GIM therapist knows that these experiences may appear anytime, also in clients suffering from severe psychological problems or disorders.

Some GIM therapists have tried to identify specific 'transpersonal imagery' (Lewis 1999) and suggest, for example, that archetypal images or symbols – like 'the wise old man', 'the witch', 'the Great Mother', mythical motives like 'The Hero's Journey' etc. – indicate a transpersonal experience. There is no doubt that experiences of this type may be profound and transformative, even spiritual, but they can hardly be transpersonal (in the sense of the word used here), for an indication of an approaching transpersonal experience is often when the image is no longer significant. The client is 'taken by the music', flows with it and experiences an extraordinary beauty and wellbeing. It is like a door opening to new and unknown layers of consciousness. The dialogue is suspended for a while, and the therapist's role is to assist the client in having the full, unexpected experience of 'something totally different' (Ingemann Nielsen 1986). This is most often done by being a silent witness – only music 'talks'.

Bruscia (2000) draws attention to the fact that transpersonal experiences are not limited to receptive music therapy, but that they probably are more rare in active music therapy, where a lot of things are happening in the 'external world' of the client. A transpersonal experience is an experience of what Bruscia calls 'the implicit order' (see Chapter 1.3). It cannot be formulated in precise words, and it cannot be repeated or replicated in music. It cannot be planned or induced, but may happen when the client is ready for it, and both client and therapist are fully open to the music. 'Spiritual' and 'transpersonal' are not identical, but may be two aspects of the same: spiritual experiences may be characterized by the client's feelings of being connected or united with something bigger than himself/herself: music, beauty, nature, God, Buddha, cosmos … In the transpersonal experience there is no longer any observing ego, no image and imager, no music and listener. Every duality is dissolved, and this is what makes the experience a paradox. Unity *is*.

4.8 International Perspectives in Clinical Areas

The clinical application of music as therapy has varied from one country to another. As stated previously, one can see a broad differentiation between a more behavioural model of music therapy in a significant portion of both training courses and clinical situations in the USA, compared with a more psychoanalytical and psychotherapeutic approach in Europe. There has been a long history internationally of an exchange of information and the dissemination of methods of music therapy that has occurred consistently at international conferences. At the European Congress of Music Therapy in Cambridge (1992), Aalborg (1995), Leuven (1998) and Naples (2001), and the World Congress of Music Therapy in Spain (1993), Hamburg (1996) and Washington (1999), seminars and collective papers identified several music therapists from different countries working within a similar clinical field, maybe using a variety of different methodologies, but collecting together their results and resources to indicate the effectiveness of music therapy with a particular client population. The development of international co-operation to date has also relied on certain factors:

1.   area of focus, such as clinical population, music therapy method, area of research. Music therapists may form joint working groups (e.g. preparing European supervision training) or found international societies (e.g. the European GIM Society)

2.   presentation of material at conferences where contact is possible with professionals from different countries working in a similar clinical field with a similar methodology

3.   publication in learned journals and edited volumes of the method and results of music therapy applied to specific populations through specific methodologies.

International co-operation through the literature

The most effective way to research the range of music therapy practices and how they have developed at an international level is to read edited volumes of chapters or papers from international conferences of music therapy. The most prolific sources for these are the International Society for Music and Medicine Conferences, which has published several books including *Music in Medicine* 1, 2 and 3, and both the World Conferences and European Conferences. As well as those, some significant practitioners in the field of music therapy have attempted to collect together a compilation of chapters within specific clinical fields in order to document an international perspective on music therapy practice. Many of these compilations are, to date, mostly documented in English and the main ones will be listed below. A short review of the content of selected ones will be included, while reference is made to some of the others that can guide readers to resources of literature that have a specific and specialized focus. The ones we would like to offer reviews on are:

Aldridge, D. (ed) (1998) *Music Therapy in Palliative Care. New Voices.* London: Jessica Kingsley Publishers.

Bruscia, K. (1987) *Improvisational Models of Music Therapy.* Springfield, Illinois: Charles C. Thomas.

Bruscia, K. (ed) (1991) *Case Studies in Music Therapy.* Gilsum, NH: Barcelona Publishers.

Heal, M. and Wigram, T. (eds) (1993) *Music Therapy in Health and Education.* London: Jessica Kingsley Publishers.

Dileo-Maranto, C.D. (ed) (1993b) *Music Therapy: International Perspectives.* Pennsylvania: Jeffrey Books.

Wigram, T. and De Backer, J. (eds) (1999) *Clinical Applications of Music Therapy in Developmental Disability, Paediatrics and Neurology.* London: Jessica Kingsley Publishers.

Wigram, T. and De Backer, J. (eds) (1999) *Clinical Applications of Music Therapy in Psychiatry.* London: Jessica Kingsley Publishers.

Wigram, T., Saperston, B. and West, R. (eds) (1995) *The Art and Science of Music Therapy: A Handbook.* London, Toronto: Harwood Academic Publications.

Professor David Aldridge has edited a volume on music therapy in palliative care, with contributions from clinicians and researchers from the whole world. It has the subtitle *New Voices,* reflecting the fact that most of these experienced clinicians have not published in their own name before. The authors are from Norway, Germany, England and Australia, and their articles are based on many years of experience within areas like child oncology, women with breast cancer, people who have AIDS or chronic degenerative diseases, and hospice patients. In 2000 Aldridge edited a parallel volume on music therapy in dementia care.

The first, and perhaps most significant book produced by Dr Kenneth Bruscia of Temple University, Philadelphia, was *Improvisational Models of Music Therapy.* This is particularly significant for European practitioners in music therapy as it outlines several of the major methods of music therapy that have become internationally used, including Free Improvisation Therapy (Juliette Alvin, England), Creative Music Therapy (Paul Nordoff and Clive Robbins, America/ Australia/UK/

Denmark/Norway/Japan) and Analytical Music Therapy (Mary Priestley, England/Denmark/Germany). It is mainly a theoretical book, describing and comprehensively defining the methods by which these models of music therapy are applied.

Moving on to the clinical area, one of the significant contributions to the literature, again by Dr Kenneth Bruscia of Temple University, is *Case Studies in Music Therapy*. The book contains 42 case histories, each describing the process of music therapy over an extended period of time, and includes children, adolescents and adults, both in individual and group therapy. Authors from nine countries are represented including the USA, Canada, Great Britain, Australia, France, Republic of South Africa, Denmark, The Netherlands and Italy. Some of these case studies are incredibly long. For example, Dr Edith Lecourt has written a chapter entitled 'Off-beat Music Therapy: a Psychoanalytic Approach to Autism', in which she reports on 88 sessions of music therapy. She is documenting her work with a four-year-old boy with signs of autism and a lack of language. Lecourt reports that he was very excited by sound – captivated, fascinated and entranced by certain sounds such as the piano. Lecourt also talks about some of the 'off-beat' responses she makes to his sounds which turn into games, establishing some musical processes such as syncopation and echo effects in the interaction that develops this boy's responsiveness both to the therapist and through the music. The richness of the material within *Case Studies in Music Therapy* and its variety is evidenced within this range of chapters, including therapy work with classrooms of six- to eight-year-old hyperactive learning-disabled children (Hibben), psychodynamic improvisation therapy with a music therapy student in training (Benedikte Barth Scheiby), the boy that nobody wanted – created experiences for a boy with severe emotional problems (Herman), music therapy at childbirth (Allison) and rehabilitation of piano performance skills following a left cerebral vascular accident (Erdonmez).

Professor Cheryl Dileo's book *Music Therapy: International Perspectives* gives comprehensive information on music therapy in many countries all over the world. The national chapters are written by prolific music therapists, who present the development of music therapy from several perspectives: history, pioneers, important models and methods, clinical applications, training programs, publications, associations and organizations, and the professional status of the music therapist. As a past president of NAMT and WFMT Professor Dileo had an optimal background for involving leading music therapists in the project. Unfortunately countries like Germany and Sweden were not represented in the book, and it deserves a new edition within a few years.

The Art and Science of Music Therapy: A Handbook provides another rich anthology of material, including the landmark 'Meta Analysis' by Jayne Standley, Professor of

Music Therapy at Florida State University in Tallahassee. Chapter 1 of this book, entitled 'Music as a Therapeutic Intervention in Medical and Dental Treatment: Research and Clinical Application.', gives an important perspective through a procedure which provides a quantitative synthesis of research data through formal statistical techniques. Further research is documented in this book in the chapters by Bruce Saperston on the effects of tempo and interactive tempos on heart rate and electromyographic responses, as well as Odell-Miller's chapter on her research into the effects of music therapy on the elderly mentally ill and Skille and Wigram's chapter on the effects of vibroacoustic therapy. The focus on different client groups includes an inevitable accumulation of clinical studies and clinical reports on the effects of music therapy with autistic children, from the point of view of diagnosing this disorder (Wigram), looking at the effects of working with the children and their mothers in co-therapeutic sessions (Warwick) and a long-term case study (Howat). Further chapters on more psychotherapeutically and psychodynamically informed music therapy look at the client–therapist relationship in music therapy sessions (Hughes), the links between sounds and symbols (Priestley) and Guided Imagery and Music (Goldberg).

Three further anthologies of music therapy case material and research work have been compiled by Tony Wigram, the first in collaboration with Margaret Heal following the European Conference in Cambridge in 1992, and the other two in collaboration with Jos De Backer (Head of Music Therapy at Leuven University in Belgium and a post-graduate PhD student at Aalborg University), the titles of which are specified above. Jessica Kingsley Publishers have promoted the arts therapies and music therapy in particular and are responsible for these publications.

Music Therapy in Health and Education is a text with 22 chapters divided into two areas – clinical practice and research. Clinical areas represented include studies on autistic children, schizophrenia, eating disorders, neurology, developmental disability and general mental health, while the research section includes a literature review and a selection of applied research with clients from similar populations as mentioned above. The importance of this book is that it represents a selection of the clinical and research work presented at the 1992 European Conference of Music Therapy at King's College, Cambridge, and documents relevant clinical and theoretical approaches that are currently practised in music therapy mainly throughout Europe, but also including work from the USA and Australia. The case studies and research are good foundational reading. The book has recently been translated into Japanese.

Clinical Applications of Music Therapy in Psychiatry (Wigram and De Backer 1999b) and *Clinical Applications of Music Therapy in Developmental Disability, Paediatrics and Neurology* (Wigram and De Backer 1999a) were written to a consistent structure where each contributor was asked to define their method of work, describe how they practise music therapy, illustrate this with a case (or cases) and then document how they analyse the musical material, interpret the music, and evaluate the effect and result of their therapy. There is some evidence in the chapters in some of these books, for example *Clinical Applications of Music Therapy in Psychiatry*, where the contributors are starting to cross-reference amongst themselves as approaches become more integrated or comparable. Nygard Pedersen focuses particularly on music therapy as holding and reorganizing work with schizophrenic and psychotic patients, referencing other significant music therapists in Europe including Mary Priestley and Frederiksen. Frederiksen, Langenberg, Streeter, Steiger and others all consistently reference Mary Priestley, the originator of psychoanalytic music therapy in Europe, indicating the connection between therapists working in different European countries. Having looked for the commonalities in the literature between different professionals within one country or between countries, one can also find significant differences. Approaches to autism vary from developmental/diagnostic (Wigram) to psychoanalytical (Di Franco) to Maslovian approaches through creative music therapy (Etkin, Brown, Howat).

In addition to these texts, three significantly important CD-ROMS have been produced in the last five years to add to the wealth of literature now available at an international level in music therapy. Professor David Aldridge, of Witten-Herdecke University in Germany, has produced *Music Therapy Info 1* and *Music Therapy Info 2*. The second CD-ROM includes a wide-ranging database of over 11,000 reference papers on music therapy from the international community, as well as many of the papers from both the World Conference in Music Therapy in Vitoria, Spain, in 1993, and the European Conference in Music Therapy in Leuven, Belgium, in 1998. The American Music Therapy Association (AMTA) has recently produced a CD-ROM which includes all papers published in the three major journals in America: *The Journal of Music Therapy, Music Therapy Perspectives* and *Music Therapy*. While the majority of material on this particular compilation is American, it does occasionally include papers from specialists all over the world (American Music Therapy Association 1999).

There is a further range of compiled volumes, many of which have focused on a specific clinical area. This second list does not claim to be complete because, thanks to the passion of some music therapists for writing, volumes are constantly appearing. But it adds further titles to an already rich resource, and these texts are all worthy of exploration by clinicians, researchers or academics in these specific fields.

Aldridge, D. (ed) (2000) *Music Therapy in Dementia Care. More New Voices*. London: Jessica Kingsley Publishers.

Aldridge, D. (ed) (1997–2002) *Kairos I–VI*. Bern, Göttingen: Hans Huber.

Bonde, L.O. and Pedersen, I.N. (eds) (1996) *Music Therapy Within Multi-Disciplinary Teams.* Proceedings of the 3rd European Music Therapy Conference. Aalborg University Press.

Bruscia, K. (ed) (1998) *The Dynamics of Music Psychotherapy.* Gilsum, NH: Barcelona Publishers.

Froehlich, M. (ed) (1996) *Music Therapy with Hospitalized Children. A Creative Arts Child Life Approach.* Pennsylvania: Jeffrey Books.

Hibben, J. (ed) (1999) *Inside Music Therapy: Client Experiences.* Gilsum NH: Barcelona Publishers.

Lee, C. (ed) (1995) *Lonely Waters.* Oxford: Sobell Publications.

Loewy, J. (ed) (1997) *Music Therapy and Paediatric Pain.* Pennsylvania: Jeffrey Books.

Pratt, R.R. and Grocke, D. (eds) (1999) *MusicMedicine 3. Music Medicine and Music Therapy: Expanding Horizons.* Melbourne: University of Melbourne.

Pratt, R.R. and Hesser, B. (eds) (1989) *Music Therapy and Music in Special Education: the International State of the Art.* St. Louis: MMB.

Conclusion

Perhaps the most important thing to find in all these texts, and in many others which have not been listed here, is the value of music therapy for people with emotional, physical or psychological problems or disorders. There are a lot of 'good stories' – maybe not always supported by clearly documented evidence as might be hoped for by the scientific world, but nevertheless a testament to some enduring and consistent progress over time. What really matters is: 'Does music therapy work?' Many of the case studies documented in these books, and the research that has been undertaken, show that music therapy is very effective. The accumulation of all this evidence, particularly at an international level, is becoming increasingly important to provide a body of evidence to institutions who employ and develop the work of music therapists.

For students, potential music therapists or members of the public there is a rich collection here of wonderfully documented personal stories of achievement over incredible disability and confusion. Music therapy can help people with autism to communicate, and music-making can give them a chance to establish a meaningful relationship with other human beings, which they find incredibly difficult. Music can provide a vehicle for resolving huge and terrible emotional conflicts in people with psychiatric disorders, and music which is used appropriately and effectively in music therapy can also reduce pain and help people cope with terminal illness as they come to the end of their lives. While music itself does not cure senile dementia or other debilitating illnesses and diseases that affect both old and young people , it can alleviate those diseases to a large extent. This is evidenced in these books and in the chapters that have been written by a very important group of highly qualified and experienced music therapists.

CHAPTER 5

Music Therapy Research and Clinical Assessment

5.1 Research in Music Therapy – An Overview

Research in the broad field of music therapy has been a real focus of attention over the last forty years, and a number of clinicians and academics have obtained whatever resources they could find to initiate, carry out and report studies. A great number of these studies are documented, and can be found in the databases (Aldridge 2002) and in journals and books (see Chapter 7).

There is a wealth of information on the methods, models of investigation and techniques of analysis available in the literature. Some books offer guidelines specifically on method, in particular Ansdell and Pavlicevic (2001), Glaser and Strauss (1967), Guba and Lincoln (1994), Madsen and Madsen (1997), Smeijsters (1997a), Wheeler (1995), and articles such as those written by Aldridge (1997), Bruscia (1998), Ferrara (1984), Forinash and Gonzales (1989) and Kenny (1998). Another selection of texts includes a compilation of studies that exemplify research methods, including Langenberg, Aigen and Frommer (1996), Pratt and Grocke (1999), Pratt and Spintge (1996) and Spintge and Droh (1992). There are also valuable texts where theory, method and worked examples of research are combined such as D. Aldridge (1996b), Amir (1992), Wheeler (1995), Wigram and Dileo (1997) and Wigram, Saperston and West (1995).

Many doctoral dissertations, most of which can be followed up through Dissertation Abstracts International, and some of which are increasingly available on CD-ROMs (Aldridge, D. 1996a, 1998b, 2001, 2002), combine a careful explanation of a research method, the use of research tools (some of which may have been generated specifically for the purpose) and a detailed documentation of results and discussion.

Typically, in Europe, music therapists receive only limited training in research methods as part of their training, when compared, for example, with clinical psychologists. This does not dampen their enthusiasm for research, and now more methods of applied clinical music therapy research are well described in the literature to help starter researchers.

The most useful and comprehensive book for learning various different models of music therapy research is the edited volume by Wheeler, *Music Therapy Research* (1995). The contributors in this volume give clear frameworks to understand the principles, formulation of research questions, methods of research, and methods of collecting and analysing data. The guidelines, practical methods and theories of these elements are clearly formulated for both the *quantitative paradigm* (Bruscia 1995a; Decuir 1995; Hanser 1995; Hanser and Wheeler 1995; McGuire 1995; Dileo-Maranto 1991; Prickett 1995) and *qualitative paradigm* (Aigen 1995a, 1995b; Bruscia 1995b, 1995c, 1995d, 1995e; Forinash 1995). The methods are exemplified with short examples, both in the qualitative chapters and the quantitative. For example, in Hanser and Wheeler's chapter on 'Experimental Research', a study by Haines (1989) is reported where the researcher looked at the effects of music therapy on the self-concepts of emotionally-disturbed adolescents. The experimental group received music therapy for six weeks, while the control group had verbal therapy and parallel activities. Their self-concepts were evaluated at the beginning and at the end of the treatment period, and no significant differences were found between the two groups.

The focus of research in music therapy has varied significantly depending on what the researcher intends to measure. Generally speaking, there is a very wide range of parameters which one can measure to evaluate both the process of music therapy and the outcome of music therapy. In terms of the process of music therapy, one could investigate any of the following parameters:

1. The nature of the client–therapist relationship.

2. The client's personal experience of music therapy.

3. The therapist's personal experience of music therapy.

4. Changing quality of music in the dynamic interaction over time.

5. Perception of others (parents, relatives, other professionals) regarding the process of music therapy.

6. How does therapy work?

7.   What is the relationship between the music and the patient as a whole person?

In terms of evaluating outcome, therapists have chosen either physical or psychological forms of measurement, or both. At a rather general level, changes after a period of therapy, or a single therapy session, can be categorized under the following headings:

Outcome of physiological measures

1.   improvement or deterioration in the physical state of the client

2.   improvements or developments in the way the client is coping with physical problems such as pain, physical disability, physical incapacity

3.   changes in physiological responses such as heart rate, blood pressure, respiration, muscle activity, electrodermal (level of arousal), electroencephalograph (brain activity), skin temperature etc.

Outcome of psychological measures

1.   improved or developed self-esteem

2.   improved self-perception and insight

3.   resolution of conflicts, emotional issues or psychological difficulties

4.   improvement or development in social interaction, social communication, self-expression

5.   improvements in the patient's capacity to manage his/her life.

To take an example, many music therapy researchers have used heart rate as an indicator of change as it has implications regarding the process of attention, cognitive processing, and awareness of the environment. Researchers have speculated that the heart has an influence on consciousness or awareness. The impact of heart rate is dynamic and fluctuates between suppressing and liberating the left and right sides of the brain. David Aldridge, in his book *From out of the Silence: Music Therapy Research and Practice in Medicine*, reports that when heart rate increases it is indicative of cognitive processing and a rejection of the environment; when heart rate decreases, there is a switch to environmental attention. The cardiovascular system reflects a person's intention to receive information. If this is so, music therapy is a sensitive tool for discerning the physiological state of a person as a whole. He reports on a study by Bason and Celler (1972) where it was found that it was possible to influence the heart rate of a patient by externally matching the pulse of their heart rate. From this, we can conclude that studies on the influence of music on heart rate must involve the matching of the music to the individual patient. This also makes physiological sense as different people have varied reactions to the same music. He also refers to the work of Haas *et al.* (1986) which showed that listening, coupled with tapping, synchronizes respiration patterns with musical rhythm, further emphasizing that active music playing can be used to influence physiological parameters.

Michael Thaut (1985) has also been very active in evaluating the effects of music on children with gross motor dysfunction, where he found that they performed with significantly better motor rhythmic accuracy when aided by auditory rhythm and rhythmic speech. His work developed into treatment of neurological disorders such as Parkinson's disease, where he also had significant success in using pulse and rhythm to regularize and improve gait (walking patterns) and from this it can be inferred that musical rhythms can be used for their therapeutic influence on physiological parameters.

Quantitative and qualitative research

Quantitative research includes concepts such as hypotheses, manipulating independent variables, measuring change with dependent variables, collecting data that can be measured in some way, often comparing the effects of an intervention on a treatment group with a control group who receive no treatment, a placebo, or an alternative treatment, and applying statistical analysis to search for significant differences. Qualitative research involves formulating research questions that investigate phenomena, taking a broad view and focus, operating in a more flexible research frame, studying and interpreting human behaviour as a phenomenon, and sometimes theory building (Grounded Theory) as a main part of the process. Measurement in quantitative research is concerned with evaluating whether the effect of music therapy is valid, reliable and significant. Qualitative methods more typically involve exploring the process of what goes on in music therapy, answering questions such as: Why is music therapy effective? How does music therapy work? What is the therapist doing? What happens within the client–therapist relationship?

Both quantitative and qualitative research methods are used in music therapy, and both paradigms are essential for the future understanding of music therapy. What's the point of producing a study which shows that an intervention is effective, if you cannot explain how to administer the intervention, or what components or elements there are within the intervention that cause it to be effective? It is like administering a medication without listing the chemical properties of the pills involved. Likewise, what is the point of exploring, defining and describing a process of therapy in great detail if there is no analysis of the outcome of that intervention? This can be likened to saying, 'This is a way of doing music therapy … but there is no guarantee it will work!' Nevertheless, both methods are carried out independently and there is a history of independent studies of both paradigms in music therapy.

There have unfortunately been some artificial or inappropriate distinctions that have driven a wedge between qualitative and quantitative approaches, such as quantitative research is only concerned with outcome, and qualitative research is to do with the process. In fact, both paradigms are interested in answering research questions, defining and describing the process, documenting outcome and analysing data. Both qualitative and quantitative research frequently involve observing, analysing, evaluating and interpreting human behaviour, and both approaches are interested in the way music therapy functions as a treatment. Most importantly, both paradigms demand rigour, and have rules and methods that need to be understood and used appropriately. When determining the paradigm that is most appropriate, it is far more relevant to establish the focus of the research question first, before deciding on an appropriate research method.

Applied behaviour analysis as a method of research

Whilst music therapists working within a psychotherapeutic or psychodynamic context would not wish to be identified as 'behaviourists', nevertheless much of their everyday work is concerned with exploring the origins of human behaviour, and attempting to work through issues which influence behaviour. Therefore, the methods of evaluating and analysing human behaviour in relation to therapeutic progress rely on both an exploration of the origins of behaviour, as well as an effective process by which the negative influences arising out of those origins, or the current negative influences at present at work, are challenged and neutralized in order for somebody to 'move forward'. Psychotherapeutic approaches rely on the concept of therapy as a process of movement or change, with a heightened awareness in a person to gain insight into the nature and origin of their difficulties and incorporate them into a more positive or progressive construct for the future.

However, at a foundational level, therapists in both America and Europe have used applied behaviour analysis to evaluate their work because it is particularly applicable to single subject research design. Single subject designs are used when the purpose of an investigation is to test hypotheses about the behaviour of a single individual or group and examine the effect of a particular strategy in music therapy. This is different from experimental group design, where the intention is to compare subjects or groups by examining the central tendency and variability of many observations. Single subject research applies the same rigorous standards to examining intra-subject changes over time but under different conditions. It is often more helpful for music therapists working individually, because instead of looking at the average response of many individuals to music therapy intervention, it looks specifically at one subject or one group, sometimes with and without music therapy. It is also useful because it doesn't rely on the presence or use of a control or comparison group. In clinical settings, the use of control groups can provoke many questions about the ethics of such a practice. First of all it's very difficult to match groups in order to set up a control group where the data would be comparable and in most clinical environments the number of subjects who share the same diagnosis is quite limited.

Single subject designs, such as are used in applied behaviour analysis, examine the functional relationships between music therapy or other treatments, and the particular behaviour which is present in the client that might be under investigation or of particular focus.

Suzanne Hanser, in her chapter on applied behaviour analysis in the book *Music Therapy Research: Quantitative and Qualitative Perspectives*, edited by Barbara Wheeler (1995), gives useful and clear examples of the different types of applied behaviour analysis, including reversal design, multiple baseline design and multiple treatment or multi-element design. She cites an example of a young boy who is prone to emotional outbursts in school, including crying, tantrums and angry behaviours. The first step in applied behaviour analysis, as in many types of research, is to establish a baseline of behaviour. For music therapists, this process will be undertaken typically in any clinical intervention where before they start working they want to identify characteristics of the client's behaviour, the issues that the client is working with or the client's physical and emotional difficulties. In the baseline that Suzanne Hanser described in this chapter, she recorded emotional outbursts for one week both in work, in the classroom and during playtime, and angry behaviours were the most common and frequent, in excess of five per day.

The music therapist begins sessions with the client, focusing on playing the guitar and using the client's favourite songs. Also involved in the work is helping the child learn how to use the guitar. The music therapy sessions take place during lunchtime, but the teacher continues to monitor the child's behaviours in the classroom and during playtime. The results of this show a good reduction of behaviours in the week following the baseline. In order to test out whether the music therapy itself is really effective, the researcher uses a reversal design (ABAB) where, for the third week, no music therapy sessions take place, and in the fourth week, the music therapy sessions are reintroduced. The results show that during the period of reversal (no music therapy sessions) the incidence of difficult behaviours increase, and that in a further period of intervention, the behaviours fall to a lower level than had occurred in the first intervention.

Introducing a multiple baseline design involved the introduction of music therapy at home as well as at school, which was decided in order to ensure that the intervention of music therapy makes a difference whether the sessions take place at home or at school. The results demonstrate that after music therapy begins at home, immediate changes are observable. The multiple baseline design offers considerable evidence in this case that music therapy is responsible for behaviour change at home as well as at school.

This is a good example of an outcome form of evaluation, although inferences can be drawn from the nature of the therapeutic intervention. This will answer the question, 'how did music therapy have an effect?', as the focus of the therapy was to help the child learn to use the guitar and the stimulus that was used was the child's own choice of favourite songs. One can speculate that a combination of acquiring a 'popular' skill (in other words, an ability to make music using a guitar, which is valuable and related to the current genre) has facilitated the client's level of self-esteem, his/her feelings of confidence and given him/her a satisfying and effective emotional experience. The knock-on effect of this has been to reduce the incidence of aggressive or difficult behaviours. What this does not explain is what the original cause for the difficult behaviours was, although that might be assumed, and therefore this type of research is largely concerned with evaluating outcome rather than process.

Aspects of analysis and clinical research

Audio and video analysis is extensively used in clinical work, and this form of therapy 'data' has for some time been classified as a form of patient records. The use of it in research studies is extremely fruitful – and sometimes the data from video recordings is almost too rich – and there are many parameters of behaviour that can be analysed and described besides the purely auditory one. It is an ideal method of analysis of improvisational music therapy, although recording of any sort also presents researchers with ethical issues, particularly in psychiatry. If consent is obtained prior to the study beginning, then the patient/subject is aware he/she is the focus of research and this may alter behaviour and the therapeutic relationship. If, however, one waits until after the study is complete to request consent to analyse and research recorded clinical material, the patient/subject may simply refuse – and six months' to two years' work may then be unusable in the study. However, it is a medium of data that allows the researcher to study many aspects of the therapy process, although ethical issues sometimes make it difficult and sensitive to record therapy work. Holck (2002) has based an entire research study on the detailed analysis of interaction and contact between learning-disabled, communication-disordered children and therapists. De Backer (2001) in Belgium has explored evidence of symbolization in clients with schizophrenia through the analysis of musical and verbal material as recorded on video, and Elefant (2001) from Israel, studied both choice-making and the evidence of responsive, intentional behaviour in girls with Rett syndrome.

One of the pioneers in the development of qualitative research methods in music therapy is Professor Even Ruud. During two decades he has worked in an interdisciplinary way with music education, therapy and anthropology. This is reflected in the research project *Music and Identity* (Ruud 1997). Based on research interviews and musical autobiographies he has analysed the relationship between musical experiences and the formation of identity. With theoretical inspiration from self-psychology and narrative philosophy Ruud shows how music experiences contribute to the construction of identity within four spheres or 'spaces': 1. the personal room, 2. the social room, 3. the room of time and space, 4. the transpersonal room. Ruud is spokesman of a theory-based empirical research, which understands music experiences in both a personal and a cultural-historical context.

There has also been some empirical research in GIM (Chapter 3.1). An important source of inspiration has been the doctoral dissertation of the Australian GIM trainer and researcher Denise Erdonmez Grocke, whose study on 'Pivotal Moments in Guided Imagery and Music' is a major contribution to phenomenological music therapy research (Erdonmez Grocke 2000). Torben Moe (Denmark) is also inspired by Grounded Theory in his study of the development of imagery in group music therapy with schizotypal patients using modified GIM. The study documents not only that these patients experience imagery of therapeutic value, but also that they are able to work with these images in a transformation process (Moe 1998, 2000; Moe, Roesen and Raben 2000).

Dag Körlin and Björn Wrangsjö (Sweden) run a continuous study of the psychological effects of GIM. They use standardized questionnaires (SCL-90, IIP and Antonovsky's Sense of Coherence Scale). Even if no control group is involved in the research, the results indicate that most of the clients involved in the study improved during the GIM treatment (Körlin and Wrangsjö 2001; Wrangsjö and Körlin 1995).

Research publications

In the spring of 1986, three therapists working in a children's hospital in Miami published a paper in the National Association for Music Therapy (NAMT) *Journal of Music Therapy* called 'Where's the Research?' (Siegal, Cartwright and Katz 1986).

Their study was undertaken to try to find out whether the music therapists working in the South East region of the USA were participating in, or were interested in, research. Of 310 music therapists surveyed, only 141 responded, a response rate of 45%. It is worth reporting one part of the conclusions of this paper:

> Twenty-five per cent of the respondents not currently involved in research indicated the following reasons for not conducting research: no time available outside of work hours, lack of funds, and absence of research in their job descriptions. Twelve per cent reportedly had no interest in pursuing research, and nine per cent felt they were not sufficiently trained. Other reasons advanced were that facilities did not allow research, no time was available during working hours, the respondent was new at the facility, and facility populations were unstable. (Siegal *et al.* 1986)

The journals of music therapy provide one with an insight into where research is going on, and also the contributions made from various clinical fields. In America, some regular reviews have looked in the past at the content of the *Journal of Music Therapy*, published by the NAMT (Codding 1987; Decuir 1987; Gfeller 1987; Gilbert 1979; James 1985; Jellison 1973; Madsen 1978). Wheeler (1988) undertook an analysis of literature from music therapy journals that included the *Journal of Music Therapy, Music Therapy, Music Therapy Perspectives* and *Arts in Psychotherapy*. Wheeler's study was based on the model used by Decuir in 1987, with the addition of the author's name.

Codding's (1987) analysis looked at 158 articles published in the *Journal of Music Therapy* between 1977 and 1985, and produced some interesting results. In particular, she found the research mode of inquiry was predominantly experimental, and that statistical designs are more prevalent than are behavioural designs in experimental research. Also, and perhaps surprisingly, she found that more studies had been conducted in clinical than in university settings.

Gfeller's (1987) study, entitled 'Music Therapy Theory and Practice as Reflected in Research Literature', noted themes in music therapy practice in America, including:

1. The prominence of behavioural and psychoanalytic theories as influencing clinical practice. Eleven per cent of the articles indicated the practice or effect of music therapy was linked to psychoanalytic theory, and 20 per cent linked to behavioural theory

2. The value of music to enhance self-esteem, to socialize and to energize through rhythm

3.   Lack of studies with elderly and physically handicapped compared with the number of people working in these fields

4.   Low incidence of articles on work in adult psychiatry

5.   Low incidence of articles concerning music's influence on physiological change, but with increasing interest in this area (in fact only 9 per cent of the total 243 articles referred to the physiological influence of music)

6.   Databased studies make up one half of the surveyed articles and are much more prevalent in the field of learning difficulty and non-handicapped than in the psychiatric population.

Wigram (1993a) made a comprehensive analysis of articles published between 1987 and 1991 from five main journals of music therapy, comparing the proportion of research articles to clinical case material and general papers (see Table 5.1).

Table 5.1: General categorization of articles in five music therapy journals (1987–1991) (Wigram 1993a)

Journal	Clinical	Research	General
Arts in Psychotherapy	61	3	36
Journal of British Music Therapy	47	19	33
Journal of Music Therapy	21	62	17
Music Therapy	41	3	56
Music Therapy Perspectives	40	11	49
TOTALS	210	98	191

Ninety-eight articles were identified as research, compared with 210 clinical papers and 191 general papers. This tells us that music therapists write more about their clinical work and music therapy theory than research. As can be seen, the majority of the research articles (65%) are in the *Journal of Music Therapy*, traditionally the main American publication concerned with research. The same analysis by Wigram showed that most research was going on in the fields of special education, music therapy training courses and general medicine, and that only a small percentage was being undertaken in psychiatry, geriatrics and sensory or physical disability.

Table 5.2 shows the results of an analysis categorizing the types of articles published in three journals of music therapy between 1998 and 2001: *Journal of*

Music Therapy (*JMT*) (USA); *British Journal of Music Therapy* (*BJMT*) (UK) and *Nordic Journal of Music Therapy* (*NJMT*) (Scandinavia). All of these journals have blind reviews and articles are refereed by editorial boards that include leading academics, clinicians and researchers in the field. The objective of this short overview is to identify the proportion of published papers that come within the field of research, when compared with other areas, and what types of research those articles report.

Table 5.2: Percentage of articles falling into research, clinical and other categories in three music therapy journals between 1998 and 2001.

Journal Research, clinical or other type of article	*Journal of Music Therapy* 1998–2001 %	*British Journal of Music Therapy* 1998–2001 %	*Nordic Journal of Music Therapy* 1998–2001 %
Clinical qualitative research	10	5	9.4
Clinical quantitative research	34	0	6.25
Non-clinical research	34	12.5	4.7
General theory and music therapy theory	14	37.5	46.9
Research about music therapy education	6	0	1.6
Clinical: psychiatry	0	4.1	10.9
Clinical: learning disability	0	8.3	10.9
Clinical: paediatrics	2	8.3	1.6
Clinical: older adults	0	4.1	3.1
Other	0	20.8	4.7

As might have been expected, the *Journal of Music Therapy* has the highest proportion of research articles, and of those, the predominant number are quantitative (34%). The articles classified under non-clinical research (34% in total) are also predominantly quantitative studies.

The clinical music therapy research studies do not always report a significant effect, but often indicate results that are in the right direction, and recommend future research with larger samples. Besides many studies on different clinical populations including older adults (Ashida 2000; Groene 2001; Johnson, Otto and Clair 2001; Koger and Brotons 2000; Silber 1999; Zelazny 2001) psychiatric patients (Smeijsters and van den Hurk 1999), patients with neurological disorders (Baker 2001a, 2001b; Haneishi 2001; Hurt *et al.* 1998), oncology patients (Burns 2001; Waldon 2001) and people with developmental disability (Ford 1999), there are excellent reviews and meta-analyses (Gregory 2000; Koger, Chapin and Brotons 1999; Wilson and Smith 2000). Specialist areas are also well represented in *JMT*, for example the Whipple's study in a neonatal intensive care unit that reported shorter hospital stay and improved weight gain in babies after parents were trained in music and multi-modal stimulation. This study comes from Florida State University where a collection of excellent studies on neonates has emerged in the last few years from Professor Jayne Standley and her research body (Standley 1991b, 1998; Cassidy and Standley 1995; Standley and Moore 1995).

The non-clinical research studies very often involve experimental research on students at universities or colleges where there are music therapy programs, evaluating for example their responses to music at an emotional level (Iwanaga and Moroki 1999), the effects of the volume of music on relaxation (Staum and Brotons 2000), the relaxing effect of music on potential stress (Knight and Rickard 2001) and the experiences of music therapy students in their clinical practicums (Darrow *et al.* 2001).

Traditionally *JMT* has documented quantitative research; however, recently, in 1998, a whole issue was devoted to qualitative research methods (Aigen 1998; Bruscia 1998; Kenny 1998), and subsequently more articles have appeared in *JMT* reporting qualitative approaches in research (Amir 1999; Lee 2000; Wheeler 1999).

The *JMT* holds pride of place as the leading journal in music therapy for reporting experimental research, providing us with resources to go to when presenting the evidence needed to underpin evidence-based practice, a subject that receives attention later in this chapter (see Chapter 5.4). There are many studies that answer that fundamental question: 'Does music therapy work?' *Music Therapy Perspectives*, the second journal published by the American Music Therapy Association (AMTA) (see Chapter 7.2), also documents research studies. This was not included in this review.

Two sources are worth mentioning for further study, and as very important starting points in a literature review. Standley and Prickett (1994) made a compilation of articles from the *JMT* called *Research in Music Therapy: A Tradition of Excellence. Outstanding Reprints from the Journal of Music Therapy 1964–1993*. This volume not only includes the original articles, but also summarizes the main elements of the studies, and their findings. One can see that the majority (32 of the 51 articles included here) are studies where recorded music was the primary tool (independent variable), and only two or three used improvisational music. This reflects the fact that improvisation is used more in Europe, and these are predominantly texts from American researchers, but also that recorded music is more easy to control as a stimulus, and studies using recorded music can be replicated.

The second source is the CD-ROM I produced by the American Association of Music Therapy: *Music Therapy Research. Quantitative and Qualitative Foundations. 1964–1998*. This compilation includes the text of every article published in *JMT*, *Music Therapy Perspectives (MTP)* and *Music Therapy* (see Chapter 7.2) between these dates, depending on one's definition of research. One could not classify all the articles in this CD-ROM as research, as there are clinical papers, position papers, theory papers, and commentaries. However a great majority are research-based, which is very different from the culture of publication found in the European journals.

In the *British Journal of Music Therapy*, the spread of publications reveals a slightly higher proportion of articles oriented towards clinical practice (Davies and Richards 1998; Oldfield and Bunce 2001; Tyler 1998) but a much greater orientation towards discussion-based articles, some of them arguing out the differences in music therapy theory and practice (Aigen 1999; Brown 1999a; Pavlicevic 1999; Proctor 1999; Streeter 1999b; Woodward 2000). There are some very interesting articles looking at the development of music therapy as a profession, and how jobs are developed (Moss 1999; Stewart 2000), and a greater proportion of articles about music therapy theory (Robertson 2000; Stige 1998a).

Primary research articles are few in number, and perhaps reflect that the development of music therapy in the UK has been clinically oriented, with only a small number of therapists undertaking research. Neugebauer and Aldridge (1998) presented their fascinating study mapping the correlation and synchronicity between heart rate and musical parameters – indicating a high degree of musical co-ordination and communication in instrumental and vocal improvisation. Edwards (1999) reported clinical effects of music therapy with children with severe burns, the data that underpinned her doctoral research at the University of Queensland. Leslie Bunt has stood in the forefront of British music therapy research for almost two decades now, and his contributions to research thinking in the UK are significant. The article in collaboration with Sarah Burns and Pat Turton (Bunt, Burns and Turton 2000) reported the process of research with cancer patients, and reflects the value of both quantitative (measures of change in salivary cortisol) and qualitative dependent measures. Aasgard (2000b), a doctoral researcher from the

Aalborg, reports on the value of songwriting in paediatric oncology and Skewes (Wigram 2002 on music therapy for bereaved adolescents).

In the *Nordic Journal of Music Therapy* there is a definite leaning towards articles and discussion on music therapy theory. Some thirty articles (46.9%), including those that are in discussion and interview sections of this publication, are concerned with theory, when compared with only 14 (21.8%) on experimental or qualitative research and a total of 17 (26.6%) on clinical practice. Theory building, metatheoretical discussions, and the attention many Europeans (and others) have been paying to developing a greater understanding of the theoretical frame and basis for music therapy should be included as a form of research.

Therefore a variety of areas of theoretical investigation are represented in articles about meaning in music, and the function of communication in music (Bruscia 2000; Hauge and Tonsberg 1998; Jungaberle, Verres and DuBois 2001; Schogler 1998; Stige 2000; Trevarthen and Malloch 2000), aesthetic aspects of music therapy (Stige 1998b), theory building (Barmark and Hallin 1999; Bonde 2001c; Kenny 1999, 2000; Ruud 2000a), processes in music therapy (Robarts 2000), and biological and other origins of musical behaviour (Dissanayake 2001; Grinde 2000; Horden 2001; Hughes 2001; Kennair 2000; Merker 2000; Stige 2000).

The research papers in the *NJMT* have focused on Guided Imagery and Music (Moe 1998; Moe, Roesen and Raben 2000), case study research (Alvin 2000), research methods and areas of inquiry (Aldridge 1999b), assessment methods (Schumacher and Calvert-Kruppa 1999), music therapy methods (Ahonen-Eerikäinen 1999; Wigram 1999c), experimental studies (Baker 2001b; Gold, Wigram and Berger 2001; Korlin and Wrangsjö 2001; Merker, Bergström-Isaacsson and Witt Engerström 2001). The NJMT also follows a line of argument or discussion, for example on the IAPs, or on the series of articles written about a classic case study of Edward, a child with developmental disability, anxiety and very active behaviour. There is also the discursive line, where contributors can elaborate on a specific area of discussion using an electronic discussion forum. Editors control the quality of input, but papers into this part of the *NJMT* don't go through the usual refereeing procedure. The contributors refer in point form to discussions raised by other contributors, allowing a free-flowing and focused exchange of ideas internationally. It is a very useful way of developing a discussion.

However, some tendencies can be observed in the European journals already mentioned, and also in *Musiktherapeutische Umschau*, the main German journal:

- Articles based on qualitative research methods have become more common.

- More articles than before are published within psychiatry and geriatrics.

- Music therapy theory and research is under the influence of and inspired by the development within 'new musicology', anthropology and ethnography.

The many literature databases and other bibliographic services have made it much easier to establish an overview of the research literature. See Chapter 7.3 for further information on this.

5.2 Development of a Research Training Program – The Aalborg University Model with Examples from Research Studies

There are many attractions to develop from clinical practice into the field of research – be it clinically based, philosophical, or historical. However, research is often a lonely business, and frequently underfunded or not included as a funded part of a contract within the clinical field. Therefore, as can be seen from overviews of the studies that have been undertaken, particularly in the USA, research typically takes place in universities, or where the university is the funder or the base for the researcher. This is where the resources may be, and also where a research qualification such as a Master's or PhD is awarded. Universities promote research, and measure how much is going on amongst their own staff.

Music therapy professors at universities have promoted research in a strong and dynamic way over many years, and many have PhD level researchers on site, including Temple University, Philadelphia; Florida State University, USA; New York University, USA; Melbourne University, Australia; Oslo University, Norway; Witten-Herdecke University, Germany; Anglia Polytechnic University, UK; City University, UK; University of the West of England, UK; and Jyvaskula University, Finland; just to name some of them.

In this chapter, we would like to show the model that was developed, and the initiatives that we followed, in order to establish a research milieu at Aalborg University in Denmark – where there are now seven students currently registered for a PhD and several who have already finished. It is not the only model, and the styles of undertaking PhD research vary from one country to another. However, the Aalborg model has included certain important elements that we would like to stress in our attempt to promote both high quality research and, at the same time, a collaborative atmosphere where researchers come to feed and learn from international experts, and also from each other.

Historical development of the research program in Music Therapy at Aalborg University

The Research School in Music Therapy was begun in a small way in 1994, and has been carefully nurtured within the Faculty of Humanities where it stands alongside seven other research programs. In the first three years of the PhD program (1994–1996), the PhD training program had a close connection to the Nordic Research Network Group in music therapy, which focused on research in clinical music therapy practice. Members of this group still maintain regular contact.

There is a network of Danish and international experts within different relevant program areas. In Denmark, these researchers represent Aalborg Psychiatric Hospital, Risskov Psychiatric. Internationally, Lemmensistituut and Leuven University (Belgium), Universität Witten-Herdecke (Germany), Melbourne University (Australia), S:t Görans Sjukhus Stochholm (Sweden) and Jyväskylän Yliopisto (Finland) are represented. Through the NorFa network, funding was made available to undertake research meetings and activities over three years, focusing on single case design research (although this did not preclude discussion and initiatives using other models). Academics and research students from Scandinavian universities met twice a year, and international experts in research such as Bruscia, Aldridge, Stern, Smeijsters, Ruud and Wrangsjö were invited to lead workshops and give lectures. The research school has therefore been developed on a strong foundation, and has attracted researchers from all over Europe with the intention of promoting new scientific areas within music therapy.

In 1997 funding was provided by the Faculty of Humanities for the awarding of scholarship grants to students from Denmark and abroad to undertake PhD level research while continuing their clinical work. This initiative has resulted in the registration of seven students in the last four years from Denmark, Norway, Belgium, Austria, Israel and Australia, who are at different stages of completion. At the present time, this program is the only European PhD research school specializing in music therapy. The PhD program at Aalborg University actually awards a PhD in Music Therapy, unlike many other programs where the qualification is in music or music education. This means that the research focus is exclusively on music therapy, primarily aimed at applied clinical research.

The Research School is centred within the science of music therapy, promoting both process and outcome research. PhD projects may be based on both theoretical and empirical clinical work. Research which focuses on clinical work must include a considerable element of theoretical and methodological study. The program currently meets the needs of Danish, Scandinavian and many other international students, and English is the working language.

To date, the Research School has provided a research milieu for a limited number of students, given the present level of funding for courses and research activities. In the short time it has been established, three Danish and two German researchers have successfully defended PhD theses, and seven more are working towards completion. This Research School has already established an enviable international reputation as a research milieu for music therapy in the world, taught courses in state-of-the-art research methods and research tools.

Central areas of research

The goal of the Research School is to train researchers with sufficient clinical, theoretical and musical knowledge to assure scientific rigour as well as a genuine musical aesthetic dimension.

The program promotes research within two main areas:

1. The fundamental principles of research into music therapy, including theories and methods to describe, analyse, interpret and evaluate method and process in music therapy. The special areas that will be promoted in this research are the investigation of musical parameters and the characteristics of interaction that result in therapeutic progress through effective treatment. Music therapy research is a comparatively young but rapidly developing discipline. PhD students must have a complete and up-to-date knowledge of the specific theoretical and metatheoretical aspects in this scientific area, in order that the research projects can be validated in the international arena.

2. Research within the clinical area, in particular research methodology, is directed towards both process and outcome research. Clinically applied research relates to the importance placed on the practical dimension in Danish and European Master's programs in music therapy, and leads directly to scientific reflection in Master's theses. On this basis the PhD training enables the development of a scientific body of knowledge (both nationally and internationally). Clinically based research is increasingly demanded by healthcare organizations deciding on the allocation of resources for a variety of medical/therapeutic interventions. Evidence-based practice calls for a hierarchical range of evidence to be presented supporting the efficacy of an intervention. The research milieu in the Music Therapy Research school at Aalborg University aims to promote the accumulation of such evidence and scientific knowledge.

The Aalborg PhD Research School started from a qualitative perspective, involving case study analysis, connected to the psychodynamic approach taught in Master's program in Europe. Over recent years contact with English and American research milieus has led to an increase in quantitative research. An eclectic advisory board of supervisors from Sweden, Norway, Germany, the USA and the UK has allowed the Research School to incorporate both paradigms. Applied clinical research is actively encouraged, alongside theoretical and historical studies.

In the present research milieu, both qualitative and quantitative research is undertaken, investigating process and outcome. Qualitative research methods are taught including phenomenology, grounded theory, case study research and other related methods. Quantitative methodology is taught including experimental design, applied behaviour analysis, comparison studies, descriptive statistics, basic use of parametric and non-parametric statistics, and other aspects of experimental method and design.

We actively encourage clinical research focused on evaluating effects on patients when one or more of four principal techniques of music therapy are used – clinical improvisation, receptive music therapy, songwriting or performance. Incorporated disciplines in music therapy practice also include music psychology, music in medicine and music education.

The Research School runs courses twice a year including the following subject areas:

1. the challenge of undertaking doctoral level research: formulating research questions and hypotheses; reviewing and analysing existing literature; defining an appropriate method; collecting data; analysing data, writing results; discussing the implications of research with reference to clinical applicability and limitations

2. methodology of qualitative and experimental (process and outcome) research; specific music therapy research design – e.g. phenomenological, case study and outcome research

3. qualitative methods, specifically related to clinical music therapy practice

4. music as a symbolic language (theories of semantics, interaction and communication)

5. focus on existing research in music therapy presented by guest professors to exemplify good research practice to the students. Guest teachers from Scandinavia, Europe, the USA and Australia have been invited to teach research methods on these courses.

INTERNATIONAL COLLABORATION AND NETWORKS

Formal agreement has been established between the Research School in Music Therapy at Aalborg University and University Witten/Herdecke Faculty of Medizin (Germany), and Melbourne University, Faculty of Music. The PhD program is supported by the European Music Therapy Confederation (EMTC) and the European Research Platform (ERP). The EMTC is a formally constituted body representing 23 countries in Europe, collaborating on the development of music therapy training, registration and research in Europe. The ERP has a role in developing and optimizing research collaboration in Europe. Aalborg University is represented in this group.

The PhD training program is linked to both the Master's program in Music Therapy and the Music Therapy Clinic – centre for treatment and research. The Music Therapy Clinic is a research clinic specialized in empirical clinical research, established as a collaborative project between Aalborg Psychiatric Hospital and Aalborg University.

There is also a strong link between the MA program and the Research Clinic at the Psychiatric Hospital, the innovative concept of which is that the university professors/teachers are an integrated part of staff teams with psychiatrists and psychologists on a daily basis at the hospital. This means that the research at the clinic grows out of a natural clinical setting, and informs the teaching of the music therapy students in the university. The Master's program at Aalborg University is oriented towards research-based teaching. The Research Clinic also publishes new methodologies and results of the research biennially in a series of books. So far, two volumes – *Music Therapy in Psychiatry I and II* have come out.

PREPARATION TO UNDERTAKE RESEARCH – SMALL- OR LARGE-SCALE PROJECTS

Over the years, it has become apparent that a great deal of time (and money) can be saved if adequate preparation is made to undertake research. First of all, the person intending to undertake research, whether it be a small-scale project, or something as major as a PhD study, needs to demonstrate knowledge, experience and competency. Not everyone wishing to go into research has undertaken an education in research methods and design, let alone collected previous experience. This may not be a barrier – as courses and supervision in research methods are offered by universities such as Aalborg. But to avoid wasting precious resources, all research proposals are evaluated by the International Board of Supervisors under the following criteria in order to confirm the potential value of the research, and the competence and knowledge of the researcher:

Evaluation of initial proposal

1. Formal academic background/music therapy qualifications.

2. Substance of the project and relevance to music therapy.

3. Well-stated focus and hypothesis.

4. Knowledge of related research.

5. Theoretical assumptions.

6. Relationship between theory/method of research and theme of the project.

7. Practical value of the project.

8. Professional/academic background of applicant – international orientation.

9. How realistic is the project proposal?

10. Other comments.

Perhaps the most critical issues are whether the researcher has carefully thought through the research question he/she wishes to investigate, and the potential method by which he/she intends to do so. This will also reveal the extent to which he/she has reveiwed the available literature, and learned something from others.

Six months (or one year part-time) into the program students are required to submit an extended proposal for approval by the Board of Supervisors. Every six months thereafter students are required to submit a research report and document their research activities to ensure they are working to their time-line, and that the standard is at PhD level. This is vital in maintaining the research process with scholarship students located all over Europe and further afield.

Information about the PhD program/Research School is available nationally and internationally, and the school is frequently referred to at international meetings, seminars and congresses. Details of how to apply and register are placed in international journals and professional bulletins. All researchers registered in the program present papers internationally and publish in refereed journals, which effectively markets the school. Over the last six years we have always had more applications than available places. The Research School is well presented on the international website: www.musictherapyworld.de. For further information see: http://www.musik.auc.dk/edu/phd-program/index.dk.html.

Perhaps the best way of exemplifying the model that Aalborg has developed is to look at some of the research that is going on, who is doing it, and in what areas it is focused. A short overview of some of the past and present researchers' activities follows, and all are referenced in the bibliography with papers published on or around their research.

Past students

Wolfgang Mahns is a German music therapist and educator with many years of clinical experience especially within the field of special education of children (also in public schools). He has also contributed to the literature of music therapy theory (Ruud and Mahns 1991). In 1998 has was awarded the first PhD of the new Aalborg program for his dissertation *Symbolbildung in der analytischen Kindermusiktherapie. Eine qualitative Studie über die Bedeutung der musikalischen Improvisation in der Musiktherapie mit Schulkindern* (symbol formation in Analytically Oriented Music Therapy with children). Mahns investigated the question: how can senso-motoric experiences and affective expression be transformed at a pre-verbal level through the musical interaction, and how can affects be transformed into symbolic interactions? He considers the therapeutic improvisation a unity of primary processes, relational situations, musical structures and the environmental context, and they are all understood as sources of symbolic meaning developing in the musical interaction.

Gudrun Aldridge is a German music therapist trained in the Nordoff-Robbins model and with many years of clinical experience from somatic areas including people suffering from dementia. She was awarded a PhD in 1999 for her dissertation *Die Entwicklung einer Melodie im Kontext improvisatorischer Musiktherapie – dargestellt am Beispiel der Melodien 'Ein Spaziergang durch Paris' und 'Die Abschiedsmelodie'* (the development of a melody in improvisatory music therapy) (Aldridge 1998). Based on comprehensive theoretical studies in melody theory and the meaning of melody Aldridge investigated the processes leading to the formation of a patient's personal melody in music therapy improvisations based on the Nordoff-Robbins model. These processes are studied carefully in analyses of selected melodic material from two cases. The analyses proceed at various levels, from a phenomenological description of the musical material to a psychological interpretation of the therapeutic meaning of the material. The specific research design enables a combination of the interpretations of the two cases leading to the formulation of a theory on how melody develops in active music therapy improvisations.

Torben Moe is a musician and Danish music therapist with many years of clinical experience within hospital psychiatry (Sankt Hans Hospital, Roskilde). He is a GIM therapist and primary trainer. In his thesis (defended 1 March 2001) he investigates the effect of modified GIM in group music therapy with psychiatric clients. Nine schizotypical patients participated in a slow-open group over six months. The intervention was music listening in a slightly altered state of consciousness, with directive guiding and music excerpts of 7–12 minutes length. The patients reported their imagery in the group. One part of the study investigated the general level of function of the clients (measured by the GAF test, a self-report questionnaire, a semi-structured interview and supplementary questions). It was documented that all but one patient improved their GAF score and reported benefit from the therapy. The attention (98 per cent) alone reflects the importance of the group therapy for the patients. The second, main part of the study was a qualitative analysis of the patients' imagery. Moe demonstrated that all patients produced imagery and he investigated how the imagery developed during the therapeutic process. A reconfiguration of the imagery of all but one patient was documented, and this reconfiguration reflects a process of psychological development and maturation, corresponding to the self-evaluations of the patients.

Niels Jørgensen Hannibal is working as a research assistant at the music therapy clinic at Aalborg Psychiatric Hospital and teaching at the music therapy program/course at Aalborg University. He finished and defended his research project titled *Pre-verbal Transference in Music Therapy – a qualitative investigation of transference processes in music therapy* in June 2001. This project investigated the dynamics of the transference relationship within musical interaction, based on two cases with clients suffering from personality disorders. Daniel Stern's theory about pre-verbal interaction is used to describe interaction patterns in the verbal interaction before the music, the relationship during the music and the verbal interaction after the music. These relational patterns are compared to the client's core conflict relation themes, which are identified from Luborsky's and Crits-Christoph's CCRT-method. This method is an empirical psychodynamic method used to reveal conflict themes that emerge in the therapeutic relationship. The comparison shows that the interaction patterns in the music are similar to the central verbal transference pattern and that these transference patterns can be transformed in the musical interaction. The result of the investigation reveals that: 1. musical interaction in the form of clinical improvisation has a psychotherapeutic potential, because the transference relationship in the music reflects relational conflicts patterns, and 2. development in the client's relational capability can be observed in the music. Niels Hannibal has also contributed to this book with the chapter about Daniel Stern's interaction theory.

Present stipendiate students

Hanne Mette Ochsner Ridder has been working clinically with music therapy since 1989, mainly with residents suffering from dementia at a gerontological care unit in Århus, Denmark. She is undertaking an experimental case study combining qualitative analyses with quantitative documentation with a focus on songs in individual music therapy with persons suffering from dementia. In the study – under the supervision of David Aldridge and Inge Nygaard Pedersen – Ridder examines responses and communicative signals elicited in persons with dementia in sessions where familiar and meaningful songs are sung. Six persons with dementia in middle to late stages showing agitated behaviour are participating in 20 individual music therapy sessions. All sessions are videotaped and nine clips representing the six participants and parts of the structure in the settings are analysed by external assessors with expertise in music therapy. In a period before music therapy, during sessions, and in a period after music therapy heartbeat is measured in five-second intervals, and staff fill out questionnaires concerning daily routines, health and agitation. There seem to be clear responses on the music therapy in five out of the six participants, which is reflected in gesture and communicative signs. One participant shows little or no musical response to the music, but shows changes in behaviour and physiological response. The expected date of completion is February 2003. Hanne Mette Ochsner Ridder has written this book's chapter on music therapy with the elderly (Chapter 4.5).

Ulla Holck is a Danish music therapist and body therapist. Her clinical work has centred around children and adolescents with autism and social and emotional problems. In her research project, under the supervision of Lars Ole Bonde, she investigated musical, mimical and gestural interactions of music therapists and children with severe communication disorders (mental handicaps and disorders within the autistic spectrum). Data collection was based on two-camera video recordings of five music therapists' work with this population. From this material Holck selected episodes which she analysed thoroughly, both in a horizontal and a vertical perspective, in order to reveal important dynamic factors in the interactions of therapist and client. In these micro-analyses of music and therapeutic interaction Holck has documented how client and therapist together develop unique patterns of interaction – called *interaction themes* – enabling a further development of communication skills. These musical, mimical and gestural interactions can be seen as clinical reflections of the infant research and theories of communication and interaction between mother and child formulated by Daniel Stern and Colwyn Trevarthen. The dissertation on *'Commusical' Interplay* was delivered in January 2002. Ulla Holck has written this book's chapter on music therapy with children with communication problems (Chaper 4.4).

Current scholarship students

Jos De Backer is Head of Studies on the five-year Master's program in Music Therapy at the Lemmens Institut and Leuven University in Belgium, and Head

Music Therapist at the University Psychiatric Clinic. He is doing a qualitative study under the supervision of Professor Tony Wigram, looking at changes in psychotic patients during music therapy. He is analysing improvisations to find out how sensory-motoric playing changes into musical form, representing the development of symbolization in these clients. His analysis also includes consideration of the therapist's role, transferences and *projective identification*, and the verbal discussions with the clients. This research is important in presenting the case for analytically informed music therapy as a relevant treatment for psychotic and schizophrenic patients. The expected date of completion is 2005 (De Backer and Van Camp 1996; De Backer and Van Camp 1999).

Cochavit Elefant is an experienced music therapy practitioner working in Israel with clients with developmental disability and Rett syndrome. She is actively involved as an assistant professor on music therapy courses in Tel Aviv and Jerusalem. She is undertaking a quantitative study under the supervision of Professor Tony Wigram, which includes qualitative analysis, to find evidence of intentional communication in girls with Rett syndrome. Seven girls, presented with 18 songs, have demonstrated not only their ability to choose, but also consistency of choice over time. Analysis of the live playing of these songs to the girls during individual therapy sessions, and their individual and collective preferences, has revealed responses to particular characteristics in the songs. This research is important in demonstrating the capacity of girls with Rett syndrome for intentional and meaningful communication through the motivating medium of music therapy. The expected date of completion is 2002 (Elefant 2001).

Trygve Aasgaard is a senior figure in Norwegian music therapy, a colleague and collaborator of Professor Even Ruud, and has worked in child oncology for many years. He is undertaking a qualitative study under the supervision of Professor David Aldridge, analysing the origins, history and context of songs that are created during therapy sessions with children with cancer. The lyrics of the songs form the main focus for the study, from the perspective of their construction, inherent ideas, meaning and context. He is looking also at the meaning of the songs to the rest of the family, and the relevance of positive and negative aspects of the songs to children who undergo difficult and often painful treatment for their illness. This research is important in the wider context of treating children with cancer, which has developed significantly over the last 15 years. The expected date of completion is 2002 (Aasgaard 1999, 2000a, 2000b, 2001).

Christian Gold is a music therapist working in Vienna with children with psychiatric disorders, emotional disturbance and developmental disabilities. He is undertaking a quantitative study under the supervision of Professor Tony Wigram to investigate the effect of long-term individual music therapy. He is measuring changes in behaviour with pre-test/post-test analysis of behaviour through the Child Behaviour Checklist, and measuring children's capacities and quality of life. He is also measuring treatment satisfaction, and is interested in overall effect size of treatment when compared with a control group who don't receive music therapy or any other form of psychotherapeutic intervention. He is collecting data from a number of music therapists working in the Vienna area in Austria. At the time of publication he had undertaken a pilot study, and had begun categorizing children into different clinical subgroups in order to correlate effect over time with clinical pathology. He is also looking for interactions in style of treatment, therapists' experience and changes in life events (Gold, Wigram and Berger 2001).

Rudy Garred is a Norwegian music therapist and educator. His project, under the supervision of Lektor Lars Ole Bonde, is a philosophical investigation of the concept of dialogue in Creative Music Therapy. He wants to explain if and how 'dialogue' can be a basic concept in the understanding of the role of music in Creative Music Therapy, and how the dialogic perspective may have consequences for clinical practice. The concept of dialogue is essential in the understanding of the client–therapist relationship as an existential 'meeting' (Garred 1996), and through studies in existential philosophy and music therapy theory Garred expects to uncover dynamics and dimensions in this phenomenon. His work is theoretically inspired by, amongst others, Martin Buber and Gabriel Marcel. The project lasts until 2003 (Garred 1996, 2001).

Felicity Baker is an Australian music therapist and Co-ordinator of the Music Therapy Program at University of Queensland, Australia. She is undertaking a quantitative study under the supervision of Professor Tony Wigram to establish whether singing improves the speaking intonation of people with brain injury who have monotone voices. The project also aims to establish what processes underlie these improvements – emotional changes, changes in physical tension and neurological changes. Following a 15-session singing program, she will analyse five case studies for changes in mood, posture and facial expression, vocal pitch control, intonation contour and singing performance using a Visual Analogue Scale, Multi-Speech software program (Kay Elemetrics) and various musical tests that she has designed. She hopes to show that singing not only stimulates neurological change, but that changes in mood and physical tension also play a role in improving the normality of intonation patterns. The project is expected to be completed in 2004.

5.3 Assessment and Clinical Evaluation in Music Therapy

Because music therapy has developed theory out of empirical practice, attention to the importance of assessment has been limited. But the indicator for a therapeutic treatment in other professions relies on effective and systematic assessment, and an area of Wigram's research has been directed to diagnostic assessment in child development and disability. There are many different forms of assessment we should be developing at a more scientific level to establish *reliability* and *validity*. These elements are hallmarks of the standardized assessments in psychology, speech and language therapy and neurology. This is the area where we can find a loose and rather weak interface between the humanistic model of music therapy and the natural science model found in medicine, psychology and other paramedical professions including occupational therapy, speech and language therapy and physiotherapy. The question most will ask is whether it is either possible or desirable for music therapy to attempt to formulate, and then maybe impose (through music therapy educations) some form of standardized model of assessment. Some educators like their students to grow and each develop their own style, a classic formula for generating a 'reinvention of the wheel' phenomenon. Individual differences in therapists' personality and skills make a uniform approach to music therapy practice unlikely.

However, assessment criteria could be more standardized. In the natural sciences, a new battery of tests, or criteria for evaluation, is sent out for trial. When standardized, the protocol is then used with confidence as a reliable tool. Why has this never really happened in music therapy? One explanation is that the administration of the standardized tool in the natural science professions is usually quite strict and there is little room for flexibility or creativity. What you get is what you test, and no more. This concept of a protocol of administration would be uncomfortable and alien to the style of most European-based music therapists, although there is more common ground for it in the USA. But not all assessment protocols are based on tests, and there are emerging models where the quality of what is happening is also evaluated through a freer and more flexible assessment.

Forms of assessment and data gathering

Table 5.3: Forms of assessment and evaluation	
Assessment model	**Function**
Diagnostic assessment	To obtain evidence to support a diagnostic hypothesis
General assessment	To obtain information on general needs, strengths and weaknesses
Music therapy assessment	To obtain evidence supporting the value of music therapy as an intervention
Initial period of clinical assessment in music therapy	To determine in the first two to three sessions a therapeutic approach relevant to the client
Long-term music therapy assessment	To evaluate over time the effectiveness of music therapy

(Wigram 1999c)

The collection of data will vary widely within and between these different models of assessment. There are very few 'general' models, let alone 'standardized' models, of assessment in our profession that have been developed for any of these assessment functions. Evaluation or assessment scales developed to date have focused on a variety of aspects of the music therapy process, including musical interaction (Pavlicevic 1995), response, relationship and musical communicativeness (Nordoff and Robbins 1977), diagnosis (Raijmaekers 1993), psychological function (Sikström and Skille 1995), cognitive, perceptual, motor and visual skills (Grant 1995), sound-musical profiles (Di Franco 1999), and the analysis of improvised music (Bruscia 1987) to name but a few.

While these scales or criteria for assessment typically rely on subjective opinion, and typically trials involving observer reliability or verification have not taken place, they are often detailed and well thought out with appropriate clinical applicability for a specific population. However, apart from the Nordoff and Robbins scales, I am not aware of any systematic and widespread use of any one of these models, which is a great shame considering the extent and detail of some of the parameters that can be used. Typically, therapists will collect one or more of the following types of data in order to make their evaluation in any one of these models of assessment. The term behaviour is used here as a descriptor of all types of behaviour – physiological, emotional, cognitive, unconscious etc. – and includes an understanding of human behaviour from psychotherapeutic, medical and behavioural traditions.

Table 5.4: Data gathering in assessment and evaluation	
Musical data	(Examples of musical events/musical characteristics)
Musical behavioural data	(Examples of clients' behaviour without musical description)
Behavioural data	(Characteristics of general behaviour in music therapy)
Interpretative data	(Interpretation of clients' musical and general behaviour supported or not supported by musical or behavioural data)
Comparative data	(Comparison of clients' behaviour in music therapy with information from other situations)

In order to advance our ability to provide more specific evidence of what happens in music therapy in order to substantiate our interpretation of behaviour and changes in behaviour, *analysis of music* is a natural starting point to formulate criteria for systematic assessment. This can also provide a more reliable and substantive body of evidence in the required interface between the humanistic approach and our colleagues from the natural sciences.

Assessment and evaluation tools

QUANTITATIVE ASSESSMENT TOOLS

The experimental research and clinical evaluation in the USA have for many years employed a variety of test instruments. In a recent article by Diane Gregory (Gregory 2000) in the *Journal of Music Therapy*, 183 articles in the journal during this period were research studies, 92 of which included a test instrument. She found a total of 115 different test instruments that were used in the evaluation of the effectiveness of music therapy. These were primarily psychological or psychometric methods of evaluation and, of the 92, only 20 were concerned with evaluating musical function. Of these 20, 50 per cent were concerned with evaluating musical skills or musical performance. Gregory commented that the variety of tests documented provided an all-encompassing range of client populations and a broad view of human behaviour which might be included in the practice of music as therapy.

It's clear from such a review of the literature that few tools have been developed that are specifically concerned with the evaluation of music therapy process and outcome from a music therapy point of view. There is a wider range of more specific assessment modalities used to evaluate therapeutic change and development in children and the learning-disabled population. Brian Wilson and David Smith from Western Michigan University in the USA made another survey of music therapy assessment in school settings (Wilson and Smith 2000).

They found, for example, a variety of developmental instruments to look at, e.g. improved communication in children with autism, such as the study undertaken by Cindy Edgerton (1994) who rated communicative and social behaviour in terms of musical interactiveness in improvised music-making. Others have assessed behaviour during music therapy or compared it with behaviour in other environments. Some therapists want to measure the effect of music instruction on rhythmic skills, and those specific studies are undertaken to, for example, investigate the relationship between the degree of disability and vocal range.

Some of these assessment protocols are linked to perceptual skills and cognitive development in order to evaluate whether music therapy can have an influence at a developmental level. However, in Wilson and Smith's review (2000), they noted that of the 41 studies that had used a music-based assessment with children with disabilities, only 16 of those were 'named' assessments and only three of those were used in more than one study. This lack of replication makes it difficult to generalize results beyond those of the original sample. It raises an important question for music therapists as to whether an assessment tool can be developed which is standardized and replicable with any level of reliability and validity.

QUALITATIVE ASSESSMENT TOOLS

From a very different point of view, music therapists working in qualitative research have tried to develop a more phenomenological and experiential model for evaluating changes that occur in music therapy sessions over time. Colin Lee has developed a method of analysing improvisations in music therapy which involves a nine-stage process. The first stage requires a holistic listening to the improvisation several times in order to obtain a sense of the whole of the piece of music that is being made and to look at those particular musical elements, properties or structures that are the most significant. Stage two involves the responses of the therapist to the music, whilst stage three requires the client to listen to their music and identify moments that they see as important. The fourth stage, used by Lee in his PhD study on the effects of music therapy with clients with HIV, involves taking improvisations to different experts, such as a musician, psychotherapist or another music therapist, and asking them to listen to an improvised section of a therapy session and identify significant points in the music as well as describing it. The final four stages of Lee's process involve a detailed transcription of the music, notating it and then analysing it to look at the structure and line of the music (Lee 2000).

BRUSCIA'S IMPROVISATION ASSESSMENT PROFILES

Another model of assessment was developed by Ken Bruscia during the 1980s and is called Improvisation Assessment Profiles (Bruscia 1987). Here, the therapist can analyse the music from the point of view of different psychological constructs, as well as musical constructs, such as variability, autonomy, salience, integration, congruence and tension. The relationship of the different elements of music, such as rhythm, melody, harmony and others, is looked at in some detail through these different profiles, and scales are used of musical parameters in order to identify salient and important aspects in music-making. A developmental use of this model has been undertaken by Wigram in his work in assessing and diagnosing children with communication disorders (Wigram 1991c, 1992b, 1995a, 1999a, 1999b, 1999c, 1999e, 2000a, 2000b). Analysing musical excerpts from improvised therapy sessions, particularly using the profiles of Autonomy to look at the interpersonal experiences that are going on between the therapist and the client, and Variability to look at the degree of rigidity or freedom present in the music of the client, have been of particular value in identifying musical elements and musical behaviour that can support or deny a hypothesized diagnosis.

LOEWY'S PSYCHOTHERAPEUTIC ASSESSMENT METHOD

Joanne Loewy (Loewy 2000) has developed a model for music psychotherapy assessment. She comments that though the music serves as a primary means of understanding the process of the moment, it is the words that can be assigned to describe the musical experience that will help the therapist to interpret its significance. The words will represent the clinical work in medical records and reports on the patient's process. Loewy has described 13 areas of inquiry that are relevant for music therapy assessment, looking at the awareness of the self, others and of the moment, thematic expression, listening and performing, the collaboration between client and therapist, degrees of concentration, range of affect, investment and motivation, the use of structure, integration, self-esteem, risk taking and independence. She differentiates the individual areas of inquiry into subgroups relating to the relationship, the dynamics, levels of achievement and cognition.

HINTZ GERIATRIC ASSESSMENT METHOD

Geriatric music therapy clinical assessment has been explored by Michelle Hintz from Temple University in the USA, looking at an assessment of musical skills and related behaviours. Her assessment addresses five main areas: expressive musical skills, receptive musical skills, behavioural/psychosocial skills, motor skills and cognitive memory skills. She is working on the basis that both active music-making and responses to music can be evaluated to look at levels of responsivity in the client, and their process in therapy. Unlike many assessment procedures, it involves scoring, which is a method common to other professions such as speech and language therapy and clinical psychology (Hintz 2000).

ASSESSMENT FOR DIAGNOSTIC PURPOSES

Many therapists define the process of assessment not in terms of a tool, but in terms of the development of a therapeutic interaction over the first two or three sessions. Some therapists have used assessment for primarily diagnostic purposes, either to explore evidence in music therapy sessions of the nature of the personality of the client or to look more carefully at their pathology and underlying difficulties.

Tony Wigram and Amelia Oldfield in the United Kingdom have both (separately) developed a model of assessment with children where they have defined a process during a session giving specific details about some of the activities they engage children in. This can include a choice of instruments, playing tonal music and atonal music, developing rhythmic interactions, singing and many other diverse elements.

Paul Nordoff and Clive Robbins, pioneer music therapists who worked in the United Kingdom, the USA, Australia and some Scandinavian countries, have written up assessment tools including scales of musical responsiveness, client–therapist relationship etc. Their tools have been taught and used by music therapists training in this particular methodology (Nordoff and Robbins 1977).

Janet Graham has recently written up a case study using the Nordoff-Robbins scales in the book *Assessment and Evaluation in the Arts Therapies* (Wigram 2000b), and uses the different Nordoff-Robbins scales to illustrate her work with a 26-year-old man with severe learning disability and autistic spectrum disorder. He was referred to develop communication skills, to encourage interaction and reduce isolation, and to offer him an opportunity for self-expression. She described the assessment period of three sessions, each lasting 20 minutes, and reported that in the initial sessions, the client was very anxious and very difficult to persuade to enter the music therapy room. Initiating musical engagement and defining it on the Nordoff-Robbins client–therapist relationship in musical activity scale, Graham showed that at the beginning of the session he was unresponsive and didn't accept approaches, but as the session progressed he moved up to level 3 on the scale, where he could engage in limited responsive activity. Because Nordoff-Robbins' methods involve the detailed analysis of musical material on their tapes, Graham was able to document, through her index sheet in the first session, the musical development of simple rhythms in the client (Graham 2000).

SPECIFIC TOOLS AND SCALES

Juliette Alvin gave us a criteria for describing listening responses, instrumental responses and vocal responses that looks at both musical and psychological process in a qualitative way (Bruscia 1987). Edgerton developed a quantitative tool. Paul Nordoff and Clive Robbins, as mentioned previously, developed different scales: the 13 categories of response, the child–therapist relationship, musical communicativeness and Musical Response Scales III. Amelia Oldfield has developed a diagnostic assessment method. Mercedes Pavlicevic developed her Musical Interaction Ratings (MIRs) for her research in schizophrenia: a nine-point scale for describing the nature of interpersonal and intermusical relatedness. Karin Schumacher and Calvert-Kruppa (1999) have recently published their tool – the Analysis of the Quality of the Relationship (AQR). Anne Steen-Møller has developed a method for describing five levels of contact (see Chapter 4.2).

These evaluation methods are specific to what happens in the music therapy situation. Two of them use quantitative methods of evaluation, while the majority use qualitative. But they nevertheless are a systematic way of recording and documenting aspects of change that occur in the therapy. There are other standardized tools, such as the Child Behaviour Checklist or the Susan Spence Social Skills Questionnaires, that can be used to look more generally at behaviour and emotional problems.

Example

As an example of music therapy assessment, we can look at a case study of a 7-year-old child with autistic spectrum disorder. (This case is part of a larger article on evidence-based practice published in the *British Journal of Music Therapy* (Wigram 2002).) In this area, music therapy has a unique contribution to offer, as autistic children and adults have core impairments in:

- social interaction
- social communication
- imaginative play.

There is also normally the presence of rigid, repetitive patterns of activity, stereotypical play, an adherence to routine, and a significant difficulty in coping with change.

Case study: Joel

Joel was referred to Harper House for assessment to evaluate his strengths and difficulties. He was diagnosed autistic, but the clinic referring him were uncertain about how autistic he was.

He was described with the following problems:

- no use of non-verbal behaviour to regulate social interaction
- does not use direct eye contact
- bad at relating to other people – and other children
- does not share enjoyment
- lack of socially imitative play
- stereotypical, ritualistic behaviour.

Speech and language therapy

In the speech and language therapy assessment, Joel had poor concentration, and did not take the initiative in verbal communication. There was evidence that he understood instructions, but in a test called Clinical Evaluation of Language Fundamentals (Pre-School) he achieved an age level of 3.1 years.

Cognitive psychology

In the cognitive psychology assessment, a Kauffman ABC, Joel achieved an intelligence quotient equivalent of 79. This indicated that his overall intellectual ability was within the normal range, although poorly developed. He had well below average scores in the achievement subtests of arithmetic and reading/decoding.

Music therapy

Joel was reported to be responsive to music. Music therapy assessment was recommended to see if there were potential strengths that would not be found in other assessments. The session lasted 50 minutes, and the table that follows describes 13 events in the therapy session, giving a description of Joel's behaviour and way of making music (see Table 5.5). In the right-hand column are the corresponding relevant 'expectations' that can be proposed for future music therapy intervention.

Defining the expectations of treatment might be considered difficult, risky, even impossible, by some in the field of music therapy. This very much depends on the clarity with which the child presents their strengths and weaknesses, and the focus of therapy. It will also depend on the previous experience of the therapist and the confidence with which he/she is able to predict potential outcome, based on previous cases with a similar presentation.

However, what is described below illustrates a method of defining the potential value of music therapy for a child, giving criteria that describe how the therapy will help the child overcome the difficulties inherent in his/her pathology, and that provide a clear explanation to other professionals involved, such as doctors, therapists and teachers, of the function of music therapy.

Table 5.5: Table showing the events in therapy, response and interaction of Joel, and the expectations of therapy			
	Events in therapy assessment	Response and interaction with Joel	Relationship to expectations of therapy
1	Speech and language therapy assessment:	Joel has poor concentration, he is distracting himself, and there is a lack of initiation	Answer Questions Understand language
2	Piano duet	I am accompanying and supporting Joel matches tempo and rhythm Joel starts to reference me by looking	Development of awareness Development of concentration Activating intersubjective behaviours
3	Piano duet 2	Pentatonic improvisation Joel references more and more He moderates tempo and volume with me: from f to p, from allegro to adagio Piano descends chromatically Joel takes over melody Joel starts moving his body Joel initiates change – kicking his legs	Shared and understood experiences Tolerance of change Flexibility Entrained responses Motivated interaction

	Events in therapy assessment	Response and interaction with Joel	Relationship to expectations of therapy
4	Continues piano	Starts to vary – asks to stop Recognizes a musical cadence: stops	Development of organization Shared experience
5	Drum duet	Variable and interactive Stable tempo – great sense of timing Can play in phrases Uses crescendos	Developed sense of self Relationship building Intersubjective behaviour
6	Drums and piano	Watching and working *with* me Feels and plays the timing in the music Breaks his own patterns	Empathic synchronicity Organization and structure Spontaneous initiation of contact
7	Dropping drumsticks on the drum	Copies what I am doing Starts using language with cues Laughing when I fail to catch the stick	Development of meaningful gestures Shared emotions Development of memory Shared experience
8	Asking him to copy rhythmic patterns	Watching me carefully He is laughing at my reaction when he deliberately does it wrong Starts a repetitive pattern of behaviour – but related to me	Awareness, attention Empathic synchronicity Relationship building
9	Imaginative game: going to sleep, waking up and having breakfast	Joel understands the idea of the game Simultaneously shares my 'Ugghh' when I pretend to eat the drumstick Drinks the 'imaginative' cup of tea	Imaginative play Shared emotions Understood experience Intersubjective behaviour

	Events in therapy assessment	Response and interaction with Joel	Relationship to expectations of therapy
10	Piano and drums	Joel started on the piano, then moved to the drums and cymbal He became independent, allowing me to accompany him	Developed and increased sense of self Containment of emotional expression
11	Microphone duet	Joel accompanies himself on the piano Develops vocal turn-taking with me More and more spontaneous language Imaginative: ends with 'I'll kick your bottom!'	Development of communicative vocalization Emergence of language in songs Developed sense of self
12	Joel singing with me on piano	Joel makes up his own words He takes a solo role Role-playing a style of singing	Emergence of language in songs Development of communicative vocalization Containment of emotional expression Increased sense of self
13	'Hello' interaction	Joel starts saying 'hello' to the speaker. I respond. He takes the microphone and sings 'hello'. He develops this, getting excited. It is like a recitative. His timing of phrases in musical structure is very developed.	Intersubjective behaviour Spontaneous initiation of contact Shared and understood experience Empathic synchronicity – shared emotions

During this session, Joel demonstrated many potentials. He could share, take turns, initiate, use verbal language spontaneously, concentrate for long periods – for example, the first period of time he played on the piano lasted 13 minutes without stopping – and during this time he demonstrated he could share emotions, indicating emotional synchronicity. He could also follow musical cues, anticipate, structure, go into imaginative play, and anticipate the way I was thinking and reacting.

This doesn't mean he was not autistic. There are many factors to take into account, and apparently interactive and social behaviour in this session may be atypical. However, it can indicate that in music therapy interaction the individual behind the autistic pathology was allowed to come out – and demonstrate his potential.

Conclusion

Music therapy assessment has an important and unique contribution to make to the diagnosis, assessment and treatment of physical, psychological and emotional illnesses, handicaps and disturbances. Music therapy provides an important part of the picture. Both in terms of the potential for free play, and also for more structured and directed play, music therapy offers a unique space for a client to demonstrate their strengths, perhaps more than their weaknesses, and this can add considerably to the material evident from a full assessment. In all clinical areas, the need for an assessment is recognized as the first stage in determining the 'indication' or appropriateness of therapeutic intervention. Music therapists have developed some tools for this and, through research, are further developing skills and tools in this area. While there is still no standardization of assessment tools, those that have been developed offer some very effective and appropriate ways of analysing and recording change in music therapy. The study by Gregory (2000) also revealed that in music therapy research (and to some degree in clinical practice) other relevant and standardized tools or forms of assessment can be drawn upon to evaluate the effect over time of music therapy on a wide variety of populations.

5.4 Evidence Based Practice in Music Therapy

Evidence Based Practice (EBP) is increasingly applied in order to determine what interventions should be funded, and can be understood as an approach to healthcare that promotes the collection, interpretation and integration of valid, important and applicable patient-reported, clinician-observed and research-derived evidence. In order to meet the requirements of EBP, clinical effectiveness must be demonstrated. Clinical effectiveness is the degree or extent to which the desired outcome is achieved when an intervention, which is known to be efficacious, is applied to a population. This brings us right back to the argument at the end of the previous section regarding the ability to predict expectations of treatment. Health authorities are concerned with the evidence that can support the expectations presented by a discipline or individual therapist. This demand has undoubtedly come in partly as a result of the increasing costs of healthcare, but also because of the increasing incidence of consumer preference – the general public is much more informed now, the field of medicine and therapy is no longer a mystery, and people would like to know whether an intervention is going to help them before they start, rather than find out afterwards that it was a 'shot-in-the-dark'.

Primarily, the clinicians (and the researcher behind the clinicians) are being called upon to show that they are making appropriate, up-to-date interventions, and that there is some evidence that those interventions are effective. What is less than satisfactory, but sometimes the case, is that out-of date interventions are administered, with no evidence they will help, and sometimes even administered ineffectively.

What, then, are the types of evidence that can be offered to support music therapy as an intervention?

- *Direct evidence* can be provided through the clinician's assessment, intermediate evaluation and staged analysis of therapeutic change. Observable changes in musical behaviour are related to generalizable change. Interpretation must be supported by argument and by specific musical events or sequences of events. Meaning and intentionality has to be drawn out of significant moments in therapy.

- *Related evidence* can be sought from the literature, and from case study material provided by clinicians working in the same pathological field, but not necessarily using the same method or approach. An international database of music therapists in clinical specialisms would be of significant value in facilitating the acquisition of such related evidence.

- *Research evidence* can be obtained both from the literature and by undertaking qualitative and/or quantitative investigations. A clinical example of a patient with Rett syndrome illustrates the potential to provide *direct* and *related evidence*, and the continuing need for *research evidence*.

Traditionally illnesses and disorders have been treated by interventions that are either based on biomedical or clinical research, or on assumptions regarding beneficial effect from clinical and anecdotal report. For example, physical therapy is indicated for physical problems, speech pathology for problems related to language and communication, and psychology, psychotherapy or medication is indicated for behavioural and mental health problems. There is still limited specification by healthcare organizations of conditions for which music therapy is an indicated treatment, challenging the profession to consider a paucity in systematic assessment, evaluation and research, and a lack of documentation in scientific journals other than music therapy publications. Yet is this really a deficiency in the music therapy profession?

Quantitative and qualitative research, and case study analysis, reveals the potential of music therapy as an indicated treatment for the above-named conditions, and many more (Bruscia 1991; Nordoff and Robbins 1971; Standley 1995; Unkefer 1990; Wigram *et al.* 1995). Purchasers of healthcare vary from one to another, and are not always consistent in their demands. Some may require hard data from randomized controlled trials, while others accept evidence from a 'body of knowledge' accumulated from various clinical interventions over time.

It is this 'body of knowledge' that can provide the clinician with material evidence to support the indication, initiation and continuation of music therapy intervention.

Issues connected to experimental studies and randomized controlled trials

The includability of evidence within this hierarchical structure does merit careful consideration and argument. The Cochrane Reviews only include studies involving randomized controlled trials (RCTs). Different types of evidence are admissible, and while RCTs are considered more reliable than other forms of evidence, and are sometimes called the 'gold standard', there are frequent occasions where RCTs are not suitable or even possible.

For the efficacy of music therapy to be recognized, and for the lack of RCTs not to be used as a principal point of challenge or criticism, some points need to be taken into consideration:

1.   Studies measuring the effects of music therapy using recorded music within an RCT model are documented in *Research in Music Therapy: A Tradition of Excellence* (Standley and Prickett 1994).

2.   Music therapy practised in Europe predominantly involves techniques of active, improvisational music-making. Studies using this method are difficult to control and impossible to replicate. This is particularly so with the autistic and learning-disabled population. RCTs are not appropriate as methods of investigation for some populations, and it is often impossible to match subjects in order to create a control.

3.   Music therapists have comparatively small case-loads of any one pathology, and are not paid to undertake research. Most of their efforts over the last 35 years of development have focused on providing clinical services, recording case material and reporting on cases.

4.   To support the RCTs that have been undertaken, Music therapy practitioners and researchers have collected a substantial number of case studies in journals and edited books.

5.   In the United Kingdom, as part of the process to be included in an Act of Parliament, evidence was presented to the Council for Professions Supplementary to Medicine in 1990/1991 on the efficacy of music therapy. This evidence, together with the criteria and standards by which music therapists are trained, examined and practise clinically, was then evaluated by medical, paramedical and nursing institutions and organizations. As a result, music therapy was granted state registration by an amendment to the 1960 Profession's Supplementary to Medicine (PSM) Act of Parliament.

6.   If RCTs are the only criteria for funding treatments, then other disciplines such as psychiatry, psychotherapy, physiotherapy, speech and language therapy and occupational therapy will find it equally hard to provide evidence.

7.   Treatment for the learning-disabled and psychiatric populations is not governed alone by evidence of change, improvement or cure from experimental research. Maintaining stability and preventing deterioration is important to prevent even more costly care. Quality of life, motivation and interest in the environment is equally important.

RCTs are only one type of evidence that can be submitted and considered under EBP, albeit perhaps one of the most persuasive ones. Table 5.6 illustrates a list of different types of evidence that can be sought to put together that body of knowledge and underpin EBP.

Table 5.6 Hierarchical structure for Evidence Based Practice and its relationship to music therapy research and clinical records

Title	Type of evidence	Found in music therapy
Systematic review	This is a review where evidence has been systematically identified, appraised and summarized according to predetermined criteria. This is sometimes referred to as an 'overview'	Standley (1995) is a good example of this
Review	A review is a summary of the available literature	Very commonly found in the opening sections of Master's and PhD theses. This needs to be more easily available to music therapy clinicians
Randomized controlled trials (RCTS)	This is a research experiment (trial) where subjects are randomly assigned to two groups – one experimental group, receiving treatment, and one control group receiving an alternative treatment, placebo or no treatment	There are some RCTs in music therapy research, but also relevant arguments why they can be inappropriate (Aldridge 1993)
Case control studies	Where patients with a particular disorder are matched with controls	There are few examples in music therapy literature
Case series	These are retrospective studies that look at clinical records	There are no examples in music therapy, but we have considerable potential for collecting evidence in this way
Case reports/case studies	This is an individual study of a case	This is the most common type of evidence found in music therapy, and provides us with much of our clinical evidence
Qualitative studies	These studies are natural and holistic. They emphasize processes, and are oriented to investigate and explore people's subjective experiences, perceptions and concerns	This form of evidence has become increasingly popular in music therapy, and is so valuable in explaining process as well as outcome
Expert opinion	This involves experts in a particular clinical speciality giving an opinion	Not commonly used in music therapy. We have our own 'experts', but the effect of renowned and credible experts from different disciplines can be seen from the evidence given by Professor Oliver Sacks to the US Senate Hearing on Older Americans.

Music therapy expects to achieve observable and measurable change in clients. There is a large body of evidence from clinical reports showing change and development in patients over time in the literature. It is clear that health institutions, schools and community-based units run by social services continue to employ music therapists because their method of therapy with patients is effective, and results can be seen in a variety of areas.

In addition to the more complex process by which research evidence is gathered, analysed and presented to underpin EBP, methods of reporting clinical work are important. The method by which music therapists present the results of their work has evolved and developed in order to describe the process and outcome of therapy. This is based on a formula where a number of important elements have to be included.

Here is an example where the referral for therapy has highlighted emotional issues in an isolated and withdrawn client.

- *Needs of the client* (defined by initial assessment and the requirements of a multidisciplinary team or teachers' group):

  To resolve internal conflicts, find the resources to express emotional feelings, overcome a feeling of isolation.

- *Objectives and goals of therapy*

  1. Work through a process of looking inside myself
  2. Explore my relationships
  3. Externalize feelings and thoughts.

- *Treatment methodology*

  1. Free improvisation using chosen instruments, tonal and atonal
  2. Improvised songwriting
  3. Listening to music and discussion.

- *Expectations of treatment*

  1. The patient will develop significantly greater self-esteem and confidence
  2. The patient will overcome anxiety and withdrawal in social situations
  3. The patient will gain insight into his/her own behaviour.

- *Evaluation criteria*

  1. Pre-therapy/post-therapy standardized measure of self-esteem
  2. Analysis of changes in musical expressivity

3. Analysis of changes in self-perception found in verbal discussion

4. Patient self-report.

- *Descriptions of events in the therapy process*

    This material is presented in the form of a narrative report, with described or notated musical examples. Therapy frequently occurs in phases, and the therapist defines the process and progress of the treatment over time in stages, giving examples from each stage (one, two or more sessions for each stage).

- *Outcome of therapy*

    This is a documentation based on the results of the *evaluation criteria*, correlated with the *objectives and goals of therapy* and the *expectations of treatment.*

- *Recommendations for further intervention*

    Financial resources for lengthy or even infinite periods of therapy are limited, and music therapists make recommendations for further periods of therapy based on revisions to the *needs of the client* and the *objectives and goals of therapy.*

The information that is provided by a music therapist within these general headings may be more quantitative, or more qualitative, or a combination of both, depending on the focus and approach used in the therapy work. To date, music therapists have typically written narrative reports on a patient's therapy sessions, with occasional but inconsistent reference to one source of raw data – musical material. This style has developed over time due to the need to 'translate' the potential jargon of musical and music therapy language into a terminology and clinical frame that other professions can understand. Therefore the interpretation of what occurred in the music therapy session has often been documented, without enough description of the actual event. So when an adult with acute anxiety plays in an emotional way on a set of drums, the report might read '… Christian expressed both frustration and anger in his music when playing the drum-set, and the therapist musically supported and acknowledged his emotional needs'. This gives us a concept of the issues that are emerging in the therapy process, but not how they emerge, or how the therapist works with them. The important, additional details to include in this example are:

- *Context*: a description of Christian's typical way of playing – musical examples

- *Event*: a description of the music that was interpreted to represent frustration and anger – musical example

- *Supportive data*: details of any verbal material from Christian that supports the interpretation of this music as representing anger and frustration

- *Contextual frame*: what this means in terms of 1. Christian's insight into his problems, 2. a change, a breakthrough or a new direction in the process of therapy, 3. whether the event can be connected to, or correlated with, any other important events happening at or around that moment in Christian's life

- *Role of music and role of therapist*: to give a more precise definition to the process of the therapy, particularly defining the musical elements and the therapist's musical/therapeutic function in facilitating this event.

Related members of a multidisciplinary team – doctors, psychiatrists, nurses, other therapists, teachers, specialists – can see an important therapeutic event has occurred, and a patient they are also concerned with may have made a significant shift in their process. What also needs to be explained is how this happened – otherwise music therapy as a process, and also in terms of outcomes, will be perceived as a rather magical and mystical therapeutic intervention.

This has presented music therapists with a challenge that has been increasingly addressed in recent years – how best to document their work so that it is understandable by other professionals and the public. Understanding musical and music therapy language is not seen as hard – and although one might not expect other professionals to understand *accelerando* or *ritardando*, everyday terms to describe musical material, such as faster, slower, with accents, monotone, louder, softer, pausing, rhythmic, without rhythm, are included in reports to give more specificity. Some music therapists notate the improvisations, or at least short themes or fragments of improvisations, in order to provide the raw material from the therapy, much the same as an art therapist might attach a picture drawn by a client to a report. Psychologists will attach the data form giving the raw scores in order that the data from which their interpretation is drawn is presented in support. In the literature, music therapists have presented their 'data' as verbal descriptions of musical material, musical notations, or verbal descriptions of behaviour (without reference to musical data).

More recently, in order to provide the actual material from which an analysis and interpretation is made, music therapists have attached tapes and CDs of musical improvisations to reports and publications. Related professionals, relatives of patients and members of the public then have the opportunity to hear the therapy work directly, while following the explanation and interpretation of the therapist in the text. Video examples have also been included in lengthier works. The form of presentation depends significantly on the context of the work, and to whom the report is being addressed. However, as all other professions with whom music therapists work have a discrete professional language or 'jargon' that needs to be learned and understood by others, music therapists similarly can and do describe the process and outcome of their therapy work in music therapy 'jargon'. The language of music as an art medium, and music therapy as a therapeutic medium, is in many ways universal, and can be followed and understood.

Conclusion

Clear and comprehensible documentation of clinical work remains a challenge for music therapists, a challenge to interface and correlate the artistic, scientific and clinical processes involved in the therapy. This is the process by which further evidence will be gathered and documented that meets the criteria of Evidence Based Practice.

CHAPTER 6

Music Therapy Training – A European, Bachelor's/ Master's Model

Introduction: The Training of a Music Therapist

'Music therapist' is not a protected professional title in European countries. Indeed, as anyone can call himself/herself an 'architect' without having completed a recognized course, it is possible to work as a 'music therapist' without having a certificate from a recognized training program. And of course it is possible to be a fine music therapist without having formal qualifications – that was the situation of most of the pioneers mentioned in Chapters 1 and 3. However, it is not possible to become a qualified music therapist without years of training, and because of the massive development of theoretical understanding, research and clinically applied skills over the last 40 years, anyone attempting to practise music therapy without having undergone a recognized training course would be uneducated, unskilled, uninformed and professionally irresponsible.

Music therapy training has also diversified in its development, and three typical models of formalized training have emerged over the last three decades.

1. *A full training program comprising Bachelor's and Master's level*

This is the model on which the training program at Aalborg University is based. Since 1996 the training is composed of a three-year Bachelor's program and a two-year Master's program. The formal requirements are a Danish upper secondary school leaving examination ('studentereksamen') or equivalent. Musical qualifications and motivation are examined in an entrance test (see Chapter 6.2). Licence to practice is granted when the full, five-year qualification is achieved. Three to four year bachelor educations are typical in Germany, Australia, the USA and Canada. Research Master's qualifications are optional courses in Australia and the USA.

2.   *A specific music therapy training course on top of a Bachelor level course in a relevant field*

This is a classic model found in many European countries (Norway, Sweden, Great Britain, Germany, France), sometimes at music conservatoires (i.e. Oslo, Stockholm, Guildhall), but also based in colleges of higher education and universities as a post-graduate study (England, Ireland, Italy, Spain). Students are often music teachers, musicians or healthcare workers with the necessary musical qualifications. The training course may last one or two years, in some programs with the possibility of qualifying at Master's level.

3.   *Short music therapy courses for professionals in related fields*

Many music teachers, nurses, occupational therapists etc. include music and musical activities in their work with pupils, clients or patients. In most countries short courses are arranged for these professionals by music therapy organizations or associations. The purpose is not to train participants as music therapists, but to teach techniques, methods, theories and interventions relevant in a particular field.

Overviews of international training programs of all three types can be found at www.hisf.no/njmt/associations.html.

The rest of this chapter is an introduction to the music therapy training program in Aalborg University – its philosophy, requirements and contents.

6.1 The Music Therapy Program at Aalborg University

The Music Therapy Program at Aalborg University meets the expectations and areas of professional competence described in the 1996 definition of music therapy by the World Federation of Music Therapy (see Chapter 1.2). In the psychotherapeutically oriented approach common in Europe, the primary task of the music therapist is to create a contact, to understand and support the client, and to help the process of interpretation through musical experiences and verbal discussions. By this means, the therapist facilitates the psychotherapeutic process. The music therapist, the client and the music are all important elements in this process.

The training program at Aalborg started in 1982, and is the only recognized training program in Denmark. This five-year, full-time, Master's level program qualifies the student in the use of music therapy at a scientific and clinical level to work independently for treatment and overall development. Students are also trained to work within multidisciplinary teams, both internally in their university program, and externally by means of practical placements in institutions in Denmark or other countries where they can receive supervision. The program gives equal weight to academic study, personal development, musical training, scientific research methodology and clinical skills.

The program was founded on a broad psychodynamic and humanistic basis, with a rather eclectic approach, since the founder Inge Nygaard Pedersen was a musicologist who also trained at the Music Therapy Mentor Course in Herdecke (Germany). This international two-year course included basic training in Creative Music Therapy (the Nordoff-Robbins tradition) and Analytical Music Therapy (taught by Mary Priestley).

These two models are very different in their understanding of man as well as music, so Inge Nygaard Pedersen and her colleague Benedikte Scheiby brought inspiring and fertile epistemological controversies to the new program in Aalborg: is man primarily a spiritual or a social being? Is music primarily an aesthetic expression following its own specific rules, or is music a symbolic expression of human emotions and psychological states?

During the first ten years the Aalborg program had an orientation primarily towards the German/Central European music therapy tradition, which is essentially psychodynamic and humanistic-existential. During the 1990s the scope of the training program broadened; the Anglo-American tradition of behaviourism and positivism is included in the curriculum. Thus the program acknowledges the current multi-paradigmatic situation within the field of music therapy. The students need to know that different clinical models, theoretical traditions and research paradigms have had, and continue to have, influence on the music therapy profession, and that these different perspectives may inform clinical practice as well as theoretical understanding of music in/as therapy.

However, the Aalborg program's concept of music and man is humanistic, and the psychodynamic tradition (as outlined broadly in Chapter 2.3) is still considered the important and primary focus and philosophy. It is the most relevant framework for a theoretical understanding of a variety of pathologies and client problems, and as a basis for the development of a therapeutic identity. A humanistic world-view includes the understanding of man as a body–mind–soul entity. These three 'levels' and perspectives on life are considered universal, however man is never independent of his specific cultural and social environment. This world-view includes a specific understanding of health and treatment: the acknowledgement of man's inherent self-healing resources, which can be stimulated and supported by therapy. Health and disease are not dichotomous either/or conditions. We believe that health involves a complex interplay of body, mind and soul. Therefore, health is better

understood as a continuum, on which the individual may place himself/herself differently, depending on how he/she copes with life's many crises, threats, stressful
and important events on each of the three levels. Bruscia (1998, Chapter 10)
presents a broad discussion of this – salutogenic – understanding of health and gives
the following definition:

> Health is the process of becoming one's fullest potential for individual and eco-
> logical wholeness. (p.84)

A humanistic understanding of music means that music is considered a man-made, a
culturally and socially grounded means of self-expression, communication and
interpersonal exchange. Music and sound may be considered a stimulus, i.e. on the
level of the body, but this is a very limited understanding of the phenomenon. On
the level of the soul, music may be understood as a divine and universal source of
knowledge; however, the question about the meaning of music is much broader. On
the level of the mind, music is a phenomenon of consciousness (Bastian 1987).
Meaning is produced in the process of musical creation (composing, improvising) as
well as in the process of musical reception (listening with body, mind and soul).
These two processes of meaning production are not identical, as music is always
ambiguous, unable to express precise, denotative meaning like language. This is not
considered a limitation, but a specific property of music that makes it an invaluable
therapeutic tool. A humanistic understanding of music acknowledges that musical
meaning is produced in a process and a context where the prerequisites of the participants play an important part. This does not mean that a client must have formal
musical qualifications or training; on the contrary, the music therapist must always
base his/her interventions on the awareness of how music is experienced by the
bodies, minds and souls of the participants. Music cannot be analysed or understood
as an abstract, autonomous object, no matter if we are dealing with a great artwork
or a simple clinical improvisation (see also Chapter 2.4).

A music therapist needs a broad, undogmatic understanding of music – as well as
a knowledge of, and skills within, many types of musical expressions and experiences. This is why the Aalborg program attaches so much importance to the musical
self-experience of the student, and also to the acquisition of therapeutically flexible
musical skills. In the psychodynamic tradition, self-experience (training analysis) is
considered the basis of psychotherapeutic training. In the same way we consider the
student's experiences as a 'student client' in music therapy (individually and in
groups) a necessary foundation for his/her development as a 'student therapist'.

The therapeutic identity is developed and trained through specific curriculum
elements (self-experience training, see Chapter 6.5) and through practicum periods.
One unique training module in the Aalborg program is 'clinical group music therapy

skills', where students learn to work with the dynamics of group music therapy through role-playing different clinical populations (Wigram 1996a). In these sessions, students not only start to develop their skills and resources as therapists (as well as finding more out about their potentials and weaknesses), but they also experience and start to understand what it must be like to have a serious pathology or illness.

In the practicum periods students learn to observe experienced music therapists at work, and gradually they develop skills in organizing and conducting their own clinical work with clients in psychiatric or special pedagogical institutions (see Chapter 6.6).

6.2 Entrance Examinations

All music therapy training programs arrange a yearly entrance test for new applicants. Formal requirements and specific skills that are sought in potential students/therapists vary from one program to another, and applicants must find the necessary information, most of which is available on the world wide web (see Chapter 7.3). The Aalborg training program attaches particular importance to competent musical skills and expressive potential in singing, instrumental playing and ear training, plus the personal maturity and realistic motivation necessary for a therapy student. The applicant must sing a prepared song, by heart and without accompaniment (e.g. a Danish song, a jazz ballad or a hymn), and it should be performed in tune, with expression and in style. A prepared piano piece must be played (e.g. an Invention by Bach, a jazz ballad from Real Book), with correct notes, in an adequate tempo and with sense of style. There are musical hearing tests including discerning chord types (major or minor), the number of tones in a cluster/chord, ability to repeat back melodies and rhythms to evaluate musical memory, and melodic prolongation in different styles. Applicants are also evaluated in their piano skills in sight-reading and harmonic chordal accompaniment (although this second element can be done on guitar).

The expressive potential, imagination and skills are tested with three improvisation tasks during the entrance interview, which have both therapeutic content and an evaluation of personal and *musical creativity*:

1. Piano improvisation: a dialogue with a professor on a selected theme, e.g. 'In the jungle'. Many students have not encountered, let alone practised, free improvisation, using atonal musical form, and arrhythmic structure. The duet improvisation is revealing to see how quickly they adapt to the musical ideas proposed by the professor – both tonal and atonal.

Students also have the option to improvise alone, with a subject they can choose.

2.   Voice and body improvisation: an improvised solo on a selected poem or an image. The students are given five minutes alone to prepare and practise this element, and are allowed to use the space and objects in the room. It is a daunting part for some students – requiring a dramatic presentation, free from inhibition, and it is a moment to explore the students' creative flexibility and expressivity, as well as how comfortable they are with their voice and their body.

3.   Clinical improvisation role-plays: a dialogue on a metallophone and a marimba with a professor, who plays 'the client', while the applicant plays 'the music therapist'. Applicants are not expected to show they already have therapeutic knowledge and skill, but there is space here to demonstrate potential and an ability to respond intuitively to some of the musical 'provocation' presented to them. Many applicants in this element already show some capacities for mirroring, matching, following and accompanying – revealing instinctive abilities in empathic therapeutic techniques. A few even reveal capacities for using more courageous therapeutic strategies, such as challenging and containing.

The duration of the full test is 45 to 50 minutes, and the final element is a verbal dialogue between the applicant and the professors on the applicant's motivation and knowledge of music therapy in theory and practice. It is interesting to explore whether the applicant really has thought through why they want to pursue a career in music therapy. Many, perhaps most, have not visited or talked to a practising music therapist. Some have hardly even dipped into the literature. To the interviewers it sometimes seems as if the applicant is following a 'romantic dream' – and we do challenge them on this point. The training is long and arduous, the prize is a still relatively unknown profession, where one doesn't have a job handed to one on a plate, and the onus is on the therapist to go out and build up his/her employment. We want to be sure that *they* are sure, and so the entrance test is more than just an evaluation of skills and abilities. It is an exploration into the personal motivation of the applicant. If they have not already obtained it, recommended literature is described in handouts; it is also recommended to visit a music therapist or have personal music therapy sessions. Since the course is mostly taught in Danish, the program requires formal qualifications in Danish. The entrance test and formal requirements are described in further detail – and in Danish only – on the home page of the program: http://www. musik.auc.dk. E-mail can be sent to: studievejl@aua.auc.dk.

The training is amongst the most expensive in the humanistic faculty, but still there is only funding for a minimum of solo teaching. Thus the demands at the entrance test are high, but also realistic. Ten to twelve applicants are accepted per year, and since 1986 around 130 candidates have completed the training.

6.3 Musical Skills in Music Therapy

A music therapist must be very flexible in his or her musical expression. No two clients are alike in their musical needs, experiences, musical and expressive skills. One session may be an inferno of chaotic sounds, another session may be a quiet sharing of sad music from a CD. The music therapist needs to develop the expertise to choose the appropriate procedure and a musical expression that is concordant with the client's needs and within the therapist's competence. If client and therapist do not 'fit together', the therapist should refer the client to a colleague.

This means that the therapist must have knowledge of a broad and varied musical repertory – from classical music to jazz and rock, and to 'therapy music' – and that he/she must be able to improvise on all sorts of instruments. The therapist must be a good singer and instrumentalist and have developed skills in playing from scores, harmonic accompaniment, playing by ear and in free improvisations on, for example, a scale, mode, motif, image, mood or other 'givens'. Body, voice and piano are the most important instruments, but guitar and percussion are also frequently used.

Among the special training disciplines of the Aalborg program we will mention *intuitive music* and *graphic notation* (Bergstrøm-Nielsen 1998, 1999). The students learn how to notate and perform musical sequences and compositions without using notes or other exact notation systems (CD cut 26). In other words, notes are just one tool amongst many for a music therapist who wishes to preserve a musical dialogue or sequence in a graphic form.

The training program in Aalborg attaches great importance to improvisation, and improvisation skills are taught more and more intensively through the semesters in order to qualify the students to use these skills in clinical practice with individual patients or groups.

However, it is not enough just to develop good musical skills in song, instrumental play and improvisation. The two cornerstones of the training are the development of the musical identity and the therapeutic identity, and they need to be in balance. In the course of training the focus will be put first on one, then on the other cornerstone, so that students reach a balance of these two aspects.

Music skills in music therapy training

There is no doubt that the recognition of music therapy as a profession relies upon its reputation as a 'specialized' intervention requiring the skills of a trained and unique professional. In music therapy training courses, different emphasis is placed on musical ability, both on entry and at final examinations and qualification. In some courses there is a focus on repertoire skills, the ability to play songs using the guitar or piano, and the use of music in a functional or pedagogic way. Musical skills are evaluated through a mechanism of testing musical knowledge and competencies of performance. Other traditions work through creative improvisation, and the therapists' musical skills are continuously assessed, and they are particularly evaluated in the context of clinical application.

Musical identity

But we can't just be satisfied with some accepted standard or level of performance. We can try to set criteria for good piano, improvisation or vocal skills, and define what pieces, songs and accompaniments students should be able to play. But the *real* skill that is most needed in music therapy is the ability to be a 'musical being' in the session. We have to create a musical environment/presence/atmosphere. Our musical responses must be fine-tuned, natural, immediate, sensitive, appropriate. Our musical awareness must be wide-ranging, founded on a broad base of experience, and with at least some knowledge of the many different genres and styles of the last thousand years.

If we expect to train students to find a way of 'reaching, helping and healing' people who have a wide variety of disorders, handicaps or illnesses, then these students must have a chameleonic musical persona, fashioned around a strong and individual but flexible musical identity.

So what does this mean in practice – in terms of how we can train students? What can you learn – and what is inborn, and cannot be learned?

Because of the unique place music can have in therapy as a non-verbal form of communication, the student needs to become fluent and skilled in using music communicatively. So they need to be able to open their ears to really hear the messages in the music of their clients, and then to interpret and understand them. That is almost the first stage, following which they have to respond, or initiate interaction.

To do this, they need to be able to play with meaning, not only with musical expressivity, but also with communicative intent. Acquiring improvisation skills to be able to do this is not a magical process, based only on intuition and good fortune; it is a complex training, learning to use many different improvisation techniques from the 64 techniques described by Bruscia (1987), to methods of frameworking, developing transitions and supporting clients (Wigram 1999d, 1999g). On top of both of these essential elements is a whole structure of abilities, skills, knowledge, experience and therapeutic sensitivity.

Developing a therapeutic approach is a process – which includes the process of developing your own musical identity, which connects with your therapeutic identity, the combination of which provides you with your professional identity.

The musical training in a music therapy program takes into consideration the following necessary studies:

- music psychology
- form and analysis of musical structure – sonata, binary, ternary, rondo, theme and variations, minuet, etc.
- psychoacoustics
- anatomy of hearing
- acoustics
- repertoire
- vocal training
- use of voice with accompaniment
- body and voice
- facility with a range of Orff instruments (percussion skills training is included as a specific course)
- guitar (guitar training is included as a specific course)
- musical dictation
- auditory training
- transposition
- harmonization
- composition
- extemporization
- sight-reading
- playing from chordal scores
- listening skills
- musical history – major composers, performers

- a range of different music – classical, popular and folk
- an understanding of musical structure for emotional purposes
- program music
- compiling a tape with a selection for a specific purpose
- songwriting.

As mentioned above, the course works on the development of a musical identity in the student. This identity will already be there, and the training over five years allows the expanding and maturing of that identity so that the student gains in both musical competence and in confidence.

What is the musical identity of the music therapist and on what is it based?

Historically developed:

- inborn musical aptitude
- history of musical experiences
- family and social influences
- likes and dislikes in music – emotional reactions to music
- knowledge of different musical genres
- musical education
- identity through his/her skills and performance on his/her main instrument

Developed in music therapy education:

- improvisational flexibility
- awareness of meaning within music
- techniques for responding to client's music e.g. mirroring, matching, exaggerating, reflecting
- integration of his/her own musical history, experiences, likes.

Are we trying to develop the students' role and therapeutic personality as artists? Is that the feeling therapists have when they are in sessions: I am perceived by clients *and* by my colleagues as an artist – a musician? Do we train students to allow their own musical identity to be evident in the therapeutic relationship? We hope so!

There is often a discussion – perhaps an argument – about the need for the music therapist to have well-developed, sophisticated and expert musical skills. Students quickly become seduced by their psychotherapeutic role, by the power they gain from knowledge about things that are medical, scientific, clinical – knowledge about the history and problems of the clients with whom they are working. These elements in the training are essential for the balance, but can reduce the influence and importance of musical skill and the place of the therapists' musical identity in therapy.

So when students, at different levels of musical skill, work at instrumental and vocal skills in transposition, harmonization, extemporization, rhythmic and melodic variability, as well as enlarging and expanding their knowledge of composed music, they may question the need for this, in a way that could be an unconscious denial or resistance to accepting their own musical limitations and the need to develop.

- Why do I need to be able to do that?

- Doesn't working with free improvisation in music therapy mean I can break free from all the rules, structure, form and technical skills of conventional performance and musical training?

- Do you still expect me to practise scales, arpeggios and harmonic skills?

Well, whether we are using free improvisation or composed music in music therapy, the subtlety of how we work with musical material relies on a high level of skill and all-round knowledge.

We need to be very skilful and eclectic musicians. The music our clients bring into our sessions can range from:

- chaotic   to   structured

- simple   to   complex

- free improvisation   to   precomposed songs

- baroque   to   modern jazz

- classical   to   romantic.

Our ability to understand our clients through their music depends on our own musical sensitivity, skill and experience. Attaching meaning to clients' musical material is achieved by:

- being able to listen to their music

- being able to remember and/or notate their music

- being able to analyse their music

- being able to contextualize their music

- being able to interpret the meaning within their music.

Up to the point of contextualization, the first three stages require musical knowledge, education, skill and experience. The process described above applies *equally* to the therapists' music and, in mutual improvisation, to both the clients' and the therapists' parts taken together. The contextualization and interpretation is where the integration of music and therapy takes place, and can be unfounded and inadequate without the informed musical analysis.

In Aalborg University, time is given to asking students to describe musical material in musical terminology, to be able to vocally or instrumentally recall clients' musical themes and style of playing, and to describe their own playing as a musical response. A particular focus is given to the way musical material from the client *or* the therapist changes over time – within an improvisation or within a whole session. Transitions occur, representing change both in the music and in the pathological state of the client.

Transitions defined by Wigram (1999g) come in three main forms:

1. *'Limbo transitions'* – where the music goes into a form of limbo or a space where nothing much is happening, while waiting for a new direction, or a return to a previous state. Music in limbo transitions is often innocuous and repetitive, e.g. a rocking octave, repeated melody fragment, chord or a single note, a trill, a held chord. Limbo is a place where one is unsure of being either here or there – waiting to see where one wants to go.

2. *'Overlap transitions'* – where one maintains the musical style of playing, the elements with which one is working, and then introduces a change to one element in order to offer an alternative musical frame. For example, if one is playing pentatonic, staccato and in a common metre (slowly), one might change first from staccato to legato, then introduce a dissonant or atonal element to the music, and finally attempt to remove the pulse to create music without pulse. This last change is often the most difficult to achieve, as people can have great difficulty letting go of pulse, which sometimes can be rigid and unchanging. The overlap idea is that a new element is introduced, while maintaining the old ones, avoiding sudden change that might be too dramatic.

3. *'Seduction transitions'* – often used with clients for whom changing is difficult and frightening. The change is introduced very gradually, often just a small change such as getting ever so gradually louder, or faster, or with small accents in the music. It is like a paint chart, where the colour bands go in a single spectrum from very dark blue to very light blue, but the changing continues imperceptibly. The title for these transitions is

not intended in any way sexually, but more as a process where something very gently and positively happens, helping a patient move slightly from fixed patterns.

Developing those transitions musically can be one of the most important skills of the music therapists – and it is a *musical* skill.

There is also discussion about how directive or non-directive the music therapist can be. Words with negative connotations such as 'manipulative', 'dominating' and 'structuring' are sometimes used to describe the approach of a therapist who is more directive. This also relates to the simplicity or complexity of the music. Using more sophisticated musical skills to frame your clients' more simple music and establish your musical identity can be viewed as directive, but it can also be seen as containing, holding, inspiring and creative. The skill students need to acquire is to have such a high level of musical fluency that they can easily find a balance between following and initiating, symbiosis and independence, musical freedom and musical structure.

It is the balance of these elements, the combining of a number of different parts together to make the whole and reach the client, that can be premeditated, intuitive, adaptive, contrived, reactive, or just sensitive and flexible. In the training of music therapy students there is a need to provide some clear frames for working in music therapy, and help them sort out the elements they can use, and how they should be appropriately combined to the best effect in working with different problems.

6.4 Theoretical and Analytical Studies

The majority of music therapists work in multidisciplinary teams. In institutions and hospitals they often have doctors, psychologists, nurses or special teachers as their primary colleagues. Being, very often, the only professional music therapist requires comprehensive interdisciplinary knowledge and good skills in listening and dialogue. The theoretical teaching of a music therapy training program should provide the student with a good ballast within relevant topics and a precise under-standing of the special role, opportunities and problems of music therapy in the context of a multidisciplinary team (Bonde and Pedersen 1996). Many European music therapists are humanistic by training and inclination, and it may be a problem for them to accept, for example, the 'machine model', when they meet a medical doctor who considers somatic or psychological problems 'defects that need repair' with medicine or technological interventions (like electroconvulsive therapy – ECT). Music therapists may also have difficulties in understanding the relevance of research in music perception, or experimental research in music therapy, for clinical practice. They may think that these types of research do not reflect the core of music therapy as an art – or that the clinical situation would be harmed by a scientific investigation. They may also meet colleagues who are sceptical as regards scientific documentation of the effectiveness of music therapy.

It is the aim of the music therapy training program at Aalborg University to provide the students with sufficient knowledge of these problems and of different types of scientific thinking, theory building and practical research (paradigms). The training should make them able to establish a positive dialogue with colleagues from other professions, based on an understanding of their view of human nature, of health and disease, of therapy and treatment. The theoretical and analytical track of the training shall provide the students with the basic knowledge and stimulate them to work independently and critically with topics relevant for clinical practice.

Each of the first six semesters has its specific theoretical topic or frame. The training has two equally important elements:

- theoretical courses, where the students are given a broad introduction to and (hopefully) an overview of the field

- independent project work, where the students in small groups (two to four students) define and investigate a specific and self-imposed problem within the semester frame. The chain of topics is multidisciplinary, and gradually focus is narrowed down to the specific problems of music therapy theory and research.

Semester 1, *Psychology of Music*, is an introduction to some of the most important subjects within this interdisciplinary field: psychoacoustics, music perception and processing by the ear and the brain, neurobiological mechanisms connected with musical activities, developmental psychology of music (especially child development), theories and tests of musical skills and aptitude, the formation of musical preferences, the relationship between music and language (see Chapter 2.1).

Semesters 2 and 3, *General and Therapy-oriented Psychology and Psychiatry*: the courses are taught by clinical psychologists and psychiatrists, who guide the students through basic problems and topics of psychology (cognition, emotion, perception, memory, learning and developmental psychology) and psychiatry (psychopathologies, diagnostic systems and treatment modalities). In the second semester the theoretical courses frame a four-week observation practicum period, where a student follows a professional music therapist in her daily work. Thus theory and practice are combined in a relevant way, and the students develop clinical observation skills (see also Chapter 2.2. on theoretical foundations).

Semester 4, *Theory of Science*, may seem a very abstract and difficult subject; on the other hand it gives the student an opportunity to work with the fundamental questions of life: what is experience and how do we acquire knowledge (epistemology)? What or how is human nature, does man have a free will or is (s)he predetermined (ontology) – and how do major psychological and psychotherapeutic models answer these questions? When is knowledge true and objective – if that is possible at all? What are the hallmarks of good argumentation? Important philosophical positions and scientific paradigms are introduced and discussed, using *Philosophy of Medicine* (Wulff *et al.* 1990) as a textbook. This is also the primer of medical students, so it gives the music therapy student a good introduction to the way doctors think.

Semester 5, *Theory of Therapy*: in the introduction course the students are given an overview of important traditions of psychotherapy (see Chapter 2.2), and the relationship between psychological theories and clinical applications in psychotherapy and behavioural therapy is discussed. So-called 'non-specific factors' of psychotherapy, which are common to all psychotherapy models, are highlighted, as is the role of the therapist within different traditions and models.

Semester 6, *Music Therapy Theory and Research I*: theory of music therapy is a cornerstone of the program. Teaching is not limited to the sixth semester, but spread over all semesters, using local and international guest teachers, who present the expert clinical areas, working models, theoretical problems or research projects. In this way the students get a first-hand introduction of clinical practices and theoretical orientations. By the end of the sixth semester the student is expected to have a good knowledge of the clinical applications of music therapy, its theoretical paradigms and traditions, and basic problems in music therapy research.

Semesters 7 and 8, *Music Therapy Theory and Research II*: the students continue their studies in music therapy theory and research. They read a large number of texts (clinical papers, theoretical papers, quantitative and qualitative research methodology, philosophy and reports), and they are introduced to relevant methods of music analysis (applicable on both improvisations and precomposed music). When possible, theory and practice are combined, i.e. when the seventh semester students write a 'musical autobiography' (inspired by Ruud 1997), and in the eighth semester they participate as a group in a Guided Imagery and Music level one course. Over five days they listen to theoretical papers and participate in experiential exercises, individually, in dyads and in groups (see Chapter 3.1). Relevant test batteries and inventories from clinical psychology and music therapy research methodologies (quantitative and qualitative) are introduced, enabling the students to develop a design to be used for data collection in their ninth semester practicum (four months). The goal is not only to inform the students about standards, problems and traditions, but also to stimulate their individual, critical reflection.

Project work is used in almost every semester, as a special learning framework. Problem-solving group work is a distinctive pedagogical mark of Aalborg University and may be considered a new learning strategy. However, the wondering and questioning attitude of the learner goes back to philosophers and teachers like Socrates and Montaigne. The latter wrote an essay 'On Teaching and Bringing Up Children' (Montaigne 1996, Chapter 26), based on (amongst other things) his own, very special experiences: he learned Latin as his 'mother tongue' in a natural way, because his father considered it a good idea and instructed everybody to speak Latin to the child. The idea of learning as an active, dynamic process is formulated by Montaigne in these words: 'The teacher should, from the very beginning, let the pupil test his abilities and capacities; the pupil should be allowed to try things out, and learn to pick and choose. Sometimes he must be led by the hand, other times he will find his own way. It is not only the teacher who must introduce his ideas; he must also listen to the pupil.' Or in the words of Socrates (after Cicero): *Obest plerumque iis qui discere volunt auctoritas eorum qui dicent* ('The authority of the teacher is often an obstacle for those who wish to learn').

Project work is a way of organizing this dynamic process of inquiry. At its best, the students develop good co-operation skills, while they study a relevant professional or theoretical problem independently, thoroughly and seriously.

The *Master's thesis* is the students' 'final project'. Most students write the thesis individually – as systematic and scientifically founded reflections on their clinical work in the ninth semester practicum. The Master's thesis is also problem oriented – whether it is a case study, a theoretical discussion or based on a research design – and many of the theses are important contributions to the development of music therapy.

6.5 Experiential Training in Music Therapy – the Self-Experience Element

Experiential Training in Music Therapy as an integrated part of an MA training program

As a pre-experience for clinical work, students on the five-year full-time MA program of music therapy at Aalborg University, Denmark are, over four years, placed in the role of 'student clients' as a preparation to work with music therapy from a psychotherapeutic basis with many different client populations. Overall, this part of the training program is called Experiential Training in Music Therapy (ETMT), and the music therapy teachers working in this area are called experiential training music therapy teachers (ETMT teachers).

ETMT, as a mandatory part of music therapy training programs, has been included at several programs, especially in Europe over the last ten years. This part of training often takes place outside the program and is worked out as a personal training course (in verbal psychotherapy or music therapy) for the students separated from the group of music therapy teachers at the training program.

At Aalborg University we have ETMT training included as a mandatory part integrated in the MA program in Music Therapy, and the students are placed as student clients from the very beginning of study, where they develop basic music therapy skills at the BA level. ETMT takes place in the first and second study years taught as 'primary ETMT discipline' (see below) in the form of group music therapy (first year), individual music therapy (second year) and psychodynamic movement (first and third years). These training disciplines, we think, create a solid foundation for methodological training through the third and fourth years and also for practicum placements in the third, fourth and fifth years. We see the supervision for students in practicum as the third step of the on-going training module starting with ETMT, then methodology training (including ETMT elements) and finally practicum placements with individual and group supervision.

To place primary disciplines of ETMT training in the first years of study differs from other psychotherapeutic training programs in Denmark and many other countries, where ETMT is a post-graduate training module. We consider the ETMT training as a very important module to be integrated with the understanding of both basic and advanced psychological and music therapy theories. Often students use material from self-experienced personal development as a basis for written reports in psychology and music therapy theory.

Origin of ETMT training modules

Originally, the idea of offering ETMT to music therapy students was developed by Mary Priestley in the early 1970s. She offered individual music therapy and Intertherapy (IMT – see below) as a supplementary private training to students from different music therapy training courses, as she had missed such training elements herself in her own education at the Guildhall School of Music and Drama.

No training programs had self-experience disciplines integrated or added to their programs at that time and the idea was perceived as rather controversial by most music therapists, although some spotted its potential. Johannes Th. Eschen from Germany was in the first student pair in the IMT training by M. Priestley, and he managed some years later to integrate ETMT as a mandatory part of the two-year full-time training program: *Mentorenkurs Herdecke* in Herdecke, Germany, 1978 to 1980. This idea was transferred to the five-year, full-time MA course in music therapy in Aalborg in 1982 by Inge Nygaard Pedersen, who founded this program, and her colleague Benedikte B. Scheiby. Throughout the 1980s this training module was run on an experimental basis, undergoing a period of development, and it was carefully evaluated by the Danish Ministry of Education in 1989. The positive result of this evaluation, where ethical issues in relationship to ETMT in particular were considered, left the ETMT module as a fully integrated, mandatory part of the program – the only university program in Denmark with such an integrated form of training including equal weight on developing personal skills, musical skills, clinical skills and academic skills simultaneously.

Primary ETMT disciplines

The primary disciplines (individual and group music therapy, psychodynamic movement and, partly, intertherapy) are identified by the fact that the students have the possibility to go through a personal therapeutic process over time. Secondary disciplines (clinical group music therapy skills, and psychodynamic group leading) offer single-standing episodes for self-experience combined with methodological training.

To develop basic tools in the primary disciplines of ETMT the students are trained in the following areas:

- learning to be familiar with their personal improvisational language – especially in the music

- experiencing the power of music as a tool for reflecting on psychological resources, limitations and preparedness

- learning to be a part of on-going dynamic processes over time

- learning to deal with projections, introjections and self-containment in practice

- learning to develop and keep a high level of sensitivity and flexibility in music therapy practice

- learning how to be vitally involved, and at the same time to survive as a music therapist.

For the primary disciplines of group and individual music therapy, and psychodynamic movement, there is no formal evaluation except for the ETMT teachers to be aware of the potential for serious problems for future professional work. Through many years of training, and the accumulation of students' reports, the following working scheme of learning processes has evolved to be representational for a wide range of 'personal' stories that arise in the ETMT training:

1. Learning to see/experience intimate relations/parents in the way they are and not the way you may want them to be (distinguishing ideal from reality).

2. Learning to contain and accept pain, disappointment aggression, joy and other feelings related to intimate relationships.

(In these two steps of the learning process, conscious awareness of projections and tranferences are addressed musically and verbally.)

3. Learning to recognize oneself in 'one's own eyes' instead of in the eyes of other people.

4. Learning to act the way you feel is right for you – independently of parental censorship and of your own defence mechanisms, in a responsible way for yourself and others.

(In these two steps of the learning process, conscious awareness of introjections are addressed musically and verbally.)

5. Learning how to develop important tools for clinical music therapy practice where you contain feelings at the same time as you allow feelings to appear and to be used as information in the relationship and interaction.

(In this step of the learning process, self-containment as a music therapy tool is addressed.)

This way of understanding the therapeutic learning process is only one of several ways, and it is related to a psychoanalytic/psychodynamic way of understanding human development.

Ethical rules

Ethical rules and a respectful understanding of the process of each student involved in the training are necessary. The most important ethical rule is that the work takes place behind a locked door with no disturbances (no telephone, interruptions etc.)

Equally important are the following ethical rules:

- All ETMT teachers are subject to professional confidentiality according to the ethical code for professional music therapists, although their role as employers of the university makes them obliged to report specific difficulties which may be identified as problematical for students' further development as professional therapists.

- All sessions are recorded or videotaped in order to cope with any disagreements regarding 'serious problems' between the student client and the ETMT teacher. In this case a neutral third party (supervisor) can listen to the tapes and try to double-check the evaluation of the ETMT teacher.

- Supervision is compulsory for ETMT teachers.

In the integrated Aalborg model which has been running for 19 years, it has never been necessary to make use of a neutral third party.

Secondary ETMT disciplines

Secondary ETMT disciplines include clinical group music therapy skills, psychodynamic group leading, partly intertherapy and GIM level one. These disciplines are identified by the fact that the students are given a frame for learning methodology using each other as student clients. These disciplines build on the learning processes from the primary disciplines and they give the students a possibility to have feedback from 'experienced clients' and direct supervision from a professional music therapy teacher. Intertherapy can be seen as both a primary and secondary discipline, as it gives the students both a chance to dive into another on-going personal process and also to have feedback and supervision as the student therapist.

Intertherapy

The form of intertherapy used at Aalborg involves two-hour sessions where two students take turns in being a therapist for one another for two 40-minute blocks, under direct supervision, and subsequently 20 minutes of individual supervision for both students. The aim of intertherapy is to train and develop the students' ability to follow, to recognize and to change patterns in a dynamic process in the dual work with clients. Also, the quick shift of being in these different roles is very important for future work, where you might have to be ready for therapy work even if you have just experienced deeply emotional situations yourself.

At the end of the intertherapy training the two students feed back to one another with direct supervision on their experience of having been a client, and of their responsibility as the student therapist in this setting. Intertherapy ends up with an internal evaluation where the student presents a case, based on three to five video cuts, with an emphasis on understanding the progression of being a therapist in the case (Pedersen and Scheiby 1999).

Clinical group music therapy skills

In clinical group music therapy skills, students take turns at being group therapists (first in pairs and then individually) for a group of other students role-playing a specific client population. The student clients are given short descriptions of the history and problems of the clients they will play, and are then brought into the therapy room for a group therapy session. The student therapists are given supervision some days before the session to address their understanding of the needs of their clients, the function and process of the session they are planning, and their therapeutic role. The session is carried out in a safe space, with careful attention to boundaries, in order to create as real a situation as possible. The therapy session normally lasts between 45 and 60 minutes and during this time the group and their therapist(s) are not disturbed. It is a therapy session.

After the session, there is a lengthy feedback, with commentary from the 'clients', therapists and observers. Analysis of the process of the session is undertaken, reviewing the video made of the session, and alternative possibilities for events that occurred during the session, both musical and verbal, are discussed. The sessions are supervised, observed and contained by a qualified teacher/therapist.

This course is run during the whole of the third year and is examined by an external examiner who observes a live 'here and now' experience of the group therapy with role-playing. The students are examined on their ability to work within the group therapy process, understand the needs of the client, their role as a therapist, and how to feed back, with an analysis of and a reflection on what happened in their session.

During training, attention is given to the therapist's musical and therapeutic identity and skills and to understanding the needs of the clients. It is also given to developing methods and techniques in group work and to storing and recalling events in the session for feedback, and to developing awareness of and supervision on transference and countertransference and interpretation from coping with this specific client population (Wigram 1996a, pp.199–212).

Psychodynamic group leading

Psychodynamic group leading has a similar frame to clinical group music therapy skills but here the students take turns in being a solo group leader for a group of students who are there authentically as student clients. The aim is to train the students in counselling and music therapy techniques of work with 'normal' to neurotic clients in group dynamic forms both on a pre-structured and on a *prima vista* basis, musically and verbally. Timing, states of consciousness, voice qualities, therapeutic presence, musical facilitating, and verbal clarifications and interpretations are in focus. Authentic group dynamic problems and resources are in focus and they are a guideline for the therapist's preparation of the session. The student therapist undertakes pre-supervision before the session. The session is supervised, observed and contained by a qualified teacher/therapist. The internal examination involves the student being a group leader for half an hour for a group of music therapy students other than those from the training group. A general structure for the session is:

- to make the group present and ready

- to give clear instructions for dynamic work and clear playing rules

- to take part in or listen carefully to the musical improvisation

- to facilitate and interpret during the verbal part and relate it to the music to close down carefully. (Bonde, Pederson and Wigram 1999)

Guided Imagery and Music – level one

As a receptive part of ETMT training, the MA program at Aalborg University has also included (since 1999) level one of the Guided Imagery and Music (GIM) training as developed in the Bonny Method, USA. This course follows the guidelines of, and is approved by, the Association of Music and Imagery. The module comprises 35 hours of theoretical, practical and experiential instruction, and is normally organized as a five-day intensive workshop.

The theoretical elements are history and philosophy of the Bonny Method and current theory and core concepts of the method. Practical and experiential elements are:

- exercises in dyads – 'guide and traveller'

- group exercises based on GIM methods

- demonstration sessions by primary trainer

- creative drawing/writing based on imagery and music experiences.

This GIM module is placed as the last part of ETMT training during the MA program as it offers very powerful experiences of music listening in a deeply altered state of consciousness. There is no formal evaluation but each student is evaluated with the student's participation in the training, potential as a GIM facilitator, and readiness to proceed to intermediate level two (on a private basis) being assessed (Bonde, Pedersen and Wigram 1999). An experiential technique like GIM fits very well into the program, as it is one of the very few training programs in the world to have consistently included self-experiential courses and modules. The metatheory and theory of consciousness in GIM also go well together with the content of the courses in general and clinical psychology, psychiatry, theory of science and therapy theory.

The GIM course is now a well-integrated secondary discipline, led by primary trainer Torben Moe. Students may later enter levels two and three of the Danish GIM training program.

Conclusion

As ETMT training is very specific and includes readiness to work with personal processes in a professional educational setting we, at the Aalborg program, always carefully inform and warn the students at the entrance test about entering such a complex program. Today, students not only from Denmark but also from other Nordic countries want to join the program because of this specialized integration into the MA program. We have had very few problems of students disagreeing with the ETMT teachers' evaluation and we have been very careful in trying to solve these problems when they do occur.

Over the years, the ETMT training has affected some students, who previously had either declared or undeclared personal problems, to the degree that the emerging problems needed attention, and they needed referral to the healthcare system. In some ways this process has revealed inherent and underlying difficulties and problems that needed attention, and certainly needed addressing before the students attempted to continue training in the complex field of music therapy. However careful one tries to be at the entrance tests, and subsequently in the professional and scientific training, one can never be totally secure about what future problems may emerge during therapy work. Often students who go into a crisis (not defined as pathological) during the training may nevertheless demonstrate good potential to develop basic psychological tools to understand and musically resonate with future clients.

6.6 Clinical Training and Placements

Students in music therapy undertake clinical practice training or clinical practicums in much the same way as students in any other medical or paramedical education. Students at Aalborg University undertake the following clinical training process:

1. Second semester students undertake four weeks' observational training.

2. Students in the sixth semester undertake a two-week, full-time observational placement followed by a one day a week, 10-week clinical training practicum.

3.   Students in the eighth semester undertake a two-week observational practicum followed by a 10-week, one day a week practicum.

4.   Students in the ninth semester undertake a six months, full-time practicum placement/internship.

In the second semester, students go to many institutions throughout Denmark and sometimes abroad, in order to observe qualified music therapists working with clients and to learn more about the different pathologies and developmental disabilities with which they will ultimately be working. The objective of this placement is for students to become good at observing, documenting the needs of the clients, the objectives of therapy and what therapists do during their sessions. At the same time they are exploring their own resources by evaluating their response to the clients, taking into consideration both positive and negative reactions to the situations within which they are working. They write a project based on this work, focusing on a specific aspect of therapy work – for example, the client–therapist relationship, styles of music used in music therapy, etc.

In the sixth and eighth semesters, after their observational period, students begin to work, under supervision, with clients. Normally, these two placements are allotted to students in order to give them an experience of both the areas of developmental disability/physical handicap and psychiatry. Other placements, such as hospice/oncology work, work with children taken into care by social services, work with long-term psychiatric populations and work with refugees, can also be available for students but there are limitations over the number of qualified therapists through which they can be supervised. Students begin to build up a small case-load of one or two individual clients and a small group with whom they work one day a week during the course of the semester. They receive supervision from a qualified music therapist and a person at the institution where they are working.

Finally, students in their ninth semester undertake a full six-months placement where they begin to understand the way the institutions or educational units work, the role of other staff and their role as music therapists. This placement is supervised individually and in group supervision at the university. It forms the major part of the student's practicum experience where they begin to take on full responsibility for therapeutic work. It is examined at the university at the beginning of the tenth semester through a practical experience exam where the student is required to present a case study with audio or video examples and explain the process of the work they have been undertaking.

Students in practicum normally have to pay attention to developing the following skills and areas of understanding:

1. a clear understanding of the philosophy, function and staffing of the institution

2. a clear perspective and knowledge of the nature and clinical descriptions of the disorders, pathologies and educational disabilities of clients with whom they are working

3. the capacity to develop a clear focus on the needs of the client – general needs, pathological needs and individual needs

4. an ability to formulate objectives and goals of therapy

5. the development of appropriate musical skills within therapy to meet the needs of the client

6. the ability to take responsibility for what happens in both individual and group therapy sessions

7. the ability to evaluate and analyse what is happening in therapy and document it

8. the ability to report to their supervisor, and to the rest of the team with whom they are working, the process of their work and to seek guidance and advice on their therapeutic direction

9. the development of insight, intuition and awareness of their role as therapists, and the effect they have on a client.

The final practicum, for which the other practicums have been steering and equipping the student, is a testing ground for the student to integrate the theory, musical skills, therapeutic knowledge and personal self-confidence in order to take responsibility as a music therapist and work with the clinical population. Learning how to practise music therapy is, in many ways, more complex and presents greater problems to the student than, for example, learning how to practise medicine or occupational therapy. Music therapy students follow general guidelines, rather than specific and precise treatment techniques. There is not always a 'right or wrong' way to put into practice the theory and technique taught in training. In therapy work like this, we think more about 'progress' and 'lack of progress', and the therapist has to work more to a criteria of 'successful or unsuccessful' and 'appropriate or inappropriate' when evaluating the effect and usefulness of his/her intervention.

This can be exciting, giving the music therapist a high degree of responsibility and requiring a high level of self-critique. It can also be daunting, sometimes leaving the music therapist, and especially the music therapy student, insecure and without clear procedures or frames for intervention. As a result they can practise at the mercy of their own biases, influences and countertransference. Supervision is therefore a vital element both for music therapists in training and for qualified therapists, particularly when they are working alone or in isolation.

CHAPTER 7

Professional and Technical Resources

7.1 National and International Co-operation

National associations and societies

The development of music therapy in many countries of the world has been accompanied by the emergence of societies for people interested in music therapy and the early practitioners in music therapy, followed by the development of professional associations in some countries in order to negotiate the rights and status of practising music therapists. This varies significantly from one country to another and has also emerged in some countries as a competitive element in the development of music therapy. In countries in Europe such as Denmark, England and Germany, the first structured organization occurred in the development of societies.

In Denmark, the Danish Society for Music Therapy promoted the development of music therapy and included early practitioners such as Claus Bang and Grethe Lund, as well as incorporating professionals from other disciplines who were interested in the practice of music therapy, such as physiotherapy, occupational therapy and psychology.

In England, from 1959, the British Society for Music Therapy promoted the development of the discipline through conferences, publications and a journal. Again, membership was open to professionals from all disciplines, as well as members of the public who were interested. In Germany, the German Society for Music Therapy developed in a similar fashion.

The earliest formalized society for music therapy was undoubtedly in the USA, where the National Association of Music Therapy (NAMT) began to hold conferences and publish material soon after the Second World War. The NAMT had a clear natural science profile, which one can also see in the association's journal – the *Journal of Music Therapy*. Later, the American Association for Music Therapy (AAMT) developed, and was set up by psychotherapeutically oriented music therapists, producing a journal called *Music Therapy*. In 1999, these two associations amalgamated to become one: the American Music Therapy Association (AMTA) which is now the biggest music therapy association in the world with more than 3500 members.

These early societies were typically started by pioneers who were generating the development of training courses in music therapy, and also attempting to introduce the clinical application of music therapy in a variety of settings including special schools, hospitals for people with learning disabilities or psychiatric disorders, and the community.

While in some countries this resulted in a cohesive and integrated approach to the development of the profession, in other countries competitive elements crept in, which has resulted in the flourishing of increasing numbers of 'societies' or 'associations' within the particular country. For example, in Italy there are, to date, something approaching 34 different societies of music therapy, and in the South American countries, one can also find numerous emerging societies in Brazil and Argentina. The reason for this can be identified through examining philosophical or practical differences between pioneers, and also considering differences in professional disciplines that were promoting the development of music therapy. For example, in many countries, particularly in Europe, two different professional groups caught hold of the potential of music therapy and tried to develop it. One group could loosely be categorized as the psychotherapeutically oriented clinical professions of psychiatry and psychology. In these professions, qualified practitioners have followed a track whereby music therapy can be developed within the clinical and philosophical frameworks that already exist and, as an adjunct, their existing practices. The other major group that can loosely be defined is music teachers, music specialists and music pedagogues. This group has promoted the concepts of music therapy much more within an educational and special educational framework.

This explains, to some extent, where there is often divergence and disagreement in many countries in Europe and further afield in the development of both the theory of music therapy and the clinical practice of music therapy. Certainly in southern European countries, the practice of therapy is regulated in law and confined to a large degree to professionals who have qualified either in psychiatry or psychology. Therefore, music specialists and teachers cannot, at this point in time, work within clinical treatment programs and identify their role as that of therapists. In fact, in some countries in Europe, the title 'music therapist' does not exist and although students go to train on music therapy courses in universities, colleges of further education and in many cases privately, that does not establish them with the title of music therapist and they have to seek employment under other professional disciplinary titles in order to introduce music therapy as part of their working practice.

Therefore, the political development necessary to promote music therapy as an independent profession has varied significantly from one country to another. In the UK, Denmark, Belgium, The Netherlands and Germany, the title 'music therapist' exists for the purpose of employment, and positions as music therapists are both available and advertised. However, in many other countries, in order to practise music therapy a person obtains employment as a social worker, day-care helper, psychologist, occupational therapist or psychotherapist in order that music therapy can be used as a method of intervention. In the UK, music therapists are state registered and the profession controlled by an Act of Parliament.

NATIONAL ASSOCIATIONS

Since 1970, there has been a considerable movement in many countries to form professional associations such as the Musikterapeuternes Landsklub (MTL) in Denmark, the Association of Professional Music Therapists in Great Britain and the Professional Association in Music Therapy in Germany. These associations have only opened membership to qualified music therapists and, at the time they were formed, also included pioneer practitioners who had not undertaken qualifications. Currently, most of these organizations undertake the following specific work:

1. maintaining a register of qualified music therapists

2. identifying and approving courses in music therapy

3. negotiating with health, education and social service institutions for the status and salary of music therapists

4. establishing codes of ethics to which music therapists must adhere in their clinical practice

5. promoting and advertising positions of music therapy

6. establishing supervisory systems for practising music therapists (not in all countries)

7. liaising with other professional associations, including other arts therapies associations and professional groups.

Both the societies and professional associations, independently and often together, have organised conferences, colloquia, seminars and workshops at national level to promote the profession, present the results of clinical work and offer short foundation courses to interested members of the public. In many countries, for example,

England, the USA, Canada and Australia, an annual conference from between two to four days is typical in order to offer members of the profession a milieu in which they can present the results of their clinical work, research or aspects of education and training within music therapy. These can range in size from very large conferences, such as one might find in the USA where more than 1000 delegates are normally expected, to small conferences, such as can be found in England and Denmark where between 50 and 100 delegates are more typical. The societies and associations have also promoted publication of music therapy material, particularly through the development of scientifically credible and well-formulated journals of music therapy. Details of this are reported in Chapter 5.2.

INTERNATIONAL CO-OPERATION THROUGH CONFERENCES AND POLITICAL ORGANIZATIONS

Since 1976, contact between countries has resulted in international conferences in music therapy. 1976 saw the first world conference in music therapy which took place in Paris followed by Buenos Aires (1978), Puerto Rico (1981), Paris (1983), Genoa (1985), Rio de Janeiro (1990), Vitoria, Spain (1993), Hamburg (1996) and Washington DC (1999).

At the time of writing, the next world congress is planned for Oxford University in Great Britain in 2002.

WORLD FEDERATION OF MUSIC THERAPY (WFMT)

Several key figures in the international music therapy community, including Dr Rolando Benenzon (Argentina, President 1985–1990), Dr Ruth Bright (Australia, President 1990–1993), Barbara Hesser (USA), Professor Tony Wigram (Denmark/England, President 1996–1999), Professor Cheryl Dileo (USA, President 1993–1996), Gianluigi di Franco (Italy), Dr Denise Grocke (Australia, President 1999–2002) and several others have promoted the development of a World Federation of Music Therapy since the world conference in Paris in 1983. This has emerged over time thanks to the pioneering efforts of these people and other professionals involved at national level and subsequently consists of a body involving more than 40 countries and 100 organizations.

The World Federation of Music Therapy is a non-executive organization which promotes world congresses in music therapy and offers guidelines and advice on training in music therapy, research, ethics, registration and political recognition. Each of these areas is represented by a Commission in the WFMT, with a Chair and international members. WFMT publishes a newsletter, which is in the process of becoming electronically produced, and is currently developing a web page on the website developed at Witten Herdecke University by Professor David Aldridge: www.musictherapyworld.net. The World Federation of Music Therapy is primarily concerned with developing international co-operation, establishing good standards in clinical practice, research and training in music therapy, and with promoting a world congress every three years at a high scientific level.

The WFMT has produced a global 'definition' of music therapy (see Chapter 1) and the Commission for Ethics has produced model guidelines for the ethical practice of music therapy, which can be used as a model to work with by countries around the world, notwithstanding local conditions and rules.

The Commission for Education and Training undertook a major survey of music therapy educations in 1992 to 1993 which was analysed, documented and subsequently published by the University of Melbourne (Erdonmez 1996). Recent symposia have also brought forth some model guidelines for music therapy education, although this is a significantly heterogeneous field for which it is almost impossible to find enough uniformity, except at a very general level, on which one can base a generic model of music therapy training.

EUROPEAN MUSIC THERAPY CONFEDERATION

In 1989, a European Music Therapy Committee was established with Professor Tony Wigram as the first Co-ordinator/President (1989–1998). He developed this organization over the next nine years from an initial beginning of five involved countries (UK, The Netherlands, Italy, Spain and Sweden) to its current status of more than 24 representatives from European countries, also including Mediterranean countries such as Malta and Israel. Every country in Europe and many countries from the former Eastern bloc are represented in the European Music Therapy Confederation (EMTC), which meets every three years for a major conference. Triennial conferences have taken place in The Netherlands (1989), England (1992), Denmark (1995), Leuven, Belgium (1998) and Italy (2001).

The EMTC was primarily formed following European directives that required countries in the EU to establish a system by which professionals qualified in post-graduate professions could have their qualifications recognized and therefore work in member states of the EU. Therefore, the EMTC has an on-going dialogue to agree registration, standards of training and ethical codes of practice within the EU. There are many complications to a process involving the recognition of professional qualifications, because the length, quality and examination procedures vary widely from one country to another – some at undergraduate level, some at post-graduate. While some courses are based in universities and colleges of higher education, there are also many privately run courses. Establishing a European form of registration with minimum standards is a goal of the EMTC.

The EMTC is, like the WFMT, a non-executive organization, and representatives sitting on the board of the EMTC are responsible for communicating with all music therapy organizations, associations and societies within their national country, communicating decisions in both directions and maintaining a fluent and on-going dialogue in music therapy within the whole of Europe and further afield. Following Professor Wigram, the presidents of the organization have been Gianluigi di Franco (1998–2001) and Jos De Backer (2001 to present). Information about the EMTC is also available on the website: www.musictherapyworld.net.

A similar organization, the South American Music Therapy Confederation, exists in South America, and acts as a central liaison for the many music therapy organizations prevalent throughout South America, particularly in Brazil and Argentina. It organizes occasional conferences.

Conclusion

Because music therapy is a small profession, there has undoubtedly been a greater need for international co-operation and support and consequently the international conferences, both at European and world level, have resulted in a satisfactory degree of recognition between countries and professionals of music therapy clinical practice research. As both the EMTC and the WFMT have grown, so has the need within various countries to establish a more integrated and unified framework of activity. For example, in Italy, even though there are well over 34 different associations and/or societies, some of these have now formed into a national confederation (CONFIAM) that seeks to regularize and develop agreements between the multiplicity of independent societies and associations.

Unity is a vital element in music therapy for its future development. In comparison, psychotherapy has fragmented into a multiplicity of different philosophies, organizations and practices. Despite the fact that it is undoubtedly clear that these different practices are individual and recognizable, the lack of unity nevertheless causes problems. While there will be different philosophies and approaches in music therapy, the underpinning theories and approaches to clinical practice can achieve a level of unity that is important when music therapy faces up against political, medical, academic and scientific institutions.

To access details of music therapy organizations, associations and societies in Europe, an overview of European associations with electronic links to their websites can be found at: www.musictherapyworld.net and www.hisf.no/njmt/associations.html.

7.2 Journals of Music Therapy

A selection of international journals

Musiktherapeutische Umschau (Germany)

Profile: The journal is published by the German association DGMT. The subtitle 'Music Therapy in Research and Practice' is informative. The German journal includes 8 to 12 original, peer reviewed articles plus debate and book reviews. One or two issues a year are thematic (e.g. music therapy in oncology). Many case studies and reports from clinical practice.

Number of issues: 4

Language: German

Subscription (price and e-address): DM 81/105 (student/normal subscriber)

Website: www.musikterapie.de/english/service.htm

British Journal of Music Therapy (Great Britain)

Profile: English journal published by the British Society for Music Therapy (BSMT) and Association of Professional Music Therapists. Included in the journal are research articles, case studies, theoretical articles, brief reports, news and commentary.

Number of issues: 2

Language: English

Subscription (price and addresses): Subscription is included in membership of BSMT: £23/£38/£55 (student/normal subscriber/institution). Older issues: £5. Subscription and older issues: Denise Christophers, 25 Rosslyn Avenue, East Barnet, Hertfordshire, EN4 8DH, UK tel. +44 (0) 20 8368 8879.

Website: www.bsmt.org/j-index.html

Journal of Music Therapy (USA)

Profile: The oldest American journal has been published since 1964; it is now published by the American Music Therapy Association (AMTA). Until 1998 the journal's profile was quantitative research in the effects of music and music therapy. Now the journal also includes qualitative research and theoretical papers.

Number of issues: 4

Language: English

Subscription (price and e-address): $105

Website: http://otto.cmr.fsu.edu/memt/jmt/index.html

Music Therapy Perspectives **(USA)**

Profile: The second American journal has a broader target group and focuses on evidence-based practice. News columns include new music technology and international perspectives.

Number of issues: 2

Language: English

Subscription (price and e-address): $95 + shipping

Website: www.allenpress.com/catalog/aindex.shtml

Journal of the Association for Music and Imagery **(USA)**

Profile: Special journal/yearbook with six to ten articles on the Bonny Method of Guided Imagery and Music in theory, clinical practice and research. Published by the Association of Music and Imagery (AMI).

Number of issues: 1

Language: English

Subscription (price and addresses): $22 + shipping (earlier volumes $17 + shipping). Jim Rankin, Secretary to the AMI, PO Box 4286, Blaine, WA 98231-4286, USA.

Website: www.bonnymethod.com/ami/resources.htm

The Australian Journal of Music Therapy

Profile: Published since 1990. Accepts papers that make an original contribution to the field of music therapy including: research studies; original reports of clinical work such as case studies or group projects; original perspectives on material previously published, such as position papers reviewing the literature in specific areas of music therapy practice which include new perspectives or implications and reviews of books that have been published in the last three years.

Number of issues: 1

Language: English

Subscription: $AUD45, plus shipping

Website: www.austmta.org.au

Canadian Journal of Music Therapy

Profile: A published, refereed journal that accepts research papers, clinical papers and position papers. Types of manuscripts that are considered for inclusion: empirical studies, review articles, theoretical articles, brief reports and case histories. The journal is published in English and French. All submissions must be original work, not previously published.

Number of issues: 2

Language: English and French

Contact: Editor: Theresa Merrill

Nordic Journal of Music Therapy

Profile: The Nordic journal has been published since 1992 in a collaboration between the Scandinavian countries. Each issue contains three or four original, peer reviewed scientific articles, plus a 'classical article' with a historical introduction, reports from clinical practice, reviews and informations on events. The website includes an open debate 'Forum', an extended 'Review' section and many other facilities.

Number of issues: 2

Language: English (occasionally reviews/reports in Scandinavian languages)

Subscription (price and address): EUR 20/25/35 (student/normal subscriber/institution).

Website: www.hisf.no/njmt/ (many articles available online).

E-JOURNALS

Some of the journals already mentioned give free access to selected articles that can be downloaded from their website (see above).

The year 2001 saw the emergence of two purely electronic journals.

Music Therapy Today e-magazine:
www.musictherapyworld.net/MMMagazine/index.html

Voices:
www.voices.no

INTERNATIONAL NEWSLETTERS

The international federations of music therapy, e.g. EMTC and WFMT publish newsletters with information on their work and important news from member countries. Go to www.musictherapyworld.net.

Newsletters are also published within the cultures of specific music therapy models. Examples are the *N/R Newsletter*, with information on Creative Music Therapy (the Nordoff-Robbins model), and the *AMI Newsletter*, with information on the Bonny Method of Guided Imagery and Music.

A more general electronic newsletter is *MusicTherapyENews*: http://www.onelist.com/group/MusicTherapyEnews.

7.3 Music Therapy and the Internet

During the last five years, the Internet has become part of everyday life in the Western world – and e-mail is often not only the quickest, but also the only reliable connection between East and West.

In a few years the computer, the sequencer and music software programs like Cubase, Finale or Sibelius will be standard equipment in therapy rooms and in music therapists' everyday life. However, many music therapists are still negative or just sceptical towards 'the digital world' – without really knowing its potentials.

Bertold Brecht was not only a major writer of the twentieth century; he was also one of the first intellectuals to see the enormous potential of the new electronic media of his time: the radio. Brecht's radio theory from the 1920s stated that this new media had an interactive, i.e., genuinely democratic potential. For many years, only radio amateurs made a reality out of this. The idea of public service radio and public access to media (primarily through the telephone) had a major breakthrough as late as the 1970s, and since then it has developed into trivial as well as exciting radio/TV programs and other interactive media – we still witness new variants of this.

Brecht would probably have loved – and criticized – the Internet, had he still been with us. It contains crap, cruelty and commercial interests, of course – but it is also a challenging and exciting interactive media and experience. You can send personal messages, statements, information and questions out into the world, and you can receive other people's responses: video, audio and cross-modal.

What you have to learn is to distinguish between options and to select what you need. The hypertext link from one page/site to another is a sophisticated yet simple way of exploring the possibilities. Click yourself into new information and interactive dialogue with colleagues, institutions and organizations from other countries. Try not to get lost in the infinite web of connections: remember always what you came for (if not just for fun – or 'surfing' as it is called with an interesting metaphor)!

This text can also be found on the Internet: the *Nordic Journal of Music Therapy* has established an important, easily accessible, and free service – go to http://www.hisf.no/njmt/. Here you will find links to many of the addresses mentioned below. You will also find 'A Mini-Manual for Music Therapy Students and Researchers to the EndNote Bibliographic Database'.

Examining websites and online services of music therapy

On the following pages we will ask three questions:

1. *How do I find the best music therapy websites?*

   Look at the 'Selected web addresses for different purposes'.

2. *How can you use the world wide web/the Internet to search literature?*

   Look at the 'Recommended strategy for literature search'.

3. *Where can I find interesting listservs on music therapy?*

   Look at the 'Listservs and newsgroups' list.

SELECTED WEB ADDRESSES FOR DIFFERENT PURPOSES

The criteria for selecting the websites mentioned have been as follows: it should give access to all sorts of relevant material, be easy to use, have interactive features, be updated regularly, include many links – and it should be free and non-commercial.

Based on these criteria our 'first four choices' would be:

- The website of the World Federation of Music Therapy, situated at the University of Witten-Herdecke, Germany: www.musictherapyworld.net. This website is comprehensive, well edited and includes a world (!) of material: databases, an article library (papers can be downloaded in different formats), an e-journal on research and clinical practice, information on new books, WFMT and EMTC plus links to training programs, research programs, journals etc.

- The website of the *Nordic Journal of Music Therapy*: www.hisf.no/njmt/. A carefully edited website including selected full-text articles, a discussion forum, e-reviews of new books, links to music therapy journals, training programs and international organizations. It now also includes the international e-journal *Voices*.

- The website of the Music Therapy program in Aalborg University: www.musik.auc.dk. A newly redesigned website including all information about the training program and the international PhD program. It also gives access to the institute e-journal *col legno* including music therapy papers (in English) and a series of monographs (in English) on subjects taught only in this program.

- The website of the American Music Therapy Association: www.musictherapy.org/. The website of the American music therapists' association covers or links to information on all sorts of relevant activities in the USA.

RECOMMENDED STRATEGY FOR LITERATURE SEARCH

The recommendations below are based on several years of experience with literature search in databases, including those referenced. In the following table you can see the results of a general search and three specific searches in seven databases:

Table 7.1: Results of a general search and three specific searches in seven databases

Database Name	Number of music therapy journals included	Search 1: Music therapy (total)	Search 2: Rett syndrome	Search 3: Hospice Palliative care	Search 4: Guided Imagery and Music
EndNote	10+	3887	20	79	491
CAIRSS	8+	2226	5	13/21	21
RILM	6+	2220	5	18/14	34
PsycINFO	7+	1544	2	6/13	68
MEDLINE	5+	953	7	19/38	28
Ingenta	7+	574	2	5/18	11
Auboline	10+	454 (books)	1 (book)	2/5 (books)	13 (books)

A short introduction to all seven databases in this survey (November 2001) is given below. But what is clear is that the specific music therapy database – the EndNote 'Music Data' library – is superior in most cases. An overall recommended search strategy would be to conduct systematic searches in the first four or five. UnCover/Ingenta is a service that allows you to order article, by fax or online, but it is quite expensive, unless you have access to it from a university or institution library. Auboline is the database of the University of Aalborg (including a link to the institute library of the music therapy program), where a large collection of music therapy books are available.

The most important databases and services – why, where and how to find and use them:

1. The EndNote database/libraries

Where: Computers in Aalborg, Herdecke, Oslo. Updates on MT info CD-ROMs I–IV.

In a different format the database can also be searched in www.musictherapyworld.net.

Advantages: Comprehensive; MT specific; all bibliographic info; incl. abstracts.

Disadvantages: Few books included; also rare journals listed.

2. CAIRSS (web address: http://imr.utsa.edu/CAIRSS.html)

Computer-Assisted Information Retrieval Service System, developed by Don Hodges, University of San Antonio, Texas.

Where: From any computer with access to the Internet.

Advantages: Comprehensive and up to date within music and MT. Abstracts. Citations can be e-mailed (to yourself) from screen. Text download facility.

Disadvantages: Almost no non-English literature; requires Java or Telnet.

Comments: CAIRSS has been improved immensely.

3. RILM (Repertoire Internationale de Literature Musicale) database/ CD-ROM

Where: Aalborg University Library (www.aub.auc.dk). Check your own library.

Advantages: Comprehensive; music specific; all bibliographic info; incl. abstracts. Citations can be e-mailed (to yourself) from screen.

Disadvantages: No systematic MT coverage; not always up to date.

Comments: The database is improving quite fast. Only access via intranet or with password.

4. PsycINFO (PsycFIRST)

Where: Aalborg University Library (AUB) and most University libraries in the world.

Advantages: The best database within clinical psychology; all bibliographic info; incl. abstracts. Citations can be e-mailed (to yourself) from screen.

Disadvantages: Not much German/Nordic literature.

Comments: PsycFIRST covers the three most recent years.

5. MEDLINE

Where: AUB and most university libraries in the world.

Advantages: The best database within medical fields; all bibliographic info; incl. abstracts. Citations can be e-mailed (to yourself) from screen.

Disadvantages: No systematic coverage of MT. Not much German/Nordic literature.

Comments: Find a free online access to MEDLINE. It is not necessary to have a password.

6. Ingenta (previously UnCover) (web address: www.ingenta.com)

Where: From any computer with access to the Internet.

Advantages: Comprehensive and up to date. If you have a password/profile, articles can be ordered by fax or online. Many additional services. Citations can be e-mailed (to yourself) from screen.

Disadvantages: No abstracts; almost no non-English literature; not MT specific.

Comments: Private ordering is expensive. Your library may provide support.

7. Auboline and the database(s) of Aalborg University Library

Where: Also available by net: www.aub.auc.dk.

Advantages: AUB has a good collection of MT books and journals.

Disadvantages: Auboline has no abstracts; journal search only by databases.

Comments: Try the 'virtual libraries' (under 'Databases'), including RILM. Check also the MT library at Institut 10 (search base: AUM).

Other important databases

AskERIC: http://ericir.syr.edu/

UTSA libraries: www.lib.utsa.edu/index.html

The Library of Congress: http://www.loc.gov/

Other selected web addresses/URLs

If you want to buy books or CDs from electronic bookstores or publishers:

MMB Music: http://www.mmbmusic.com (many links)

Jessica Kingsley Publishers: www.jkp.com

Barnes and Noble: www.barnesandnoble.com

MT journals and other relevant electronic journals

Music Therapy Today e-magazine:
www.musictherapyworld.net/MMMagazine/index.html

Voices: www.voices.no

MusicTherapyEnews: http://www.onelist.com/group/MusicTherapyEnews.

To subscribe to *Music Therapy Enews*, go to
http://groups.yahoo.com/group/MusicTherapyEnews, click on 'Subscribe', and
follow the link and instructions for 'New Member'.

Musiktherapeutische Umschau: www.musiktherapie.de/

Psyche: http://psyche.cs.monash.edu.au/

Try your local virtual library!

Example: Aalborg University Library gives teachers and students access to many
electronic journals and services. Try also:

http://www.lib.utsa.edu/index.html (Unviersity of Texas at San Antonio
Libraries). Gives access to many electronic reference sources (incl. CAIRSS,
MEDLINE).

http://www.human-nature.com/free-associations/glover/bibliography.html
  Gives access to many special bibliographic informations.

LISTSERVS AND NEWSGROUPS

A listserv is a list of electronic mail addresses. When you subscribe you can receive
and send (copies of) e-mails from/to other members of the list. The communication
includes information about courses, practicum placements and jobs (in the USA),
stupid questions, clinical dialogues, literature discussions etc. – you will learn how to
select what you need.

Right now (November 2001) there are two specific MT listservs. The 'Music
Therapy Listserv' is open to all people interested in the area. A new listserv,
MT-PRO, is beginning now and will only be open to professional music therapists
worldwide.

Where to register the Music Therapy Listserv:
  http://www.musictherapy.org/listserv.html.

To join the listserv, send an e-mail to the list owners: Alexandra Mesquita-Baer (alex.baer@starband.net) or Lynne Hockenbury (LynneHock@aol.com).

Where to get information about and register MT-PRO:
  http://users.multipro.com/clark/mtpro/ – and follow instructions to subscribe.

About 'Netiquette': list ethics and practical advice can be found at:
  http://ukanaix.cc.ukans.edu/~dirkcush/net.html.

7.4 Books and CD-ROMs

This book includes many references and a comprehensive bibliography. In Chapter 4.8 we presented a selection of edited volumes including international contributions on selected clinical topics. In this chapter we will give short introductions to selected important books and other releases on music therapy in theory and practice.

Books

Aldridge, David (1996) *From out of the Silence: Music Therapy Research and Practice in Medicine*

Dr Aldridge holds the chair of qualitative research at the Faculty of Medicine at the private university of Witten-Herdecke (Germany). An English professor in Germany is not a common phenomenon, and Dr Aldridge is an extraordinary figure in the international music therapy culture. He is a true bridge-builder, embracing and connecting Anglo-American and Central European perspectives and experiences, the arts therapies and professionals from different sections of the health sector. His broad outlook is documented in the hundreds of articles he has published in professional journals and in several edited books and CD-ROMs.

The book from 1996 is a comprehensive and extremely informative book. Based on scientific case studies and literature reviews, Dr Aldridge documents how music therapy can be an effective intervention within several medical areas: dementia, Alzheimer's, inflammatory bowel disease – and developmental disability. He outlines the principles of building an interdisciplinary research culture within medicine in such a way that professionals with different backgrounds and paradigms can work together in mutual respect, and he gives a survey of methodologies suitable for music therapy research.

In continuation of this book Dr Aldridge and his colleagues at University of Witten-Herdecke have published the KAIROS series – four volumes in German so far – documenting results, methods and procedures from clinical practice. The volumes are thematic.

Dr Aldridge has edited two books on music therapy in palliative care and dementia care (Aldridge 1998a, 2000), both with contributions from clinicians and researchers from many countries. He is also research supervisor of the PhD program at Aalborg University (Denmark) and an eager spokesman for international research collaboration. One of his most important international initiatives is the release of four CD-ROMs with databases, international congress reports (Vitoria, Spain 1993; Leuwen, Belgium 1998; Washington 1999) dissertations, articles, video clips and other material: *Music Therapy Info 1* (1996c), *Info 2* (1998b), *Info 3* (2001) and *Info 4* (2002). The contents include databases with bibliographic information on tens of thousands of articles, books and other papers on music therapy and related topics. The CD-ROMs are practical results of Dr Aldridge's ideas of exploiting modern information technology in the service of clinicians and researchers. Another example is the international website www.musictherapy world.net.

Bruscia, Ken (1987) *Improvisational Models of Music Therapy.*

Bruscia, Ken (1998a) *Defining Music Therapy* (2nd edition).

Bruscia's 1987 book is introduced in Chapter 4.8. It belongs – together with *Case Studies in Music Therapy* (Bruscia 1991) – to the basic literature of any professionally trained music therapist. In the early 1990s Dr Bruscia, who is Professor of Music Therapy at Temple University, Pennsylvania, took the initiative to Barcelona Publishers, which has developed into one of the most important international providers of music therapy literature.

In 1998 Barcelona Publishers released the 2nd edition of a classic book: Dr Bruscia's comprehensive overview of music therapy definitions, first published in 1989. The new edition is an almost total revision, including many new chapters and ideas. In this book we are inspired by Dr Bruscia's systematic account of levels and practices of music therapy, introduced and used, for example, in Chapters 1.2, 3.8 and 3.9.

Decker-Voigt, Hans-Helmuth and Knill, Paulo (eds) (1996) *Lexikon Musiktherapie.*

This great German handbook replaced the widely spread *Handbuch Musiktherapie* from 1983. Leading German clinicians, researchers and other experts write about their expert fields, and the professional level of the one- to eight-page articles is high. The lexicon suffers from one problem: it is organized alphabetically, not systematically, and the component references represent very different types of topics and levels of problems, as can be illustrated with the entries in letter A (translated into English): Resistance – Affect – Active music therapy – Ambulant music therapy – Ambulant treatment of eating disorders – 'Being different' (a concept within *morphological music therapy*) – Anthroposophical music therapy – Appeal of music instruments – Filing and documentation of therapeutic material – Associative improvisation. The handbook is not a means to achive a systematic overview, and the best entrance to the goldmine of information in this book is to use the index of keywords.

Kenny, Carolyn Bereznak (1989) *The Field of Play: A Guide for the Theory and Practice of Music Therapy.*

In this book Kenny asks if it is possible to develop a language capable of describing the experience of music therapy and – based on such a language – to create a theoretical model reflecting the process of musical interaction in a precise way, at the same time being understandable for professionals with a different background. She attempts to give an answer by developing a holographical model called 'the field of play'. The field is defined by four elements (rituals, an altered state of consciousness, power and energy), all connected with ancient healing processes. Kenny develops her model within an existential-phenomenological and hermeneutical framework, and she includes the inevitable paradoxes of any attempt to translate sensory experience into verbal language. The holistic model of description is extensively discussed, but Kenny keeps reminding us that theoretical constructions and models can only be useful for music therapy if they are based on the experience of beauty in clinical work and on love of the profession. Dr Kenny was trained as a clinician and a researcher in the USA, but today she helds a position at the Simon Fraser University in Vancouver, Canada.

Pavlicevic, Mercedes (1997) *Music Therapy in Context. Music, Meaning and Relationship.*

This book deals with important questions in the theory and practice of music therapy: how is the clinical improvisation in music therapy different from free improvisation in a variety of styles? How does the cultural background influence the clinical improvisation and process? What is the function of words and verbal language, when the therapeutic relationship is based on music? The book is in three parts. Part One reflects on the question of meaning in music: important theories are discussed and related to the therapeutic context. Part Two is an investigation of the relationship between human emotions and clinical improvisation, and Pavlicevic develops her concept of 'dynamic form'. In Part Three psychodynamic theory is related to interpersonal events in music therapy – Dr Pavlicevic was trained as a Nordoff-Robbins music therapist. Today she works clinically and teaches in London and the Republic of South Africa.

Ruud, Even (1998a) *Musikk som kommunikasjon og samhandling.*

Ruud, Even (1999) *Music Therapy: Improvisation, Communication and Culture.*

Dr Ruud, who is Professor in Music Therapy in Oslo, Norway, has published a great number of books and articles during more than 25 years, not only in music therapy but also in musicology, music anthropology and music education. His doctoral thesis from 1990 is a reference work in Scandinavian music therapy, and still the most comprehensive and complete text on the topic in a Nordic language. It reviews and discusses the history of music therapy, the most important models, methods and procedures, the major clinical areas, but also the philosophical, theoretical and scientific foundations of music therapy, including an analysis of the understanding of music in music therapy and of music therapy as a means of communication and an interaction potential.

Dr Ruud's work in the last ten years is reflected in a text anthology in English, giving a fine overview of his contributions to the theory and metatheory of music therapy. Ruud belongs to the critical and social constructionist tradition, according to which the meaning of music is always situated in a local and specific context. This context and the meaning of music (therapy) must be studied using qualitative research methods, demanding basic self-reflexive skills of the researcher. Following this line the result may not be so many 'positive stories' about the benefits of music therapy. On the other hand these qualitative narratives are characterized by careful documentation, detailed description and rigorous interpretations of what is actually happening in the therapy room – and in the interplay of music therapy and the world outside the therapy room.

Smeijsters, Henk (1997) *Multiple Perspectives. A Guide to Qualitative Research in Music Therapy.*

Smeijsters, Henk (1999) *Grundlagen der Musiktherapie.*

The Dutch music psychologist and professor of music therapy has played an important role in the development of an international dialogue within the theory and research of music therapy. Dr Smeijsters publishes in Dutch, German and English, and the two books mentioned here are major contributions to the literature in the 1990s. *Multiple Perspectives* gives a critical overview of qualitative research methodologies and traditions, and their application to music therapy. The presentation format is composed of a presentation of the methodology in general (e.g. phenomenology, Grounded theory, morphology, hermeneutics), a presentation of one or two examples of a music therapy application, and finally a critical discussion. Dr Smeijsters also discusses the most important advantages and disadvantages of quantitative and qualitative research methods, which he considers complementary – including many common features.

Grundlagen der Musiktherapie represents Dr Smeijsters' personal contribution to the theory of music therapy, including examples of its application to clinical practice. He suggests that the concept of analogy should be considered a core concept, common to psychotherapeutical and special educational music therapy (see also Chapter 3.9). Analogy, indication criteria, treatment and evaluation are interwoven in this theory, which Dr Smeijsters applies to selected clinical populations: depression, schizophrenia, autism and developmental delay.

CD-ROMs

Aldridge, David (ed) (1996, 1998b, 2001, 2002) CD-ROM: *Music Therapy Info* Volumes 1 to 4.

The four CD-ROMs with the common title *Music Therapy Info* are presented in the text above. Professor Aldridge has also released a CD-ROM with video cases:

Aldridge, David (ed) (1998) *Music Therapy with Children.*

AMERICAN MUSIC THERAPY JOURNALS ON CD-ROM

In 1999 the American Music Therapy Association (AMTA) released a CD-ROM containing all articles published from 1956 to 1998 in the three major American journals: *Journal of Music Therapy, Music Therapy Perspectives* and *Music Therapy.*

The majority of the material is American, but the CD-ROM also contains papers written by non-American specialists (see also Chapters 7.2).

CHAPTER 8

A Glossary and Lexicon
of Music Therapy

Active music therapy

Music used purposefully or clinically requiring the active participation of the client(s). The process of music-making in a clinical session, either with precomposed, improvised or extemporized music. The relationship is built through the meaning of the sounds within the shared musical experience.

Allocentric/allopathic

Allocentric: having one's awareness directed towards 'the opposite', something missing or not present. Allopathic use of music: a way of healing, harmonizing or curing using music with a complementary quality, e.g., using lively, up-tempo music with depressive clients and clients in low spirits. In other words: A is a contrast principle, complementary to the principle of homeopathy. See also 'the ISO-principle'.

Analytical Music Therapy

Active, psychotherapeutic method, developed by the English music therapist Mary Priestley in circa 1970. It is based on the symbolic use of musical, non-verbal improvisations, where the client sings or plays on self-chosen instruments in musical dialogues with the therapist. A 'playing rule' or a symbolic theme related to the problem of the client is decided before the improvisation and is discussed and reflected upon after the improvisation. Today the method is called Analytically Oriented Music Therapy (AOM).

Applied Behaviour Analysis

Principal method of analysis for behavioural psychology or behaviour oriented therapy approaches. Typically used in investigative research, taking as a reference point and goal the behaviour that is to be evaluated. The process involves establishing a baseline, observing (and usually measuring) the behaviour that is being treated by the therapy, and then evaluating the effect of the therapy over time.

(Clinical) Assessment

Clinical assessment is a process of evaluating a client's history and presenting problems in order to assess his/her therapeutic needs. Assessment can be undertaken within different domains – biographical, physical, behavioural, cognitive, functional and psychodynamic (amongst others) depending on the expertise and orientation of the clinician. Therapeutic assessment involves both a holistic and a specific evaluation of a client (or group of clients).

Behavioural Music Therapy

Behavioural methods involving the influence of music on human behaviour, where responses are monitored to musical listening or musical activity. Music is used to increase, decrease, modify or reinforce carefully defined target behaviours in order to have a significant effect on a person's adaptation, education or development.

Clinical

A term which refers to the identification and attention to symptoms or other aspects of an illness. It can also refer to an approach where one is scientifically detached and strictly objective. The term is used in music therapy in reference to clinical improvisation (see below).

Clinical improvisation

Widely used method of *active music therapy* in Europe. Generally, the use of musical improvisation with a specific therapeutic purpose in an environment facilitating response and interaction. A musical relationship is gradually built through shared repertoire and exchange of musical expressions. The theoretical basis is that the spontaneously produced sounds created within a musical framework represent aspects of personality at conscious or unconscious levels. Recordings of improvisations within a treatment or therapeutic intervention form a clinical record of the client's therapeutic process. Main models of improvisational music therapy are defined in Bruscia (1987): *Improvisational Models of Music Therapy*. Clinical improvisation is, therefore, a procedure where instrumental or vocal improvisations are directed towards certain aims to obtain relevant evidence related to certain symptoms, to pathological or psychological problems.

Compliance
Originally means pliant or an inclination to give way to the will of others. In clinical concepts it is a term that refers to the client's willingness to co-operate, which is dependent on many different psychological factors.

Coping
An English term, which has been transferred to the professional terminology of Danish psychotherapy as a term for the client's ability to manage his/her mental problems. It is an important aim for therapy work to develop the client's ability of coping by use of coping mechanisms or coping behaviour. This refers to ways of behaving and intrapsychic processes that help the client to better manage situations of crisis and symptoms of somatic illnesses.

Countertransference
Countertransference was defined by Freud as the process through which the unconscious conflicts and motives of the therapist are activated by the contact experienced with the client, and are then transferred to the client. He considered countertransference as a disturbing and negative element in therapy. In later psychoanalysis (since Heimann) countertransference is defined on a broader basis including being considered as a positive tool through which the therapist can gain significantly more insight into the personality and unconscious conflicts of the client.

Creative Music Therapy (the Nordoff-Robbins model)
A method of music therapy developed during the 1960s by the American composer and pianist Dr Paul Nordoff and the English child specialist Clive Robbins. The method has now expanded to be practised in England, Germany, the USA, Australia, Japan, South Africa and Scandinavia. The method originally started for the treatment of handicapped children, but has now extended to adults, and other clinical areas. The goals are the development of the client's self-expression, creativity and communication potential. In the classic model, a team of two therapists (pianist and co-therapist) work in individual therapy using clinical improvisation (piano singing and percussion) as a medium to involve the client in a musical process that can achieve therapeutic objectives. In group music therapy, sometimes specially composed songs and musical play are used.

Death instinct

Freud's concept of operating with two complementary ideas – life and death instincts (Eros and Thanatos). This can be understood as a speculative generalization of the differences between sexuality and libido. A death instinct is understood as a biologically inborn desire or tendency to go back to an earlier, more primitive position, e.g., from an organic to an inorganic state of being, whereas an inverse life instinct is to build up greater and more complex structures.

Dissociation

Separation, splitting, disintegration or elimination of single elements of a totality. The term is used in psychology as a definition of a defence mechanism, where the client splits off the emotions which are connected to memories or to the patient's stories of traumatic experiences.

Entrainment

A synchronization of physiological rhythms of the body (heart frequency, pulse, brain waves) and external rhythmical stimuli created through live or recorded music that can be modified in tempo. The music therapist can obtain a specific physiological effect by matching the client's pulse in the music and subsequently influence the pulse in the direction he/she wishes. The American music therapist Mark Rider has developed a therapeutic procedure on this principle combined with a theory called 'homeodynamics' (Rider 1997, 1999).

Free Improvisation Therapy (the Alvin model)

Method of music therapy developed by Juliette Alvin in the 1950s. The therapist gives the client complete freedom to improvise as he/she wishes without any rules, structure or themes. Developmental approach where musical instruments are of central importance as part of the client–therapist relationship.

Guided Imagery and Music (the Bonny Method)

A receptive music therapeutic model developed by the American music therapist Helen Bonny in the 1970s. It was originally designed especially to create a framework for self-developmental work with spiritual and transpersonal experiences. The client ('traveller') listens to carefully selected classical music in a slightly altered state of consciousness, and he/she experiences physical, mental or existential problems in the form of imagery in many modalities. The images are reported as metaphors in an on-going dialogue with the therapist ('guide'). The combination of music and imagery has proved effective within many different clinical areas.

Homeostasis
A flexible, physiological state of being in balance (equilibrium); the striving towards equilibrium by the organism, always seeking to re-establish the initial condition (like a thermostat). Originally the term comes from biology and defines the striving of the organism to maintain stability in spite of the changing conditions of the surroundings.

Interaction
Co-operation or interplay between two or more participants. The term is used in psychology, identifying several patterns of interaction between mother and infant. In therapy it identifies the interplay between the therapist and the client.

Intertherapy
Training discipline for music therapy students, developed in Analytical Music Therapy by Mary Priestley. There are three participants: a supervisor/therapist who contains the experiences, and two students who take turns in the roles of therapist and client.

Intuitive music
A group improvisation form, where the music is created in the 'here and now', based on intuition or on a few principles or rules. No scores are used, but often written instructions or graphic noted ideas are used for the musical process.

ISO-principle
Two complimentary treatment principles (I and C) of music therapy and for the application of music in therapy. According to the I principle, music matching the mood of the client must be used (e.g. sad music for a client in low spirits). According to the C principle, music with a contrasting quality must be selected (e.g. lively, cheerful music for a client in low spirits) (Benenzon 1997).

Mandala
'Ring' or 'circle' in Sanskrit. An image or painting in a circular or almond-shaped form, well known in spiritual and religious traditions from many cultures, symbolizing unity and wholeness. M is used as an expressive arts tool in conjunction with some music therapy models, e.g. Guided Imagery and Music, where the client is given an opportunity to recall and express his/her experiences during the 'music travel' in another modality.

Morphological music therapy

Morphological music therapy was developed by a group of German music therapists (among others Eckhard Weymann and Rosemarie Tüpker), who based their model on W. Salber's morphological psychology. Salber claims (with Goethe) that the psyche is generating and transforming forms ('Gestalts') all the time, and that everyday life and art can be seen as 'prototypical areas of treatment'. Gestalt formation and transformation takes place in six discrete processes: 1. Aneignung (appropriation), 2. Umbildung (metamorphosis), 3. Einwirkung (influence), 4. Anordnung (arrangement), 5. Ausbreitung (unfolding), 6. Ausrüstung (equipment). Morphology has also defined four 'treatment steps': 1. Leiden können (being able to suffer), 2. Methodisch werden (becoming methodical), 3. Anders werden (becoming different), 4. Werkstellen (implementation). Finally, Morphology has developed a research procedure in four steps: wholeness – internal regulation – transformation – reconstruction (see Exner 1998a; Smeijsters 1997a; Tüpker 1988).

Music healing

The use of musical experiences to heal mind, body and spirit, to induce self-healing and to promote wellness. Active techniques include breathing, vocalizing, toning, chanting; receptive techniques include listening, entraining, resonating, imaging or physically reacting to music, musical vibrations or electric musical signals.

Music in Medicine

Music is used to influence the patient's physical, mental or emotional states before, during or after medical, dental or paramedical treatment. Methods include preparation for medical intervention, and enhancing/facilitating the process of treatment. Publications: *Music Medicine Vol II & III*, International Society for Music in Medicine; Dileo (ed) (1999) *Music Therapy & Medicine*.

Musical behaviour

Action or conduct of a person engaged in music-making or music listening. In music therapy, this represents both a person's reaction to music, and also aspects of their personality, character and pathology in active music-making or receptive listening.

Musical creativity

The ability to produce musical sounds in a way or combination that is characterized by originality of thought or inventiveness, and is original to the person producing them. This ability can be either innate or developed over time through musical education or musical experiences.

Musical psychodrama

Musical psychodrama is a group method of work inspired by Gestalt therapy, where clients use music (instrumental, vocal) in the dramatized recreation of dreams, fantasies or episodes from a life history. It is based on the psychodrama approach by Joseph Moreno, a method including role-playing, where the identification of the dynamic of the group is used for therapeutic objectives.

Music psychotherapy

A generic term for therapy methods where music (active or receptive) and the therapeutic relationship are used to work with, and to improve, the psychological condition of the client. The therapy can be ego supportive, personality developing or transpersonally oriented. The therapy aims at improving consciousness of mental conflicts, self-insight and psychological development. The methods can be psychodynamic, existential or transpersonal.

Musical relationship

The development of a musical relationship between a client or group of clients and a therapist is the foundation of the improvisational methods of music therapy used in Europe. This concept can include many different forms of musical relationship; however, the primary focus is based on shared musical experiences that have meaning for the clients and therapists involved.

Musicality

The concept goes back to the end of the nineteenth century and is closely related to the new and expanding tradition of experimental research in the human perception of music. There have been many (also conflicting) theories of Musicality during the twentieth century, reflecting differing ideas of the nature of Musicality and how it can be researched, measured, tested and applied to educational or therapeutic purposes. Important researchers and theorists are Carl E. Seashore (a representative of positivist 'tone' psychology), James L. Mursell (the Gestalt approach), Robert W. Lundin (behaviourism) and John Blacking (anthropology) (see Jørgensen 1982: *5 Musikalitetsteorier/4 theories of musicality*). Many researchers of the positivist-experimental paradigm have developed tests of Musicality (also called 'musical aptitude', 'music capacity', 'musical talent' or 'music intelligence'), e.g. Seashore, Wing and Bentley. Using standardized inventories they have interpreted the test results of a person in order to compare them with established group norms, or to predict the relevance and eventual outcome of formal music teaching. Many of the elements of these classic tests are still included in entrance tests high level for music training programs (including music therapy), e.g. musical memory, interval identification, chord analysis.

In contemporary cognitive music psychology there is consensus that Musicality – defined as musical knowledge and performance skills – is not significantly modified by genetic or physical factors (e.g. race and sex); in other words the potential ability of creating and experiencing music is a common and universal human competency. However, it can be developed to a lesser or greater extent, dependent on how music is defined, valued and promoted in the specific milieu or culture of a person. Musical skills can be developed through practise with or without formal training – in the latter case as 'situated learning' of music, still common in many non-Western cultures. In Howard Gardner's (1997) influential contemporary theory of 'multiple intelligences', Musicality is defined as musical intelligence, one of seven (or more) specific intelligences. This theory has been adapted for educational purposes in many countries.

Numinoso
The Numinoso is a concept of 'something experienced as totally different' (Ingemann Nielsen 1986). It may refer to the Divine in a very broad sense, or it can be a very intensive experience of Unity or Wholeness. Spiritual and transpersonal therapy approaches strive to help the client to establish and maintain contact with the Numinoso.

Object relations theory
The relationship between a subject and his/her inner and outer 'objects' which can, for example, be a person, an animal or a thing. The theory of Freud combines the objects to the drives which means that they are either real or improvised tools for gaining satisfaction. In later psychoanalytic theory the subject's interaction with inner and outer objects is emphasized. Melanie Klein describes the split of the 'bad' and the 'good' object as a core phenomenon of the oral phase. Here the child is not able to distinguish between 'the breast' and 'the mother'. Winnicott developed the term 'transitional object' as a term for the object the child is attached to in the difficult phase of learning to distinguish between inner (improvised) and outer (physical, independent) objects.

Organum
Musical part-song based on the principle that two or more melodic parts move in parallel (note-to-note), either in a fixed interval (e.g. fifths or octaves), or more freely in a mixture of parallel and counter movement.

Pathology

The branch of medicine concerned with the cause, origin and nature of disease, including the changes occuring as a result of disease. Pathology is also a term used to denote the manifestation of a disease, and can be applied as a description of any deviation from the normal.

Pleasure principle

In classic psychoanalysis, Freud contrasts the principle of pleasure and the *reality principle*. According to Freud the earliest mental function is a co-ordinated striving for gratification and withdrawal from the unpleasant tension and affect of pain and/or pleasure. The reality principle, which is developed later, gradually modifies the pleasure-seeking, pain-avoiding operations and replaces immature wish fulfilment with more appropriate adaptive behaviour. The pleasure principle is connected to the id and the reality principle to the ego and the superego.

Primary and secondary processes

In classical psychoanalysis, primary processes are understood to be the earliest and most basic ways of psychological functioning. Primary processes are connected to the id and include early, pre-logical types of symbols, where different drives are mixed up and where no sense of time and space exists. Primary processes are found in the dreams of adults, in inner imaginations, fantasies – and as pathology by psychotic people. The secondary processes are connected to the ego and are developed gradually as a realistic, logical and rational relationship towards oneself and the surroundings. One can observe the growth of perceptions, emotions, thinking processes and social responsibility in this phase of development. In a later psychoanalytic tradition (G. Ammon, School of Berlin), the term tertiary process exists which is understood as the quick alternation between primary and secondary processes. A tertiary condition can be observed just before falling asleep, or when engaged in creative working processes. Tertiary processes often arise in experientially based psychotherapy as is typical in European music therapy. In Stern's interpersonal theory concerning the psychological development of an infant, the two (primary and secondary) processes are turned around; it is maintained that the infant is social and rational just after birth, while the ability to symbolize develops later.

Projective identification

In classical psychoanalysis, the term for a defence mechanism where the subject projects split-off parts of himself/herself into another object (e.g. another person in order to control or destroy the object).

Psychodynamic movement

A method for training music therapists within the analytical tradition. Psychodynamic movement is the term for musical, group-dynamic activities with the body as the primary instrument ('box of resonance'), where the body and voice function as the primary channels of expression.

Receptive music therapy

A generic term for models where music listening is applied for clinical purposes in individual or group therapy. In Guided Imagery and Music, the client listens to carefully selected, classical music in a slightly altered state of consciousness, enabling an exploration of problems, memories and emotions in the form of metaphoric imagery. In the group method 'Musical Life Panorama' (I. Frohne Hagemann 1990), the musical history of the client creates a sound board for working through emotions and for the exchange of memories. In other methods the favourite music of the client is applied, or the music therapist sings/plays to the client. Receptive music therapy always involves listening and the (receptive) musical experience is the starting point of the therapeutical dialogue.

Reliability

A term used mainly in quantitative research and clinical evaluation that requires a tool or system of measurement to give consistent results when used in different or replication studies where the circumstances of the study are similar.

Resistance

A professional term in psychoanalysis and psychotherapy identifying a client's conscious and unconscious unwillingness that repressed conflicts should come into consciousnes.

Supervision

A teaching form where experienced clinicians (psychologists, music therapists, psychotherapists) supervise students or less experienced therapists (supervisees). The supervisee is expected to present a case or a specific problem to be supervised. Also refers to supervision of research studies.

Theory of humours

A classic doctrine of health and disease based on the theory of four bodily fluids or 'humours': blood, phlegm, yellow bile and black bile. According to this theory, health was a matter of harmonic balance between the humours, while disease reflected an imbalance between them. Music was considered a therapeutic tool capable of influencing, even restoring the balance. Historically the doctrine goes back to circa 400 BC, and it was foundational in medical theory right up to the eighteenth century.

Transference

Transference was defined by Freud as the process where the client, in the therapeutic situation, replays a contemporary version of lost childhood memories or regressed unconscious fantasies. The therapist becomes the object of the transference and can be identified by the client with the same traits and reactions as a meaningful person from the client's past. For this reason the therapist often presents himself/herself in a neutral way in order to keep his/her own personality back or even 'out of sight'.

Transitional object

The English psychoanalyst and object relations theorist Dr Donald Winnicott developed the term 'transitional object' as a term for the special object (e.g. a 'nipple cloth', a flap of a quilt, a little melody) to which a child in the oral phase (by the age of 4–12 months) is attached. It is in the difficult phase where the child has to learn to distinguish between itself as a subject on the one side and inner (improvised) and outer (physical, independent) objects on the other side.

Turn-taking

A skill at being able to intuitively follow a (sometimes unspoken) rule of changing between active playing and then waiting or listening to another (others). This is developed both in games and in different types of communicative interaction – for example, between mother and child, or between client(s) and therapist.

Validity

A term used in different ways that primarily is concerned with the verifiability, and believability, of the results that are achieved from research or clinical evaluation. To establish validity it is necessary to demonstrate that the tool of assessment or evaluation actually measures what it is supposed to measure. Other forms of validity include *content validity, criterion-related validity, construct validity, internal validity* and *external validity*.

Vibroacoustic therapy

A form of receptive music therapy employing the physical properties of sound and vibration. Pulsed, sinusoidal, low frequency sound between 30 Hz and 80 Hz is combined with relaxing and predictable music and is played through speakers built into a bed or chair. Patients lying on a vibroacoustic unit experience a gentle, internal vibration in different parts of their body, depending on the frequency used. Research to date has revealed effective treatment of physical disorders such as cerebral palsy, muscle tension and spasm as well as alleviation of pain.

Bibliography

This list contains articles and books referenced in the different chapters.

Aasgaard, T. (1999) 'Music Therapy as Milieu in the Hospice and Paediatric Oncology Ward.' In D. Aldridge (ed) *Music Therapy in Palliative Care. New Voices.* London: Jessica Kingsley Publishers.

Aasgaard, T. (2000a) '"Musik-Umfeld-Therapie" in Hospizen und auf Pädiatrischen Onkologiestationen.' In D. Aldridge (ed) *Kairos IV. Beiträge zur Musiktherapie in der Medizin.* Bern: Verlag Hans Huber.

Aasgaard, T. (2000b) '"A Suspiciously Cheerful Lady." A Study of a Song's Life in the Paediatric Oncology Ward, and Beyond ...' *British Journal of Music Therapy 14*, 2, 70–82.

Aasgaard, T. (2001) 'An Ecology of Love: Aspects of Music Therapy in the Pediatric Oncology Environment.' *Journal of Palliative Care*, 3, 177–181 (and companion CD-ROM segment 6).

Ahonen-Eerikäinen, H. (1999) 'Different Forms of Music Therapy and Working Styles of Music Therapists. – A Qualitative Study.' *Nordic Journal of Music Therapy 8*, 2, 156–167.

Aiello, R. (ed) (1994) *Musical Perceptions.* Oxford: Oxford University Press.

Aigen, K. (1991) 'The Roots of Music Therapy: Towards an Indigenous Research Paradigm.' (Doctoral dissertation, New York University, 1990.) *Dissertation Abstracts International 52*, 6, 1933A.

Aigen, K. (1995a) 'Principles of Qualitative Research.' In B. Wheeler (ed) *Music Therapy Research. Quantitative and Qualitative Perspectives.* Phoenixville: Barcelona Publishers.

Aigen, K. (1995b) 'Interpretational Research.' In B. Wheeler (ed) *Music Therapy Research. Quantitative and Qualitative Perspectives.* Phoenixville: Barcelona Publishers.

Aigen, K. (1996a) *Here we are in Music: One Year with an Adolescent, Creative Music Therapy Group.* St. Louis, MO: MMB.

Aigen, K. (1996b) Being in Music: *Foundations of Nordoff-Robbins Music Therapy.* St. Louis, MI: MMB Music.

Aigen, K. (1998) *Paths of Development in Nordoff-Robbins Music Therapy.* Gilsum, NH: Barcelona Publishers.

Aigen, K. (1999) 'The True Nature of Music-Centered Music Therapy Theory.' *British Journal of Music Therapy 13*, 2, 77–82.

Aldridge, D. (1993) 'Music Therapy Research: I. A Review of the Medical Research Literature Within a General Context of Music Therapy Research.' Special Issue: Research in the Creative Arts Therapies. *Arts in Psychotherapy 20*, 1, 11–35.

Aldridge, D. (1994) 'An Overview of Music Therapy Research.' *Complementary Therapies in Medicine 1994*, 2, 204–216.

Aldridge, D. (1996a) *From out of the Silence: Music Therapy Research and Practice in Medicine.* London: Jessica Kingsley Publishers.

Aldridge, D. (1996b) 'The Development of Music Therapy Research as a Perspective of Complementary Medicine.' In S. Olesen and E. Høg *Communication in and about Alternative Therapies.* Odense: Odense University Press.

Aldridge, D. (1996c) *Music Therapy Info-CD-Rom I.* Witten/Herdecke: Universität Witten/Herdecke.

Aldridge, D. (1997) *Kairos I – Beiträge zur Musiktherapie in der Medizin.* Kairos. Bern: Verlag Hans Huber.

Aldridge, D. (1998a) *Music Therapy in Palliative Care. New Voices.* London: Jessica Kingsley Publishers.

Aldridge, D. (1998b) *Music Therapy Info CD-ROM II.* Witten/Herdecke: Universität Witten/Herdecke.

Aldridge, D. (1999) *Music Therapy with Children CD-ROM.* London: Jessica Kingsley Publishers.

Aldridge, D. (ed) (1999a) *Kairos III Beiträge zur Musiktherapie in Der Medizin.* Bern: Verlag Hans Huber.

Aldridge, D. (1999b) 'Personal Opinion: Developing a Community of Inquiry.' *Nordic Journal of Music Therapy 8,* 1, 25–35.

Aldridge, D. (2000) *Music Therapy in Dementia Care: More New Voices.* London: Jessica Kingsley Publishers.

Aldridge, D. and Aldridge, G. (1999) 'Life as Jazz: Hope, Meaning, and Music Therapy in the Treatment of Life-Threatening Illness.' In C. Dileo *Music Therapy & Medicine: Theoretical and Clinical Applications.* Silver Spring, MD: American Music Therapy Association.

Aldridge, D. (2001) *Music Therapy Info-CD-Rom III.* Witten/Herdecke: Universität Witten/Herdecke.

Aldridge, D. and Brandt, G. (1991) 'Music therapy and inflammatory bowel disease.' *The Arts and Psychotherapy 18,* 113–121.

Aldridge, D. and Fachner, J. (2002) *Music Therapy World Info CD-Rom IV.* Witten/Herdecke: Univerität Witten/Herdecke.

Aldridge, D., Di Franco, G., Ruud, E. and Wigram, T. (eds) (2001) *Music Therapy in Europe.* Rome: Ismez.

Aldridge, G. (1996) '"A Walk Through Paris": The Development of Melodic Expression in Music Therapy with a Breast-Cancer Patient.' *The Arts in Psychotherapy 23,* 3, 207–223.

Aldridge, G. (1998) *Die Entwicklung einer Melodie im Kontext improvisatorischer Musiktherapie. (Melodiudvikling i improvisatorisk musikterapi).* PhD afhandling, Aalborg Universitet.

Aldridge, G. (2000) 'Improvisation as an Assessment of Potential in Early Alzheimer's Disease.' In D. Aldridge (ed) *Music Therapy in Dementia Care. More New Voices.* London: Jessica Kingsley Publishers.

Alvin, J. (1975) *Music Therapy* (revised edition). London: John Claire Books.

Alvin, J. (1976) *Music Therapy for the Handicapped Child* (second edition). London: Oxford University Press.

Alvin, J. (1978) *Music Therapy for the Autistic Child.* London: Oxford University Press.

Alvin, J. (1978/2000) 'A Research project – Martin.' (Reprinted from J. Alvin and A. Warwick *Music Therapy for the Autistic Child.* Oxford: OUP. *Nordic Journal of Music Therapy 9,* 1, 50–59.

American Music Therapy Association (1999) *Music Therapy Research: Quantitative Foundations CD-Rom I.* Silver Spring, Maryland: AMTA Publications.

American Psychiatric Association (1994) *Diagnostic and Statistical Manual of Mental Disorders* (fourth edition). Washington DC.

Amir, D. (1992) 'Awakening and Expanding the Self: Meaningful Moments in Music Therapy as Experienced and Described by Music Therapists and Music Therapy Clients.' *Dissertation Abstracts International 53*, 8, 4361B (University Microfilms No. DEY91–34717).

Amir, D. (1993) 'Research in Music Therapy: Quantitative or Qualitative?' *Nordic Journal of Music Therapy 3*, 2, 3–10.

Amir, D. (1999) 'Musical and Verbal Interventions in Music Therapy: A Qualitative Study.' *Journal of Music Therapy 36*, 2, 144–175.

Andrews, T. (1997) *Music Therapy for Non-Musicians.* Batavia, OH: Dragonhawk Publishers.

Ansdell, G. (1995) *Music for Life – Aspects of Creative Music Therapy with Adult Clients.* London: Jessica Kingsley Publishers.

Ansdell, G. (1996) 'Talking about Music Therapy. A Dilemma and a Qualitative Experiment.' *British Journal of Music Therapy 10*, 1, 4–15.

Ansdell, G. (1997) 'Musical Elaborations. What Has New Musicology to Say to Music Therapy?' *British Journal of Music Therapy 11*, 2, 36–44.

Ansdell, G. (1999) 'Challenging Premises.' *British Journal of Music Therapy 13*, 2, 72–76.

Ansdell, G. (2001) 'Musicology: Misunderstood Guest at the Music Therapy Feast?' In D. Aldridge, G. Di Franco, E. Ruud and T. Wigram (eds) *Music Therapy in Europe.* Rome: Ismez.

Ansdell, G. and Pavlicevic, M. (2001) *Beginning Research in the Arts Therapies. A Practical Guide.* London: Jessica Kingsley Publishers.

Ashida, S. (2000) 'The Effect of Reminiscence Music Therapy Sessions on Changes in Depressive Symptoms in Elderly Persons with Dementia.' *Journal of Music Therapy, 37*, 3, 170–182.

Assagioli, R. (1965) *Psychosynthesis: A Manual of Principles and Techniques.* New York: Hobbs, Dorman.

Assagioli, R. (1969) 'Symbols of transpersonal experiences.' *Psychosynthesis Research Foundation 11*, 3–21.

Association of Music and Imagery (1999) *Training Directory.* Philadelphia: AMI Publications.

Austin, D. (1991) 'The Musical Mirror: Music Therapy for the Narcissistically Injured.' In T. Wigram and J. De Backer (eds) *Clinical Applications of Music Therapy in Psychiatry.* London: Jessica Kingsley Publishers.

Baker, F. (2001a) 'The Effects of Live, Taped and No Music on People Experiencing Posttraumatic Amnesia.' *Journal of Music Therapy 38*, 3, 170–192.

Baker, F. (2001b) 'Rationale for the Effects of Familiar Music on Agitation and Orientation Levels of People in Posttraumatic Amnesia.' *Nordic Journal of Music Therapy 10*, 1, 32–41.

Bang, C. (1979/1998) 'A World of Sound and Music.' *Nordic Journal of Music Therapy 7*, 2, 154–163.

Bang, C. (1980) 'A World of Sound and Music: Music Therapy and Musical Speech Therapy with Hearing Impaired and Multiply-Handicapped Children.' *Teacher of the Deaf 4*, 106–15.

Bang, C. (1998) 'Introduction to "A World of Sound and Music".' *Nordic Journal of Music Therapy 7*, 2, 150–153.

Barger, D.A. (1979) 'The Effects of Music and Verbal Suggestion on Heart-Rate and Self Reports.' *Journal of Music Therapy 16*, 4, 158–171.

Bärmark, J. and Hallin, M. (1999) 'Sailing between the Charybodis of Theoretical Abstractions and the Scylla of Unreflected Experiences. Some Comments upon an Essay by Carolyn Kenny.' *Nordic Journal of Music Therapy 8*, 2, 137–142.

Bason, B.T. and Celler, B.G. (1972) 'Control of the Heart Rate by External Stimuli.' *Nature 4*, 279–280.

Bastian, P. (1987) *Ind i musikken.* Kbh.: Gyldendal/PubliMus.

Baumgartner, G. (1997) 'Bewegungsfundierte musiktherapie in der gerontopsychiatrie. Ein beispiel für die anvendung der RES-diagnostik in der praxis.' *Musik, Tanz- und Kunsttherapie 8,* 105–114.

Bean, J. (1995) 'Music Therapy and the Child with Cerebral Palsy: Directive and Non-directive Intervention.' In T. Wigram, B. Saperston and R. West. *The Art and Science of Music Therapy: A Handbook.* London: Harwood Academic.

Beck, A. (1976) *Cognitive Therapy and the Emotional Disorders.* New York: International Universities Press.

Benenzon, R.O. (1982) *Music Therapy in Child Psychosis.* Springfield, Illinois: Charles C. Thomas.

Benenzon, R.O. (1997) *Music Therapy Theory and Manual: Contributions to the Knowledge of Nonverbal Contexts.* Springfield, Illinois: Charles C. Thomas.

Bergstrøm-Nielsen, C. (1998) 'Sprog som musikalsk notation: en undersøgelse af verbal notation og dens forudsætninger med særligt henblik på Stockhausens Aus den Sieben Tagen og Für kommende Zeiten.' *Col legno (elektronisk udgave på www.musik.auc.dk).*

Bergstrøm-Nielsen, C. (1999) 'Intuitive music and graphic notation at Aalborg University. On two musical training disciplines within music therapy education and their theoretical backgrounds.' *Col legno (elektronisk udgave på www.musik.auc.dk).*

Bergstrøm-Nielsen, C. and Weymann, E. (eds) (2000) *First European Symposium: Improvisation Teaching within Music Therapy Training.* Hamburg: Förderkreis des Instituts für Musiktherapie der Hochshule für Musiktherapie und Morphologie Hamburg.

Bever, T.G. and Chiarello, R.J. (1974) 'Cerebral Dominance in Musicians and Nonmusicians.' *Science 185,* 150, 537–539.

Bierbaum, M.A. (1958) *Variations in Heart Action Under the Influence of Musical Stimuli.* Unpublished Master's thesis, University of Kansas.

Bion, W.R. (1967) *Second Thoughts. Selected Papers on Psychoanalysis.* London: Maresfield (reprints).

Bolger, E.P. and Judson, M.A. (1984) 'The Therapeutic Value of Singing.' *The New England Journal of Medicine 311,* 1704.

Bonde, L.O. (1992a) 'Balladen om musikken – Profilen og segmenterne i Danmarks Radio.' *Mediekultur 18,* 1992, 65–69.

Bonde, L.O. (1992b) 'Sol- og måneskinshistorier– musikterapi i 90-årenes Europa.' *Nordisk tidsskrift for musikkterapi 1,* 1, 33–37.

Bonde, L.O. (1993) *Musikterapilitteratur. Lille bibliografi og Vejledning i litteratursøgning.* AUC, Institut 10.

Bonde, L.O. (1994) 'Oplysning – Oplevelse – Oplivelse. Fællesoppgaver i undervisning og terapi.' *Nordisk Tidsskrift for Musikk og Musikkterapi 3,* 1, 13–18.

Bonde, L.O. (1996a) 'Sound and Psyche. Impressions from the 8th World Congress of Music Therapy in Hamburg, July 14th–20th 1996.' *Nordic Journal of Music Therapy 5,* 2, 122–127.

Bonde, L.O. (1997) 'Music Analysis and Image Potentials in Classical Music.' *Nordic Journal of Music Therapy 6,* 2, 121–128.

Bonde, L.O. (1999a) 'Metaphor and Metaphoric Imagery in Music Therapy Theory: A Discussion of a Basic Theoretical Problem – With Clinical Material from GIM Sessions.' 9th World Congress of Music Therapy, Washington DC, November 17–22, 1999. Under udgivelse på CD-ROM: D. Aldridge (ed) (2001) *Music Therapy Info Vol. III.*

Bonde, L.O. (1999b) 'Music Therapy, The Internet and Other Electronic Resources – An Update.' *Nordic Journal of Music Therapy 8,* 1, 100–104.

Bonde, L.O. (ed) (1999c) *Nordic Journal of Music Therapy. 8(1) Special Issue: Music Therapy in Aalborg University.* Sandane: Høgskulen i Sogn og Fjordane.

Bonde, L.O. (2000) 'Metaphor and Narrative in Guided Imagery and Music.' *Journal of the Association for Music and Imagery* 7, 59–76.

Bonde, L.O. (2001a) 'Musikpsykologi.' Opslag i nyudgaven af *Gads Musikleksikon*. Kbh.: G.E.C. Gad.

Bonde, L.O. (2001b) 'Musik og smertebehandling.' In U. Fasting and L. Lundorff (eds) *Smerter og smertebehandling i klinisk praksis*. Kbh.: Munksgaard.

Bonde, L.O. (2001c) 'Steps towards a Meta-Theory of Music Therapy? An Introduction to Ken Wilber's Integral Psychology and a Discussion of its Relevance for Music Therapy.' *Nordic Journal of Music Therapy* 10, 2, 176–187.

Bonde, L., Nygaard Pedersen, I. and Wigram, T. (1999) *Studieordningen for Kandidatuddannelsen i musikterapi, Institut for musik og musikterapi*. Aalborg Universitet: Aalborg.

Bonde, L., Nygaard Pedersen, I. and Wigram, T. (2001) *Når Ord ikke Slår Til: En handbøg i Musikterapiens teori og praksis i Danmark*. (Music Therapy: When Words are Not Enough. A Handbook of Music Therapy Theory and Practice in Denmark.) KLIM: Århus.

Bonde, L.O. and Pedersen, I.N. (eds) (1996) *Music Therapy Within Multi-Disciplinary Teams*. Proceedings of the 3rd European Music Therapy Conference, Aalborg, June 1995. Aalborg University Press.

Bonny, H. (1989) 'Sound as Symbol: Guided Imagery and Music in Clinical Practice.' *Music Therapy Perspectives* 6, 7–11.

Bonny, H. (1990) 'Music and Change.' *Journal of the New Zealand Society for Music Therapy* 12, 3, 5–10.

Bonny, H. (1994) 'Twenty-One Years Later: A GIM Update.' *Music Therapy Perspectives* 12, 2, 70–74.

Bonny, H. (2001) 'Music and Spirituality.' *Music Therapy Perspectives* 19, 1, 59–62.

Bonny, H.L. (1975/1999) 'Music and consciousness.' *Journal of Music Therapy* 12, 121–135. Reprint *Nordic Journal of Music Therapy* 8, 2, 171–179.

Bonny, H.L. and McCarron, N. (1984) 'Music as an adjunct to anaesthesia in operative procedures.' *Journal of the American Association of Nurse Anaesthesiologists* 2, 55–57.

Bonny H.L. and Pahnke, W.N. (1972) 'The Use of Music in Psychedelic (LSD) Psychotherapy.' *Journal of Music Therapy*, 9, 3, 64–87.

Bonny, H. and Savary, L. (1973, reprint 1990) *Music and your Mind: Listening with a New Consciousness*. New York: Harper & Row.

Boxill, E.H. (1985) *Music Therapy for the Developmentally Disabled*. St. Louis: MMB.

Braben, L. (1992) 'A Song for Mrs Smith.' *Nursing Times* 88, 41, 54.

Briggs, C. (1991) 'A Model for Understanding Musical Development.' *Music Therapy* 10, 1, 1–21.

Bright, R. (1981) *Practical Planning in Music Therapy for the Aged*. New York: Musicgraphics.

Bright, R. (1997) *Music Therapy and the Dementias*. St. Louis: MMB Horizon Series.

Brotons, M. (2000) 'An Overview of the Music Therapy Literature Relating to Elderly People.' In D. Aldridge (ed) *Music Therapy in Dementia Care. More New Voices*. London: Jessica Kingsley Publishers.

Brotons, M. and Koger, S.M. (2000) 'The Impact of Music Therapy on Language Functioning in Dementia.' *Journal of Music Therapy* 37, 3, 183–195.

Brotons, M. and Prickett-Cooper, P. (1994) 'Preferences of Alzheimer's Disease Patients for Music Activities: Singing, Instruments, Dance/Movement, Games, and Composition/Improvisation.' *Journal of Music Therapy* 31, 3, 220–233.

Brotons, M. and Prickett-Cooper, P.K. (1996) 'The Effects of Music Therapy Intervention on Agitation Behaviors of Alzheimer's Disease Patients.' *Journal of Music Therapy* 33, 1, 2–18.

Brown, S. (1999a) 'Some Thoughts on Music, Therapy, and Music Therapy.' *British Journal of Music Therapy 13*, 2, 63–71.

Brown, S. (1999b) 'The Music, the Meaning, and the Therapist's Dilemma.' In T. Wigram and J. De Backer (eds) *Clinical Applications of Music Therapy in Developmental Disability, Paediatrics and Neurology*. London, Philadelphia: Jessica Kingsley Publishers.

Brown, C.J., Chen, A.C.N. and Dworkin, S.F. (1991) 'Music in the Control of Human Pain.' *Music Therapy 8*, 47–60.

Brown, S., Götell, E. and Ekman, S. (2001) 'Music-therapeutic Caregiving: The Necessity of Active Music-making in Clinical Care.' *The Arts in Psychotherapy 28*, 2001, 125–135.

Bruhn, H. (2000) *Musiktherapie. Geschichte – Theorien – Grundlagen*. Göttingen: Hogrefe.

Bruhn, H., Oerter, R. *et al.* (eds) (1985) *Musikpsychologie. Ein Handbuch in Schlüsselbegriffen*. München – Wien – Baltimore: Urban & Schwarzenberg.

Bruscia, K.E. (1987) *Improvisational Models of Music Therapy*. Springfield: Charles C. Thomas.

Bruscia, K.E. (1991) *Case Studies in Music Therapy*. Phoenixville: Barcelona Publishers.

Bruscia, K.E. (1994) *IAP – Improvisation Assessment Profiles. Kartlegging gjennom musikkterapeutisk improvisasjon*. Sandane: Høgskulen i Sogn og Fjordane.

Bruscia, K.E. (1995) 'Modes of Consciousness in Guided Imagery and Music (GIM): A Therapist's experience of the Guiding Proces.' In Carolyn Kenny (ed) *Listening, Playing and Creating: Essays on the Power of Sound*. Albany, NY: State University of New York Press.

Bruscia, K.E. (1995a) 'Topics and Questions in Quantitative Research.' In B. Wheeler (ed) *Music Therapy Research. Quantitative and Qualitative Perspectives*. Phoenixville: Barcelona Publishers.

Bruscia, K.E. (1995b) 'Topics, Phenomena and Purposes in Qualitative Research.' In B. Wheeler (ed) *Music Therapy Research. Quantitative and Qualitative Perspectives*. Phoenixville: Barcelona Publishers.

Bruscia, K.E. (1995c) 'The Process of Doing Qualitative Research: Part 1: Introduction.' In B. Wheeler (ed) *Music Therapy Research. Quantitative and Qualitative Perspectives*. Phoenixville: Barcelona Publishers.

Bruscia, K.E. (1995d) 'The Process of Doing Qualitative Research: Part 2: Procedural Steps.' In B. Wheeler (ed) *Music Therapy Research. Quantitative and Qualitative Perspectives*. Phoenixville: Barcelona Publishers.

Bruscia, K.E. (1995e) 'The Process of Doing Qualitative Research: Part 3: The Human Side.' In B. Wheeler (ed) *Music Therapy Research. Quantitative and Qualitative Perspectives*. Phoenixville: Barcelona Publishers.

Bruscia, K.E. (1996) *Music for the Imagination: Rationale, Implications and Guidelines for its Use in Guided Imagery and Music (GIM)*. Santa Cruz, CA: Association for Music and Imagery.

Bruscia, K.E. (1998) *Defining Music Therapy* (second edition). Gilsum NH: Barcelona Publishers.

Bruscia, K.E. (1998a) *The Dynamics of Music Psychotherapy*. Gilsum NH: Barcelona Publishers.

Bruscia, K.E. (1998b) 'Standards of Integrity for Qualitative Music Therapy Research.' *Journal of Music Therapy 35*, 3, 176–200.

Bruscia, K.E. (2000) 'The Nature of Meaning in Music Therapy. Ken Bruscia interviewed by Brynjulf Stige.' *Nordic Journal of Music Therapy 9*, 2, 84–96.

Bunt, L. (1987) *Music Therapy for the Child with a Handicap: Evaluation of the Effects of Intervention*. PhD thesis (unpublished). City University, London.

Bunt, L. (1994) *Music Therapy: An Art Beyond Words*. London: Routledge.

Bunt, L., Burns, S. and Turton, P. (2000) 'Variations on a Theme: The Evolution of a Music Therapy Research Programme at the Bristol Cancer Help Centre.' *British Journal of Music Therapy 14*, 2, 62–69.

Bunt, L. and Marston-Wyld, J. (1995) 'Where Words Fail, Music Takes Over: A Collaborative Study by a Music Therapist and a Counselor in the Context of Cancer Care.' *Music Therapy Perspectives* 13, 1, 46–50.

Burke, M. (1997) 'Effects of Physioacoustic Intervention on Pain Management of Post-Operative Gynecological Patients.' In T. Wigram and C. Dileo (eds) *Music, Vibration and Health.* Pennsylvania: Jeffrey Books.

Burke, M. and Thomas, K. (1997) 'Use of Physioacoustic Therapy to Reduce Pain During Physical Therapy for Total Knee Replacements in Patients over Age Fifty-Five.' In T. Wigram and C. Dileo (eds) *Music, Vibration and Health.* Pennsylvania: Jeffrey Books.

Burns, D.S. (2001) 'The Effect of the Bonny Method of Guided Imagery and Music on the Mood and Life Quality of Cancer Patients.' *Journal of Music Therapy* 38, 1, 51–65.

Bush, C. (1996) *Healing Imagery and Music: Pathways to the Inner Self.* Portland, Oregon: Rudra Press.

Butler, C. and Butler, P.J. (1997) 'Physioacoustic Therapy with Cardiac Patients.' In T. Wigram and C. Dileo (eds) *Music, Vibration and Health.* Pennsylvania: Jeffrey Books.

Cady, G.L. and McGregor, P. (1995) *Mastering the Internet.* Clameda, CA: Sybex Inc.

Campbell, D. (1991) 'Imagery and the Physiology of Music.' In D. Campbell *Music – Physician for Times to Come.* Wheaton, IL: Theosophical Publishing House.

Campbell, D. (1997) *The Mozart Effect. Tapping the Power of Music to Heal the Body, Strengthen the Mind, and Unlock the Creative Spirit.* New York: Avon Books.

Carruth, E. (1997) 'The Effects of Singing and the Spaced Retrieval Technique on Improving Face-Name Recognition in Nursing Home Residents with Memory Loss.' *Journal of Music Therapy* 34, 3, 165–186.

Casby, J.A. and Holm, M.B. (1994) 'The Effect of Music on Repetitive Disruptive Vocalizations of Persons with Dementia.' *The American Journal of Occupational Therapy* 48, 10, 883–899.

Cassidy, J.W. and Standley, J.M. (1995) 'The Effect of Music Listening on Physiological Reponses of Premature Infants in the NICU.' *Journal of Music Therapy* 32, 4, 208–227.

Chesky, K.S. (1992) *The Effects Of Music and Music Vibration Using the MVT™ on the Relief Of Rheumatoid Arthritis Pain.* PhD dissertation, University of North Texas. Unpublished.

Chesky, K.S. and Michel, D.E. (1991) 'The Music Vibration Table (MVT™): Developing a Technology and Conceptual Model for Pain Relief.' *Music Therapy Perspectives* 9, 32–38.

Chetta, H. (1981) The Effect of Music and Desensitisation of Preoperative Anxiety in Children.' *Journal of Music Therapy* 18, 2, 74–87.

Choi, B.C. (1996) 'What is the Internet? Why Should Music Therapists Use It?' *Music Therapy Perspectives* 14, 2, 98–99.

Christensen, E. (1996) *The Musical Timespace. A Theory of Music Listening.* Aalborg: Aalborg University Press.

Christie, M. (1992) 'Music Therapy Applications in a Skilled and Intermediate Care Nursing Home Facility: A Clinical Study.' *Activities, Adaptation and Aging* 16, 4, 69–87.

Christie, M. (1995) 'The Influence of a Highly Participatory Peer on Motivation Group Behaviours of Lower Functioning Persons who have Probable Alzheimer's Type Dementia: A Feasibility Study.' *Music Therapy Perspectives* 13, 2, 91–96.

Cissoko, B. (1995) *Ridende på trommen Syngende vejen frem – et shamanistisk perspektiv på Musikterapi.* Speciale, Aalborg Universitet.

Clair, A.A. (1991a) 'Music Therapy for a Severely Regressed Person with a Probable Diagnosis of Alzheimer's Disease.' In K. Bruscia (ed) *Case Studies in Music Therapy.* Phoenixville PA: Barcelona Press.

Clair, A.A. (1991b) 'Rhythmic Responses in Elderly and their Implications for Music Therapy Practice.' *Journal of the International Association for the Handicapped 6*, 3–11.

Clair, A. (1996a) 'The Effect of Singing on Alert Responses in Persons with Late Stage Dementia.' *Journal of Music Therapy 33*, 4, 234–247.

Clair, A.A. (1996b) *Therapeutic Uses of Music with Older Adults.* Baltimore, MD: Health Professions Press.

Clair, A.A. (1998) 'Music for Persons with Dementia and their Caregivers.' In C.M. Tomaino (ed) *Clinical Applications of Music in Neurological Rehabilitation.* St. Louis: MMB Music.

Clair, A.A. (2000) 'The Importance of Singing with Elderly Patients.' In D. Aldridge (ed) *Music Therapy in Dementia Care. More New Voices.* London: Jessica Kingsley Publishers.

Clair, A. and Bernstein, B. (1990a) 'A Preliminary Study of Music Therapy Programming for Severely Regressed Persons with Alzheimer's-type Dementia.' *Journal of Applied Gerontology 9*, 3, 299–311.

Clair, A. and Bernstein, B. (1990b) 'A Comparison of Singing, Vibrotactile and Nonvibrotactile Instrumental Playing Responses in Severely Regressed Persons with Dementia of the Alzheimer's Type.' *Journal of Music Therapy 27*, 3, 119–125.

Clair, A. and Bernstein, B. (1993) 'The Preference for Vibrotactile versus Auditory Stimuli in Severely Regressed Persons with Dementia of the Alzheimer's Type Compared to Those with Dementia Due to Alcohol Abuse.' *Music Therapy Perspectives 11*, 1, 24–27.

Clair, A. and Bernstein, B. (1994) 'The Effect of No Music, Stimulative Background Music and Sedative Background Music on Agitated Behaviors in Persons with Severe Dementia.' *Activities, Adaptation and Aging 19*, 1, 61–70.

Clair, A., Bernstein, B. and Johnson, G. (1995) 'Rhythm Playing Characteristics in Persons with Severe Dementia Including Those with Probable Alzheimer's Type.' *Journal of Music Therapy 32*, 2, 113–131.

Clair, A. and Ebberts, A. (1997) 'The Effects of Music Therapy on Interactions Between Family Caregivers and their Care Receivers with Late Stage Dementia.' *Journal of Music Therapy 34*, 3, 148–164.

Clark, M. (1999) 'The Bonny Method and Spiritual Development.' *Journal of the Association for Music and Imagery 6* (1998–1999), 55–62.

Clark, M. E., Lipe, A.W. and Bilbrey, M. (1998) 'Use of Music to Decrease Aggressive Behaviors in People with Dementia.' *Journal of Gerontological Nursing July/1998*, 10–17.

Clarkson, G. (1998) *I Dreamed I was Normal: A Music Therapist's Journey into the Realms of Autism.* St. Louis: MMB Music.

Codding, P. (1987) 'A content analysis of the "Journal of Music Therapy".' *Journal of Music Therapy 24*, 4, 195–202.

Cohen, N. (1992) 'The Effect of Singing Instruction on the Speech Production of Neurologically Impaired Persons.' *Journal of Music Therapy 29*, 2, 87–102.

Coutts, C.A. (1965) 'Effects of Music on Pulse Rates and Work Output of Short Duration.' *Research Quarterly 36*, 17–21.

Cowan, D.S. (1991) 'Music Therapy in the Surgical Arena.' *Music Therapy Perspectives 9*, 42–45.

Critchley, M. and Hensen, R.A. (1977) *Music and the Brain: Studies in the Neurology of Music.* London: Heinemann Medical Books.

Crowe, B.J. and Scovel, M. (1996) 'Special Feature – An Overview of Sound Healing Practices: Implications for the Profession of Music Therapy.' *Music Therapy Perspectives 14*, 1, 21–29.

Curtis, S.L. (1982) *The Effect of Music on the Perceived Degree of Pain Relief, Physical Comfort, Relaxation and Contentment of Hospitalised Terminally Ill Patients.* Unpublished Master's thesis, Florida State University.

Curtis, S.L. (1986) 'The Effect of Music on Pain Relief and Relaxation of the Terminally Ill.' *Journal of Music Therapy 23*, 1, 10–24.

Damasio, A.R. (1994) *Descartes' Error. Emotion, Reason and the Human Brain.* New York: G. Putnam's Sons.

Darner, C.I. (1966) 'Sound Pulses and the Heart.' *Journal of the Acoustical Society of America 39*, 414–416.

Darrow, A.A. and Cohen, N. (1991) 'The Effect of Programmed Pitch Practice and Private Instruction on the Vocal Reproduction Accuracy of Children with Hearing Impairments: Two Case Studies.' *Music Therapy Perspectives 9*, 61–65.

Darrow, A.A., Johnson, C.M., Ghetti, C.M. and Achey, C.A. (2001) 'An Analysis of Music Therapy Student Practicum Behaviours and Their Relationship to Clinical Effectiveness: An Exploratory Investigation.' *Journal of Music Therapy 38*, 4, 307–320.

Davies, A. and Richards, E. (1998) 'Music Therapy in Acute Psychiatry. Our Experience of Working as Co-Therapists with a Group for Patients from Two Neighbouring Wards.' *British Journal of Music Therapy 12*, 2, 53–59.

Davis, W.B., Gfeller, K.E. and Thaut, M. (1999) *An Introduction to Music Therapy. Theory and Practice.* Boston: McGraw-Hille College.

De Backer, J. (1993) 'Containment in Music Therapy.' In M. Heal and T. Wigram (eds) *Music Therapy in Health and Education.* London: Jessica Kingsley Publishers.

De Backer, J. (2001) *Music Therapy in Psychiatry. From Sensory-Motoric playing to Musical Form with Psychotic Patients.* Unpublished communication. Aalborg University, PhD courses.

De Backer, J. and Van Camp, J. (1996) 'Muziektherapie in de behandeling van psychotische patiënten.' In M. De Hert and E. Thys (ed) *Zin in waanzin. De wereld van schizofrenie.* Amsterdam: EPO Publisher.

De Backer, J. and Van Camp, J. (1999) 'Specific Aspects of the Music Therapy Relationship to Psychiatry.' In T. Wigram and J. De Backer (eds) *Clinical Applications of Music Therapy in Psychiatry.* London and Philadelphia: Jessica Kingsley Publishers.

Decker-Voigt, H.H. (ed) (1992) *Spiele der Seele. Traum, Imagination und künstlerisches Tun.* Bremen: Trialog.

Decker-Voigt, H.H. and Knill, P.J. (eds) (1996) *Lexikon Musiktherapie.* Göttingen, Bern, Toronto, Seattle: Hogrefe-Verlag.

Decuir, A. (1987) 'Readings for Music Therapy Students: An Analysis of Clinical Literature from the *Journal of Music Therapy.*' In C.D. Maranto and K.E. Bruscia (eds) *Perspectives in Music Therapy Education and Training.* Philadelphia: Temple University.

Decuir, A. (1995) 'Statistical Methods of Analysis.' In B. Wheeler (ed) *Music Therapy Research. Quantitative and Qualitative Perspectives.* Phoenixville: Barcelona Publishers.

De Jong, M.A., van Mourik, K.R. and Schellekens, H.M. (1973) 'A Physiological Approach to Aesthetic Preference-music.' *Psychotherapy and Psychosomatics 22*, 46–51.

Del Campo san Vicente, P., de Manchola, I. and Torres Serna, E. (1997) 'The Use of Vibroacoustics in Idiopathic Parkinson's Disease.' In T. Wigram and C. Dileo (eds) *Music, Vibration and Health.* Pennsylvania: Jeffrey Books.

Denney, A. (1997) 'Quiet Music: An Intervention for Mealtime Agitation?' *Journal of Gerontological Nursing 23*, 7, 16–23.

dst. (2001). Dansk statistisk årbog 2001. www.dst.dk.

Deutsch, D. (1982) *The Psychology of Music* (second edition 1999). New York: Academic Press.

Diderichsen, B. (1998) 'Psykoanalytisk psykoterapi.' In E. Hougaard *et al. Psykoanalysens Hovedtraditioner.* Kbh.: Dansk Psykologisk Forlag.

Di Franco, G. (1993) 'Music Therapy: A Methodological Approach in the Field of Mental Health.' In M. Heal and T. Wigram (eds) *Music Therapy in Health and Education.* London: Jessica Kingsley Publishers.

Di Franco, G. (1999) 'Music and Autism. Vocal Improvisation as Containment of Stereotypes.' In T. Wigram and J. De Backer (eds) *Music Therapy Applications in Developmental Disability, Paediatrics and Neurology.* London: Jessica Kingsley Publishers.

Di Franco, G. (2001) *La Voce Della Emozione.* Roma: Ismez.

Dileo, C. (ed) (1999) *Music Therapy and Medicine: Theoretical and Clinical Applications.* Silver Spring, MD: American Music Therapy Association.

Dileo-Maranto, C.D. (1991a) *Applications of Music in Medicine.* Washington: The National Association for Music Therapy, Inc.

Dileo-Maranto, C.D. (1991b) 'A Classification Model for Music in Medicine.' In C.D. Maranto (ed) *Applications of Music in Medicine.* Washington: National Association for Music Therapy, Inc.

Dileo-Maranto, C.D. (1993a) 'Applications of Music in Medicine.' In M. Heal and T. Wigram (eds) *Music Therapy in Health and Education.* London: Jessica Kingsley Publishers.

Dileo-Maranto, C.D. (1993b) *Music Therapy: International Perspectives.* Pennsylvania: Jeffrey Books.

Dileo-Maranto, C.D. (1994a) 'A Comprehensive Definition of Music Therapy with an Integrative Model for Music Medicine.' In R. Spintge and R. Droh (eds) *Music and Medicine.* St. Louis: Magna Music Baton.

Dileo-Maranto, C.D. (1994b) 'Research in Music in Medicine: The State of the Art.' In R. Spintge and R. Droh (eds) *Music and Medicine.* St. Louis: Magna Music Baton.

Dileo-Maranto, C.D. (1995) 'Reviewing the Literature.' In B. Wheeler (ed) *Music Therapy Research. Quantitative and Qualitative Perspectives.* Phoenixville: Barcelona Publishers.

Dissanayake, E. (2001) 'An Ethological View of Music and its Relevance to Music Therapy.' *Nordic Journal of Music Therapy 10,* 2, 159–175.

Dosamantes, I. (1992) 'The Intersubjective Relationship Between Therapist and Patient: A Key to Understanding Denied and Denigrated Aspects of the Patient's Self.' *The Arts in Psychotherapy 19,* 5, 359–365.

Dun, B. (1993) 'Music Therapy at the Royal Children's Hospital, Melbourne.' In A. Lem (ed) *Music Therapy Collection.* Canberra: Ausdance.

Dyreborg, E. (1972) *Musikterapi.* (Under medvirken af Claus Bang, Frode Bavnild og Carlo Svendsen). Kbh.: Gyldendals pædagogiske Bibliotek.

Eagle, C.T. (1991) 'Steps to a Theory of Quantum Therapy.' *Music Therapy Perspectives 9,* 56–60.

Edgerton, C. (1994) 'The Effect of Improvisational Music Therapy on the Communicative Behaviours of Autistic Children.' *Journal of Music Therapy 31,* 1, 31–62.

Edwards, J. (1995) '"You are Singing Beautifully": Music Therapy and the Debridgement Bath.' *The Arts in Psychotherapy 22,* 1, 53–55.

Edwards, J. (1998) 'Music Therapy for Children with Severe Burn Injury.' *Music Therapy Perspectives 16,* 2, 20–25.

Edwards, J. (1999a) 'Music Therapy with Children Hospitalised for Severe Injury or Illness.' *British Journal of Music Therapy 13,* 1, 21–27.

Edwards, J. (1999b) 'Considering the paradigmatic frame: social science, research approaches relevant to research in music therapy.' *The Arts in Psychotherapy. An International Journal 26,* 2, 73–80.

Edwards, J. (2000) 'Developing a platform for research to inform music therapy practice with hospitalised children.' Thesis (PhD). University of Queensland, Australia.

Eeg, S. (2001) *Musikprojektet på Betania. Om musik og demente.* Århus: Lokalcenter Betania.

Eklund, G. and Hagbarth, K.E. (1965) 'Motor Effects of Vibratory Muscle Stimuli in Man.' *Electroencephalography and Clinical Neurophysiology 19,* 619–625.

Elefant, C. (2001) 'Speechless yet Communicative: Revealing the Person Behind the Disability of Rett Syndrome through Clinical Research on Songs in Music Therapy.' In D. Aldridge, G. Di Franco, E. Ruud and T. Wigram (eds) *Music Therapy in Europe.* Rome: Ismez.

Ellis, A. (1975) *Reason and Emotion in Psychotherapy.* New York: Crown Publishers.

Ellis, D.S. and Brighouse, G. (1952) 'Effects of Music on Respiration and Heart Rate.' *American Journal of Psychology 65,* 39–47.

Elsass, P. (1992) *Sundhedspsykologi.* København: Gyldendal.

Erdonmez, D. (1992) 'Clinical Applications of Guided Imagery and Music.' *Australian Journal of Music Therapy, 3,* 37–44.

Erdonmez, D. (1993) 'Music: A Mega Vitamin for the Brain.' In M. Heal and T. Wigram (eds) *Music Therapy in Health and Education.* London: Jessica Kingsley Publishers.

Erdonmez, D. (1995) 'A Journey of Transition with Guided Imagery and Music.' In C. Lee (ed) *Lonely Waters.* Oxford. Sobell Publications.

Erdonmez, D. (1996) *Directory of Music Therapy Training Courses Worldwide.* University of Melbourne: Faculty of Music.

Erdonmez Grocke, D.E. (1999a) 'Pivotal Moments in Guided Imagery and Music.' In J. Hibben (ed) *Inside Music Therapy: Client Perspectives.* Gilsum, MD: Barcelona.

Erdonmez Grocke, D.E. (1999b) 'The Music that Underpins Pivotal Moments in Guided Imagery and Music.' In T. Wigram and J. De Backer (eds) *Clinical Applications of Music Therapy in Psychiatry.* London: Jessica Kingsley Publishers.

Erdonmez Grocke, D.E. (1999c) 'A Phenomenological Study of Pivotal Moments in Guided Imagery and Music (GIM) Therapy.' The University of Melbourne, 524 pages. *Dissertation Abstracts International* #9982778. (University of Witten-Herdecke, *Music Therapy Info CD-ROM III.*)

Etkin, P. (1999) 'The Use of Creative Improvisation and Psychodynamic Insights in Music Therapy with an Abused Child.' In T. Wigram and J. De Backer (eds) *Clinical Applications of Music Therapy in Developmental Disability, Paediatrics and Neurology.* London: Jessica Kingsley Publishers.

Exner, J. (1998a) 'De fire behandlingsskridt. En introduktion til den morfologiske musikterapi.' In I.N. Pedersen (ed) *Indføring i musikterapi som en selvstændig behandlingsform.* Musikterapiklinikken. Aalborg Psykiatriske Sygehus/Aalborg Universitet.

Exner, J. (1998b) 'Casestudy med fokus på parallelliteten imellem udviklingstrin inden for den terapeutiske kontakt og forandringer i givne forsvarsmønstre.' In I.N. Pedersen (ed) *Indføring i musikterapi som en selvstændig behandlingsform.* Musikterapiklinikken. Aalborg Psykiatriske Sygehus/Aalborg Universitet.

Feder, S., Karmel, R.L. and Pollock, G.H. (eds) (1990) *Psychoanalytic Explorations in Music.* Madison, Conn.: International Universities Press.

Feder, S., Karmel, R.L. and Pollock, G.H. (eds) (1993) *Psychoanalytic Explorations in Music: Second Series.* Madison, Conn.: International Universities Press.

Ferrara, L. (1984) 'Phenomonology as a Tool for Musical Analysis.' *The Musical Quarterly 70,* 355–373.

Fink-Jensen, K. (1997) *Musikalsk stemthed – et henrykt nu! Temaer og former i børns lytteoplevelser i skolen.* PhD afhandling. Kbh.: Danmarks Lærerhøjskole.

Fitzgerald-Cloutier, M.L. (1993) 'The Use of Music Therapy to Decrease Wandering: An Alternative to Restraints.' *Music Therapy Perspectives 11*, 1, 32–36.

Flatischler, R. (1984) *Die vergessene Macht des Rhytmus. TA KE TI NA – Der rhytmische Weg zur Bewusstheit.* Essen: Synthesis Verlag.

Flatischler, R. (1992) 'The Influence of Musical Rhythmicity on Internal Rhythmic Events.' In R. Spintge and R. Droh (eds) *MusicMedicine.* St. Louis: Magna Music Baton.

Flatischler, R. (1996) 'The Effects of Musical Rhythm on Body and Mind: The Interaction Field of the TA KE TI NA Rhythm Process.' In R.R. Pratt and R. Spintge (eds) *MusicMedicine II.* St. Louis: Magna Music Baton.

Flower, C. (1993) 'Control and Creativity: Music Therapy with Adolescents in Secure Care.' In M. Heal and T. Wigram (eds) *Music Therapy in Health and Education.* London: Jessica Kingsley Publishers.

Flower, C. (1999) 'Islanders: Making Connections in Music Therapy.' In T. Wigram and J. De Backer (eds) *Clinical Applications of Music Therapy in Developmental Disability, Paediatric and Neurology.* London: Jessica Kingsley Publishers.

Folker, H. (1994) 'Kohut og musikken.' *Nordisk Tidsskrift for Musikkterapi 3*, 2, 55–56.

Fønsbo, C.D. (1999) 'Musikterapi i et krigsramt land. Om etablering af en musikterapiklinik i Bosnien.' *Nordisk Tidsskrift for Musikkterapi 8*, 2, 180–185.

Ford, S.E. (1999) 'The Effect of Music on the Self-Injurious Behaviour of an Adult Female with Severe Developmental Disabilities.' *Journal of Music Therapy 36*, 4, 293–313.

Forinash, M. (1995) 'Phenomenological Research.' In B. Wheeler (ed) *Music Therapy Research. Quantitative and Qualitative Perspectives.* Phoenixville: Barcelona Publishers.

Forinash, M. and Gonzales, D. (1989) 'A Phenomenological Persective of Music Therapy.' *Music Therapy 8*, 35–46.

Foster, N.A. (1998) *An Examination of the Facilitatory Effect of Music on Recall, with Special Reference to Dementia Sufferers.* Unpublished PhD dissertation, University of London.

Freud, S. (1926) *Hemmung, Symptom and Angst.* Gesammelte Werke XIV.

Friis, B.Z. (1993) *Det indre udtryk. Dybdepsykologiske aspekter i musikterapi.* PhD afhandling, Aalborg Universitet.

Friis, S. (1987) *Musik i ældreplejen.* Kbh.: Munksgaard.

Froehlich, M. (1984) 'A Comparison of the Effect of Music Therapy and Medical Play Therapy on the Verbalisation of Paediatric Patients.' *Journal of Music Therapy 21*, 1, 2–15.

Froehlich, M. (ed) (1996) *Music Therapy with Hospitalized Children. A Creative Arts Child Life Approach.* Pennsylvania: Jeffrey Books.

Frohne-Hagemann, I. (ed) (1990) *Musik und Gestalt: Klinische Musiktherapie als integrative Psychotherapie.* Paderborn: Junfermann.

Gabrielsson, A. (1999) 'Strong Experiences of and with Music.' In:D. Green (ed) *Music Psychology.* Oxford: Oxford University Press.

Gabrielsson, A. and Lindstrom, S. (1993) 'On Strong Experiences of Music.' *Musikpsychologie: Jahrbuch der Deutschen Gesellschaft fur Musikpsychologie 10*, 114–125.

Gabrielsson, A. and Lindstrom, S. (1995) 'Can Strong Experiences of Music have Therapeutic Implications?' In R. Steinberg (ed) *Music and the Mind Machine.* New York: Springer.

Gaertner, M. (1999) 'The Sound of Music in the Dimming, Anguished World of Alzheimer's Disease.' In T. Wigram and J. De Backer (ed) *Clinical Applications of Music Therapy in Psychiatry.* London: Jessica Kingsley Publishers.

Gardiner, J.C. *et al.* (2000) 'Music Therapy and Reading as Intervention Strategies for Disruptive Behavior in Dementia.' *Clinical Gerontologist 22*, 1, 31–46.

Gardner, H., Kornhaber and Wake, W.K. (1996) *Intelligence: Multiple Perspectives*. Fort Worth: Harcourt Brace College Publishers.

Gardner-Gordon, J. (1993) *The Healing Voice: Traditional and Contemporary Toning, Chanting, and Singing*. Freedom CA: The Crossings Press.

Garfield, L. (1987) *Sound Medicine: Healing with Music, Voice and Song*. Berkeley, CA: Celestial Arts.

Garred, R. (1996) 'Musikkterapeutisk improvisasjon som "møte".' *Nordisk Tidskrift for Musikkterapi* 5, 2, 76–86.

Garred, R. (2001) 'The Ontology of Music in Music Therapy.' *Voices*. Website: www.Voices.no.

Gaston, E.T. (1951) 'Dynamic music factors in mood change.' *Music Educators Journal 37*, 42–44.

Gaston, E.T. (1968) *Music in Therapy*. New York: Macmillan.

Gaston, E.T. (1995) 'Man and music.' *Nordic Journal of Music Therapy 4*, 2, 83–98.

Gerdner, L.A. and Swanson, E.A. (1993) 'Effects of Individualized Music on Confused and Agitated Elderly Patients.' *Archives of Psychiatric Nursing 7*, 5, 284–291.

Gfeller, K.E. (1987) 'Music Therapy Theory and Practice as Reflected in Research Literature.' *Journal of Music Therapy 24*, 178–194.

Gfeller, K.E. (1992) 'Music Therapy in the Treatment of Medical Conditions.' In W.B. Davis, K.E. Gfeller and M. Thaut (eds) *An Introduction to Music Therapy: Theory and Practice*. USA: Wm C. Brown.

Gilbert, J.P. (1979) 'Published Research in Music Therapy 1973–1978: Content, Focus and Implications for Future Research.' *Journal of Music Therapy 16*, 3, 102–110.

Glaser, B. and Strauss, A. (1967) *The Discovery of Grounded Theory*. Chicago: Aldine.

Glynn, N.J. (1992) 'The Music Therapy Assessment Tool in Alzheimer's Patients.' *Journal of Gerontological Nursing 18*, 1, 3–9.

Goddaer, J. and Abraham, I. (1994) 'Effects of Relaxing Music on Agitation During Meals Among Nursing Home Residents with Severe Cognitive Impairment.' *Archives of Psychiatric Nursing 8*, 3, 150–158.

Gold, C., Wigram, T. and Berger, E. (2001) 'The Development of a Research Design to Assess the Effects of Individual Music Therapy with Mentally Ill Children and Adolescents.' *Nordic Journal of Music Therapy 10*, 1, 17–31.

Goldberg, F. (1994) 'The Bonny Method of Guided Imagery and Music as Individual and Group Treatment in a Short-term Acute Psychiatric Hospital.' *Journal of the Association of Music and Imagery 3*, 18–34.

Goldberg, F. (1995) 'The Bonny Method of Guided Imagery and Music.' In T. Wigram, B. Saperston and R. West (eds) *The Art and Science of Music Therapy: A Handbook*. London: Harwood Academic.

Götell, E., Brown, S. and Ekman, S.L. (2000) 'Caregiver-assisted Music Events in Psychogeriatric Care.' *Journal of Psychiatric Mental Health and Nursing 7*, 2, 119–125.

Gouk, P. (ed) (2000) *Music Healing in Cultural Contexts*. Aldershot: Ashgate.

Graham, J. (2000) 'Assessment and Evaluation: An Approach for Initial Clinical Assessment and On-going Treatment in Music Therapy.' In T. Wigram (2000b) *Assessment and Evaluation in the Arts Therapies: Art Therapy, Music Therapy and Dramatherapy*. Radlett: Harper House Publications.

Grant, R. (1995) 'Music Therapy Assessment for Developmentally Disabled Clients.' In T. Wigram, B. Saperston and R. West (eds) *The Art and Science of Music Therapy: A Handbook*. London: Harwood Academic.

Gregory, A.H. (1994) 'Timbre and Auditory Streaming.' *Music Percept 12*, 2, 161–174.

Gregory, D. (2000) 'Test Instruments Used by *Journal of Music Therapy* Authors from 1984–1997.' *Journal of Music Therapy 37*, 2, 79–94.

Grinde, B. (2000) 'A Biological Perspective on Musical Appreciation.' *Nordic Journal of Music Therapy* *9*, 2, 18–27.

Grocke, D.E. (1999) *A Phenomenological Study of Pivotal Moments in Guided Imagery and Music (GIM) Therapy*. PhD thesis. Faculty of Music, Melbourne: The University of Melbourne.

Groene, R.W. (1993) 'Effectiveness of Music Therapy 1:1 Intervention with Individuals having Senile Dementia of the Alzheimer's Type.' *Journal of Music Therapy 30*, 3, 138–157.

Groene, R.W. (1995) 'The Effect of Therapist and Activity Characteristics on the Purposeful Responses of Probable Alzheimer's Disease Participants.' *Journal of Music Therapy 35*, 2, 119–136.

Groene, R.W. (2001) 'The Effect of Presentation and Accompaniment Styles on Attentional and Reponsive Behaviours of Participants with Dementia Diagnoses.' *Journal of Music Therapy 38*, 1, 36–50.

Grof, S. (1987) *Introduktion til Den Indre Rejse. Selvopdagelsens Eventyr*. Kbh.: Borgen.

Guba, E. and Lincoln, Y. (1994) 'Competing Paradigms in Qualitative Research.' In N. Denzin and Y. Lincoln (eds) *Handbook of Qualitative Research*. Newbury Park, CA: Sage.

Haas, F., Distenfield, S. and Axen, K. (1986) 'Effects of Perceived Musical Rhythm on Respiratory Pattern.' *Journal of Applied Psychology 61*, 3, 1185–1191.

Hadley, S. (1998) *Exploring Relationships Between Life and Work in Music Therapy: The Stories of Mary Priestley and Clive Robbins*. PhD Thesis, Philadelphia: Temple University.

Haines, J.H. (1989) 'The Effects of Music Therapy on the Self-esteem of Emotionally Disturbed Adolescents.' *Music Therapy 8*, 1, 78–91.

Halpern, S. (1985) *Sound Health: The Music and Sounds that Make Us Whole*. San Francisco: Harper and Row.

Hamel, P. (1978) *Through Music to the Self*. Boulder, CO: Shambhala.

Haneishi, E. (2001) 'Effects of a Music Therapy Voice Protocol on Speech Intelligibility, Vocal Acoustic Measures, and Mood of Individuals with Parkinson's Disease.' *Journal of Music Therapy 38*, 4, 273–290.

Hannibal, N.J. (1998) 'Refleksion i og om musikalsk improvisation i musikterapi.' In I.N. Pedersen (ed) *Indføring i musikterapi som en selvstændig behandlingsform*. Aalborg, Musikterapiklinikken, Aalborg Psykiatriske Sygehus. 1: 141–164.

Hannibal, N. (2000) 'Overføring i den musikalske interaktion.' In C. Lindvang (ed) *Den musikterapeutiske behandling* Årsskrift 2000. Musikterapi i psykiatrien. Musikterapiklinikken. Aalborg Psykiatriske Sygehus/Aalborg Universitet.

Hannibal, N. (2001) *Præverbal Overføring i Musikterapi – kvalitativ undersøgelse af overføringsprocesser i den musikalske interaktion*. PhD projekt, AAU. Under udgivelse.

Hanser, S.B. (1995) 'Applied Behaviour Analysis.' In B. Wheeler (ed) *Music Therapy Research. Quantitative and Qualitative Perspectives*. Phoenixville: Barcelona Publishers.

Hanser, S.B. (1999/1987) *The New Music Therapist's Handbook*. St. Louis: Warren H. Green.

Hanser, S. and Clair, A.A. (1995) 'Retrieving the Losses of Alzheimer's Disease for Patients and Caregivers with the Aid of Music.' In T. Wigram, B. Saperston and R. West (ed) *The Art and Science of Music Therapy: A Handbook*. Amsterdam: Harwood Academic Publishers.

Hanser, S. and Wheeler, B.L. (1995) 'Experimental Research.' In B. Wheeler (ed) *Music Therapy Research. Quantitative and Qualitative Perspectives*. Phoenixville: Barcelona Publishers.

Hanson, N. *et al.* (1996) 'A Comparison of the Effectiveness of Differing Types and Difficulty of Music Activities in Programming for Older Adults with Alzheimer's Disease and Related Disorders.' *Journal of Music Therapy 33*, 2, 93–123.

Hargreaves, D. (1986) *The Developmental Psychology of Music*. Newcastle: Cambridge University Press.

Hargreaves, D.J. and North, A.C. (eds) (1997) *The Social Psychology of Music.* Oxford: Oxford University Press.

Hargreaves, D.J. and Zimmerman, M.P. (1992) *Developmental Theories of Music Learning. Handbook of Research on Music Teaching and Learning. A Project of the Music Educators National Conference.* R. Colwell. New York: Schirmer Books.

Harner, M. (1990) *The Way of the Shaman* (third edition). San Francisco, CA: Harper and Row.

Hart, M. (1990) *Drumming on the Edge of Magic.* San Francisco, CA: Harper-SanFrancisco.

Hauge, T.S. and Tønsberg, G.E.H. (1998) *Musikalske Aspekter i Førspråklig Samspil. En Analyse av Musikalske Elementer i Førspråklig Sosialt Samspill mellom Døvblindfødte Barn og Seende Hørende Voksne.* Skådalen Kompetansesenter, postboks 13, Slemdal, 0321 Oslo.

Heal, M. (1995) 'A Comparison of Mother–Infant Interactions and the Client–Therapist Relationship in Music Therapy Sessions.' In T. Wigram, B. Saperston and R. West (eds) *The Art and Science of Music Therapy: A Handbook.* London, Toronto: Harwood Academic.

Heal, M. and Wigram, T. (1993) *Music Therapy in Health and Education.* London: Jessica Kingsley Publishers.

Hegi, F. (1988) *Improvisation und Musiktherapie.* Paderborn: Junfermann.

Hegi, F. (1998) *Übergänge zwischen Sprache und Musik. Die Wirkungskomponenten der Musiktherapie.* Paderborn: Junfermann.

Heimann, P. (1950) 'On Countertransference.' *International Journal of Psychoanalysis 31*, 81–84.

Hevner, K. (1936) 'Experimental Studies of the Elements of Expression in Music.' *American Journal of Psychology 48*, 246–268.

Hibben, J. (ed) (1999) *Inside Music Therapy: Client Experiences.* Gilsum NH: Barcelona Publishers.

Hintz, M. (2000) 'Geriatric Music Therapy Clinical Assessment: Assessment of Music Skills and Related Behaviours.' *Music Therapy Perspectives 18*, 1, 31–40.

Hodges, D.A. (1980) 'Appendix A: Physiological Responses to Music.' In: *Handbook of Music Psychology.* Washington: National Association of Music Therapy.

Hodges, D.A. (ed) (1996a) *Handbook of Music Psychology.* San Antonio: IMR Press.

Hodges, D.A. (1996b) 'Neuromusical Research: A Review of the Literature.' In D. Hodges (ed) *Handbook of Music Psychology.* San Antonio: Institute for Music Research.

Holck, U. (1992) 'Musikterapi med socialt og/eller psykisk belastede unge.' *Nordisk tidsskrift for musikkterapi 1*, 1, 27–29.

Holck, U. (1997) 'From Practical Work. In Search for Data with a Video Camera.' *Nordic Journal of Music Therapy 6*, 1, 53–58.

Holck, U. (2002) 'Kommunikalsk' sammenspil i Muskterapi. Kvalitative Videoanalyser af Musikalske og gestiske Interaktuoner med Børn med Betydelig Funktionsnedsættelser, herunder Børn med Autisme. PhD Thesis. Aalborg University: Denmark.

Holdsworth, E. (1974) *Neuromuscular Activity and Covert Musical Psychomotor Behaviour. An Electromyographic Study.* Unpublished doctoral dissertation, University of Kansas.

Hooper, J. and Lindsey, J. (1997) 'The Use of the Somatron in the Treatment of Anxiety Problems with Clients who have Learning Disabilities.' In T. Wigram and C. Dileo (eds) *Music, Vibration and Health.* Pennsylvania: Jeffrey Books.

Horden, P. (ed) (2000) *Music as Medicine. The History of Music Therapy since Antiquity.* Aldershot: Ashgate.

Horden, P. (2001) 'Science, Magic, and Continuity in the History of Music Therapy. On "Rhythm and Health" by Charles W. Hughes.' *Nordic Journal of Music Therapy 10*, 2, 188–190.

Høstmark Nielsen, G. and von der Lippe, A.L. (eds) (1996) *Psykoterapi med voksne. Fem synsvinkler på teori og praksis.* Kbh.: Hans Reitzels Forlag.

Hougaard, E., Diderichsen, B. and Nielsen, T. (eds) (1998) *Psykoanalysens hovedtraditioner. En indføring i psykoanalytisk, oplevelsesorienteret, kognitiv, systemorienteret og integrativ psykoterapi.* Kbh.: Dansk Psykologisk Forlag.

Howat, R. (1995) 'Elizabeth: A Case Study of an Autistic Child with Individual Music Therapy.' In T. Wigram, B. Saperston and R. West (eds) *The Art and Science of Music Therapy: A Handbook.* London: Harwood Academic.

Hughes, C.W. (2001) 'Rhythm and Health.' *Nordic Journal of Music Therapy 10,* 2, 191–204.

Hunter, H. (1968) 'An Investigation of Psychological and Physiological Changes Apparently Elicited by Musical Stimuli.' *Bulletin of the Psychology of Music,* 53–68.

Hurt, C.P., Rice, R.R., McIntosh, G.C. and Thaut, M.H. (1998) 'Rhythmic-Auditory Stimulation in Gait Training for Patients with Traumatic Brain Injury.' *Journal of Music Therapy 35,* 4, 228–242.

Ingemann Nielsen, T. (1986) *Bevidstheden og det som er helt anderledes.* Kbh: Psykologisk Laboratotium.

Iwanaga, M. and Moroki, Y. (1999) 'Subjective and Physiological Responses to Music Stimuli Controlled Over Activity and Preference.' *Journal of Music Therapy 36,* 1, 26–38.

James, M.R. (1985) 'Sources of Articles Published in the *Journal of Music Therapy:* The First 20 Years, 1964–1983.' *Journal of Music Therapy 22,* 2, 87–94.

Jellison, J. (1973) 'The Frequency and General Mode of Enquiry of Research in Music Therapy, 1952–1972.' *Council for Research in Music Therapy 35,* 1–8.

Jensen, A.F. (2001) *Metaforens magt. Fantasiens fostre og fornuftens fødsler.* Århus: Modtryk.

Jensen, B. (1999) 'Music Therapy with Psychiatric In-Patients: A Case Study with a Young Schizophrenic Man.' In T. Wigram and J. De Backer (eds) *Clinical Applications of Music Therapy in Psychiatry.* London: Jessica Kingsley Publishers.

Jespersen, H.T. *et al.* (1987) *Man skal høre meget. Musikaliteten i fokus. En bog om lærere og undervisning.* Kbh.: Chr. Ejlers Forlag.

Johnson, F. (1995) 'Integrating Technology.' *Music Therapy Perspectives 13,* 2, 61–62.

Johnson, J.K., Cotman, C.W., Tasaki, C.S. and Shaw, G.L. (1998) 'Enhancement of Spatial-temporal Reasoning after a Mozart Listening Condition in Alzheimer's Disease: A Case Study.' *Neurologic Research 29,* 8, 666–672.

Johnson, J., Otto, D. and Clair, A.A. (2001) 'The Effect of Instrumental and Vocal Music on Adherence to a Physical Rehabilitation Exercise Program with Persons who are Elderly.' *Journal of Music Therapy 38,* 2, 82–96.

Jones, L. (1997) 'Vibroacoustics with Hospitalised Children.' In T. Wigram and C. Dileo (eds) *Music, Vibration and Health.* Pennsylvania: Jeffrey Books.

Jørgensen, H. (1988) *Musikkoplevelsens psykologi.* Olso: Norsk Musikkforlag.

Jung, C.G. (1933) *Modern Man in Search of a Soul.* New York: Harcourt.

Jung, C.G. (1963) *Memories, Dreams, Reflections.* New York: Pantheon Books.

Jung, C.G. (1964) *Man and His Symbols.* New York: Doubleday.

Jungaberle, H. (1999) 'Music and Metaphor – Understanding the Transmission from Music to Language in Therapy.' Paper given at the 9th World Congress of Music Therapy 'Music Therapy: A Global Mosaic: Many Voices, One Song'. Washington DC, November 17–22, 1999.

Jungaberle, H., Verres, R. and DuBois, F. (2001) 'New Steps in Musical Meaning – the Metaphoric Process as an Organizing Principle.' *Nordic Journal of Music Therapy 10,* 1, 4–16.

Kemp, P. (1994) *Tid og fortælling. Introduktion til Paul Ricoeur.* Århus Universitetsforlag.

Kennair, L.E.O. (2000) 'Developing Minds for Pathology and Musicality: The Role of Theory of Development of Personality and Pathology in Clinical Thinking illustrated by the Effect of Taking an Evolutionary Perspective.' *Nordic Journal of Music Therapy 9,* 1, 26–37.

Kenny, C.B. (1982) *The Mythic Artery: The Magic of Music Therapy*. Atascadero, CA: Ridgeview Publishing Co.

Kenny, C.B. (1989) *The Field of Play: A Guide for the Theory and Practice of Music Therapy*. Atascadero, CA: Ridgeview Publishing Co.

Kenny, C.B. (ed) (1995) *Listening, Playing and Creating: Essays on the Power of Sound*. Albany: State University of New York Press.

Kenny, C.B. (1996) 'The Dilemma of Uniqueness. An Essay on Consciousness and Qualities.' *Nordisk tidsskrift for musikkterapi 5*, 2, 87–96.

Kenny, C.B. (1998) 'Embracing Complexity: The Creation of a Comprehensive Research Culture in Music Therapy.' *Journal of Music Therapy 35*, 3, 201–217.

Kenny, C.B. (1999) 'Beyond this Point There Be Dragons: Developing a General Theory in Music Therapy.' *Nordic Journal of Music Therapy 8*, 2, 127–136.

Kenny, C.B. (2000) 'Setting the Stage for General Theory in Music Therapy – Reply to Bärmark & Hallin.' *Nordic Journal of Music Therapy 9*, 1, 64–69.

Kernberg, O.F. (1975) *Borderline Conditions and Pathological Narcissism*. New York: Jason Aronson.

Kernberg, O.F., Selzer, M.A., Koenigsberg, H.W., Carr, A.C. and Appelbaum, A.H. (1992) *Borderline og psykodynamisk psykoterapi*. Kbh.: Hans Reitzels Forlag.

Killingmo, B. (1995) 'Affirmation in Psychoanalysis.' *International Journal of Psychoanalysis 76*, 503–518.

Kennelly, J. and Edwards, J. (1997) 'Providing Music Therapy to the Unconscious Child in the Paediatric Intensive Care Unit.' *The Australian Journal of Music Therapy 8*, 18–29.

Kjærulff, P. (2001) *The Ringbearer's Diary*. Cercola (NA): Altre Menti Edizioni.

Klausmeier, F. (1978) *Die Lust sich musikalisch auszudrücken*. Hamburg: Rowohlt.

Knight, W.E.J. and Rickard, N.S. (2001) 'Relaxing Music Prevents Stress-Inducing Increases in Subjective Anxiety, Systolic Blood Pressure, and Heart Rate in Healthy Males and Females.' *Journal of Music Therapy 38*, 4, 254–272.

Koger, S.M. and Brotons, M. (2000) 'The Impact of Music Therapy on Language Functioning in Dementia.' *Journal of Music Therapy 37*, 3, 183–195.

Koger, S.M., Chapin, K. and Brotons, M. (1999) 'Is Music Therapy an Effective Treatment for Dementia? A Review of the Literature.' *Journal of Music Therapy 36*, 1, 2–15.

Kohut, H. (1957) 'Observations on the Psychological Functions of Music.' *The Psychoanalytic Quarterly, 5*, 389–407.

Kohut, H. (1984) *How Does Analysis Cure?* Chicago: University of Chicago Press.

Kohut, H. and Levarie, S. (1950) 'On the Enjoyment of Listening to Music.' *The Psychoanalytic Quarterly, 19*, 64–87.

Korb, C. (1997) 'The Influence of Music Therapy on Patients with a Diagnosed Dementia.' *The Canadian Journal of Music Therapy 5*, 1, 26–54.

Korlin, D. and Wrangsjö, B. (2001) 'Gender Differences in Outcome of Guided Imagery and Music (GIM) Therapy.' *Nordic Journal of Music Therapy 10*, 2, 132–143.

Korlin, D. and Wrangsjö, B. (2002) 'Treatment Effects of Guided Imagery and Music (GIM) Therapy.' *Nordic Journal of Music Therapy 11*, 1, (in press).

Kortegaard, H.M. (1993) 'Music Therapy in the Psychodynamic Treatment of Schizophrenia.' In M. Heal and T. Wigram (eds) *Music Therapy in Health and Education*. London, Toronto: Jessica Kingsley Publishers.

Kovach, A. (1985) 'Shamanism and Guided Imagery and Music.' *Journal of Music Therapy 22*, 3, 154.

Kümmel, W.F. (1977) *Musik und Medizin. Ihre Wechselbeziehungen in Theorie und Praxis von 800 bis 1800.* Freiburg/München: Verlag Karl Aber.

Kurth, E. (1931) *Musikpsychologie.*(reprint 1947/1969). Berlin: Olten Verlag.

Lakoff, G. and Johnson, M. (1999) *Philosophy in the Flesh: The Embodied Mind and its Challenge to Western Thought.* New York: Basic Books.

Landreth, J.E. and Landreth, H.F. (1974) 'Effects of Music on Physiological Response.' *Journal of Research in Music Education 22,* 4–12.

Langenberg, M. (1988) *Vom Handeln zum Behandeln: Darstellung besondere Merkmale der Musiktherapeutischen behandlungssituation im Zusammenhang mit der Freien Improvisation.* (From Action to Treatment: A Presentation of Specific Characteristics in the Music Therapy Treatment Situation Based on Free Improvisation.) Stuttgart: Fischer.

Langenberg, M., Aigen, K. and Frommer, J. (eds) (1996) *Qualitative Music Therapy Research. Beginning Dialogues.* Gilsum NH: Barcelona Publishers.

Langer, S.K. (1942) *Philosophy in a New Key: A Study in the Symbolism of Reason, Rite and Art.* New York: New American Library of World Literature.

Langer, S.K. (1953) *Feeling and Form: A Theory of Art.* New York: Charle Scribner's Sons.

Laszig, P. (1997) 'Netzwerken: Psychoanalytische ressourcen im World Wide Web.' *Psyche* http://psyche.cs.monash.edu.au, 1184–89.

Lecourt, E. (1993) 'Music Therapy in France.' In C. Dileo-Maranto (ed) *Music Therapy: International Perspectives.* Pennsylvania: Jeffrey Books.

Lecourt, E. (1994) *L'experience musicale, Resonances Psychoanalytiques.* Paris: L'Harmattan.

Lee, C. (ed) (1995) *Lonely Waters.* Oxford: Sobell Publications.

Lee, C. (1996) *Music at the Edge. Music Therapy Experiences of a Musician with AIDS.* London, New York: Routledge.

Lee, C. (2000) 'A Method of Analysing Improvisations in Music Therapy.' *Journal of Music Therapy 37,* 2, 147–167.

Lehikoinen, P. (1988) *The Kansa Project: Report from a Control Study on the Effect of Vibroacoustical Therapy on Stress.* Sibelius Academy, Helsinki. Unpublished paper.

Lehikoinen, P. (1989) *Vibracoustic Treatment to Reduce Stress.* Sibelius Academy, Helsinki. Unpublished paper.

Lehtonen, K. (1993a) 'Reflections on Music Therapy and Developmental Psychology.' *Nordisk Tidsskrift for Musikterapi 2,* 1, 3–12.

Lehtonen, K. (1993b) 'Is Music an Archaic Form of Thinking?' *Nordisk tidsskrift for musikkterapi 2,* 1, 3–12.

Lewis, K. (1999) 'The Bonny Method of GIM: Matrix for Transpersonal Experience.' *Journal of the Association for Music and Imagery 6,* 63–86.

Lincoln, Y. and Guba, E. (1985) *Naturalistic Inquiry.* Newbury Park, CA: Sage.

Lindvang, C. (1998) 'Musikterapeutens rolle i opbygning af psykoterapeutisk relation med skizofrene.' In I.N. Pedersen (ed) *Musikterapi i psykiatrien. Årsskrift 1998.* Musikterapiklinikken. Aalborg Psykiatriske Sygehus/Aalborg Universitet.

Lindvang, C. (2000) 'Den musikterapeutiske behandling – teoretiske og kliniske reflektioner.' In C. Lindvang (ed) *Musikterapi i psykiatrien. Årsskrift 2000.* Musikterapiklinikken. Aalborg Psykiatriske Sygehus/Aalborg Universitet. Den Psykiatriske Forskningsenhed i Nordjyllands Amt.

Lipe, A. (1991) 'Using Music Therapy to Enhance the Quality of Life in a Client with Alzheimer's Dementia: A Case Study.' *Music Therapy Perspectives 9,* 102–105.

Loewy, J. (ed) (1997) *Music Therapy and Paediatric Pain.* Pennsylvania: Jeffrey Books.

Loewy, J. (2000) 'Music Psychotherapy Assessment.' *Music Therapy Perspectives 18*, 1, 47–58.

Lord, R.R. and Garner, J.E. (1993) 'Effects of Music on Alzheimer Patients.' *Perceptual and Motor Skills* 76, 2, 451–455.

Lord, W. (1968) *The Effect of Music on Muscle Activity during Exercise as Measured by Heart Rate.'* Unpublished paper. University of Kansas.

Lund, G. (1988) *Musikterapi og skizofrene – en undersøgelse af nonverbal kommunikation.* Aalborg Universitetsforlag.

Lundin, R. (1967) *An Objective Psychology of Music.* New York: The Ronald Press Co.

Madsen, C.K. (1978) 'Research on Research: An Evaluation of Research Presentations.' *Journal of Music Therapy 15*, 2, 67–73.

Madsen, C.K., Cotter, V. and Madsen, C.H. (1968) 'A Behavioural Approach to Music Therapy.' *Journal of Music Therapy 5*, 3, 69–71.

Madsen, C.K. and Madsen, C.H. (1997) *Experimental research in music* (third edition). Raleigh, NC: Contemporary Publishing Company.

McGuire, M.G. (1995) 'Writing the Research Report.' In B. Wheeler (ed) *Music Therapy Research. Quantitative and Qualitative Perspectives.* Phoenixville: Barcelona Publishers.

McNiff, S. (1984) 'Cross-cultural Psychotherapy and Art.' *Art Therapy 1*, 3, 125–131.

McNiff, S. (1986) 'Freedom of Research and Artistic Inquiry.' *Arts in Psychotherapy 13*, 4, 279–284.

McNiff, S. (1988) 'The Shaman Within. Special Issue: Creative Arts Therapists as Contemporary Shamans: Reality or Romance?' *Arts in Psychotherapy 15*, 4, 285–291.

McNiff, S. (1998) *Art-Based Research.* London: Jessica Kingsley Publishers.

Mahns, W. (1997) *Symbolbildungen in der analytischen Kindermusiktherapie. Eine qualitative Studie über die Bedeutung der musikalischen Improvisation in der Musiktherapie mit Schulkindern.* PhD afhandling. Aalborg Universitet.

Mahns, W. and Pedersen, I.N. (1996) *Nordic Network in Music Therapy Research.* Aalborg: Institut for Musik og musikterapi.

Malloch, S.N. (1999) 'Mothers and Infants and Communicative Musicality.' *Musicæ Scientiæ* (special issue 1999–2000), 29–57.

McClellan, R. (1988) *The Healing Forces of Music: History, Theory and Practice.* Warwick, NY: Amity House.

Merker, B. (2000) 'A New Theory of Music Origins.' *Nordic Journal of Music Therapy 9*, 2, 28–31.

Merker, B., Bergström-Isaacsson, M. and Witt Engerström, I. (2001) 'Music and the Rett Disorder: The Swedish Rett Center Survey.' *Nordic Journal of Music Therapy 10*, 2, 42–53.

Michel, D. (1991) *Music for Developing Speech and Language Skills in Children. A Guide for Parents and Therapists.* St. Louis: MMB.

Michel, D. and Chesky, K. (1993) 'Music Therapy in Medical Settings: The Challenge for More Rigorous Research – especially in Music and Music Vibration Areas.' Paper to the 7th World Congress of Music Therapy, Vitoria, Spain.

Millard, K.A. and Smith, J.M. (1989) 'The Influence of Group Singing Therapy on the Behavior of Alzheimer's Disease Patients.' *Journal of Music Therapy 26*, 2, 58–70.

Milner, B. (1962) 'Laterality Effects in Audition.' In V.B. Mountcastle (ed) *Interhemispheric Relations and Cerebral Dominance.* Baltimore: John Hopkins Press.

Moe, T. (1995) 'Musikterapi med højresidigt hjerneskadede, er det muligt?' *Musik & Terapi 22*, 2.

Moe, T. (1998) 'Musikterapiforløb med en skizotypisk patinet ud fra en modifikation af metoden Guided Imagery and Music (GIM).' *Nordic Journal of Music Therapy 7*, 1, 14–23.

Moe, T. (2000) *Restituerende faktorer i gruppemusikterap med psykiatriske patienter, baseret på en modifikation af Guided Imagery and Music (GIM)*. PhD afhandling, Aalborg Universitet.

Moe, T., Roesen, A. and Raben, H. (2000) 'Restitutional Factors in Group Music Therapy with Psychiatric Patients Based on an Modification of Guided Imagery and Music.' *Nordic Journal of Music Therapy 9*, 2, 36–50.

Moe, T. and Thostrup, C. (1999) 'Mennesker med erhvervede hjerneskader – brug af musik.' *Specialpædagogik 1*, 3–10.

Møller, A.S. (1995) 'Kontaktniveauer i musikterapi med fysisk/psykisk udviklingshæmmede.' *Nordic Journal of Music Therapy 4*, 2, 99–102.

Montaigne, M.D. (1996) *Essays*. Oslo, Aschehoug.

Montello, L. and Coons, E.E. (1998) 'Effects of Active Versus Passive Group Music Therapy on Preadolescents with Emotional, Learning and Behavioural Disorders.' *Journal of Music Therapy 35*, 1, 49–67.

Moog, H. (1976) *The Musical Experience of the Pre-school Child*. (trans. C. Clarke). London: Schott.

Moreno, J. (1988) 'Multicultural Music Therapy: The World Music Connection.' *Journal of Music Therapy 25*, 1, 17–27.

Moreno, J. (1999) *Acting your Inner Music. Music Therapy and Psychodrama*. St. Louis: Magna Music Baton.

Moss, H. (1999) 'Creating a New Music Therapy Post. An Evidence-Based Research Project.' *British Journal of Music Therapy, 13*, 2, 49–58.

Motte-Haber, H.d.l. (1985) *Handbuch der Musikpsychologie*. Laaber: Laaber-Verlag.

Motte-Haber, H.d.l. (ed) (1987) *Handbuch der Musikpädagogik bd. 4: Psychologische Grundlagen des Musiklernens*. Laaber: Laaber-Verlag.

Muff, P. (1994) 'Musikterapi og udviklingshæmmede.' *Nordisk tidsskrift for musikkterapi 3*, 1, 19–20.

Muller, P. and Warwick, A. (1993) 'Autistic Children: The Effects of Maternal Involvement in Therapy.' In M. Heal and T. Wigram (eds) *Music Therapy in Health and Education*. London: Jessica Kingsley Publishers.

Müller-Busch, H.C. (1997) *Schmerz und Musik. Musiktherapie bei Patienten mit chronischen Schmerzen*. Stuttgart: Gustav Fischer.

Munk-Madsen, N.M. (2001) *Musikterapi til demente med adfærdsforstyrrelser*. Gentofte Kommune: Plejehjemmet Kridthuset.

Mursell, W. (1970) *The Psychology of Music* (second edition). N.Y.: Johnson Reprinting Co. (1937 first edition).

Myskja, A. (1999) *Den musiske medicin. Lyd og musikk som terapi*. Oslo: Grøndahl Dreyer.

Nattiez, J.J. (1990) *Music and Discourse: Towards a Semiology of Music*. Princeton, New Jersey: Princeton University Press.

Neugebauer, L. and Aldridge, D. (1998) 'Communication, Heart Rate and the Musical Dialogue.' *British Journal of Music Therapy 12*, 2, 46–52.

Newham, P. (1993) *The Singing Cure. An Introduction to Voice Movement Therapy*. London: Rider Books.

Newham, P. (1998) *Using Voice and Movement in Therapy. The Practical Application of Voice Movement Therapy Volume I*. London: Jessica Kingsley Publishers.

Newman, S. and Ward, C. (1993) 'An Observational Study of Intergenerational Activities and Behaviour Change in Dementing Elders at Adult Day Care Centers.' *International Journal of Aging and Human Development 36*, 4, 321–333.

Nöcker-Ribaupierre, M. (1999) 'Premature Birth and Music Therapy.' In T. Wigram and J. De Backer (eds) *Clinical Applications of Music Therapy in Developmental Disability, Paediatrics and Neurology*. London: Jessica Kingsley Publishers.

Norberg, A., Melin, E. and Asplund, K. (1986) 'Reactions to Music, Touch, and Object Presentation in the Final Stage of Dementia. An Exploratory Study.' *International Journal of Nursing Studies 23*, 4, 315–323.

Nordoff, P. and Robbins, C. (1971) *Therapy in Music for Handicapped Children*. London: Victor Gollancz.

Nordoff, P. and Robbins, C. (1977) *Creative Music Therapy*. New York: Harper and Row.

Odell-Miller, H. (1995) 'Approaches to Music Therapy in Psychiatry with Specific Emphasis upon the Evaluation of Work within a Completed Research Project with Elderly Mentally Ill People.' In T. Wigram, B. Saperston and R. West (eds) *The Art and Science of Music Therapy: A Handbook*. London: Harwood Academic Publications.

Odell-Miller, H. (1997) 'Music Therapy and the Functions of Music with Older Mentally Ill for People in a Continuous Care Setting.' In M. Denham (ed) *Continuing Care for Older People*. London: Stanley Thornes Publisher.

Odell-Miller, H. (1999) 'Investigating the Value of Music Therapy in Psychiatry: Outcome Related to Reasons for Referral.' In T. Wigram and J. De Backer (eds) *Clinical Applications of Music Therapy in Psychiatry*. London: Jessica Kingsley Publishers.

Odell-Miller, H. (2001) 'Music and its Relationship to Psychoanalysis.' In Y. Searle and I. Streng (eds) *Where Analysis Meets the Arts*. London: Karnac.

Olderog-Millard, K.A. and Smith, J.M. (1989) 'The Influence of Group Singing Therapy on the Behavior of Alzheimer's Disease Patients.' *Journal of Music Therapy 26*, 2, 58–70.

Oldfield, A. (1995) 'Communicating through Music: The Balance between Following and Initiating.' In T. Wigram, B. Saperston and R. West (eds) *The Art and Science of Music Therapy: A Handbook*. London: Harwood Academic Publishers.

Oldfield, A. (2000) 'Music Therapy as a Contribution to the Diagnosis made by the Staff Team in Child and Family Psychiatry – an Initial Description of a Methodology.' In T. Wigram (ed) *Assessment and Evaluation in the Arts Therapies: Art Therapy, Music Therapy and Dramatherapy*. Radlett: Harper House Publications.

Oldfield, A. and Adams, M. (1990) 'The Effects of Music Therapy on a Group of Profoundly Mentally Handicapped Adults.' *Journal of Mental Deficiency Research 34*, 2, 107–125.

Oldfield, A. and Bunce, L. (2001) '"Mummy can Play Too …" Short-term Music Therapy with Mothers and Young Children.' *British Journal of Music Therapy 15*, 1, 27–36.

Palo-Bengtsson, L., Winblad, B. and Ekman S.L. (1998) 'Social Dancing: A Way to Support Intellectual, Emotional and Motor Functions in Persons with Dementia.' *Journal of Psychiatric and Mental Health Nursing 5*, 6, 545–554.

Pavlicevic, M. (1995) 'Interpersonal Processes in Clinical Improvisation: Towards a Subjectively Objective Systematic Definition.' In T. Wigram, B. Saperston and R. West (eds) *The Art and Science of Music Therapy: A Handbook*. London: Harwood Academic Publishers.

Pavlicevic, M. (1997) *Music Therapy in Context. Music, Meaning and Relationship*. London: Jessica Kingsley Publishers.

Pavlicevic, M. (1999a) *Music Therapy: Intimate Notes*. London and Philadelphia: Jessica Kingsley Publishers.

Pavlicevic, M. (1999b) 'Thoughts, Words and Deeds: Harmonies and Counterpoints in Music Therapy Theory.' *British Journal of Music Therapy 13*, 2, 59–62.

Pavlicevic, M. and Trevarthen, C. (1994) 'Improvisational Music Therapy and the Rehabilitation of Persons Suffering from Chronic Schizophrenia.' *Journal of Music Therapy 31*, 2, 86–104.

Pedersen, I.N. (1987a) 'Musikterapi – et alternativt behandlingstilbud.' *Forskning og Samfund 7*. Kbh.: Forskningssekretariatet.

Pedersen, I.N. (1987b) *Musikterapi-en uddannelse under udvikling. Et nyt skud på stammen af universitetspædagogiske traditioner.* Upubliceret rapport. Aalborg Universitet.

Pedersen, I.N. (1990) 'Kandidatuddannelsen i musikterapi ved Aalborg Universitetscenter. Et historisk og nutidigt perspektiv.' *Dansk Akademisk Tidsskrift for Musikterapi 1,* 1.

Pedersen, I.N. (1994) 'Musikterapi i Danmark.' *Nordisk Tidsskrift for Musikkterapi 3,* 1.

Pedersen, I.N. (1997) 'The Music Therapist's Listening Perspectives as Source of Information in Improvised Musical Duets with Grown-up, Psychiatric Patients Suffering from Schizophrenia.' *Nordisk Tidsskrift for Musikkterapi 6,* 2.

Pedersen, I.N. (1998) *Indføring i muskterapi som er selvstændig behandlingsform.* (Introduction to Music Therapy as a Primary Treatment Form.) Musikterapiklinikken. Aalborg Psykiatriske Sygehus – Aalborg Universitet.

Pedersen, I.N. (1998a) 'Musikterapiens start inden for psykiatrien – lidt historie.' In I.N. Pedersen (ed) *Indføring i musikterapi som en selvstændig behandlingsform.* Musikterapi i psykiatrien. Årsskrift 1998. Musikterapiklinikken. Aalborg Psykiatriske Sygehus/Aalborg Universitet.

Pedersen, I.N. (1998b) 'Musikterapi som det første skridt i en psykoterapeutisk behandlingsform med skizofrene/psykotiske patienter – en holdende og reorganiserende musikterapeutisk metode.' In I.N. Pedersen (ed) *Indføring i musikterapi som en selvstændig behandlingsform.* Musikterapiklinikken. Aalborg Psykiatriske Sygehus/Aalborg Universitet.

Pedersen, I.N. (1999) 'Musikterapi – et nyt behandlingstilbud.' *Medicus 6.* Lægekredsforeningen for Århus Amt.

Pedersen, I.N. (2000) 'Inde-fra eller ude-fra – orientering i terapeutens tilstedeværelse og nærvær.' In C. Lindvang (ed) *Den musikterapeutiske behandling. Musikterapi i psykiatrien,* Årsskrift 2000. Musikterapiklinikken. Aalborg psykiatriske Sygehus/Aalborg Universitet. Den Psykiatriske Forskningsenhed i Nordjyllands Amt.

Pedersen, I.N., Frederiksen, B. and Lindvang, C., (1998) 'Musikterapiens indplacering i Danmark – som akademisk disciplin – som behandlingstilbud idnen for psykiatrien i DK – i en forståelse af psykiske problemer.' In I.N. Pedersen (ed) *Indføring i musikterapi som en selvstændig behandlingsform.* Musikterapiklinikken. Aalborg Psykiatriske Sygehus/Aalborg Universitet.

Pedersen, I.N. and Scheiby, B.B. (1981) *Musikterapeut-Musik-Klient.* Aalborg Universitetsforlag.

Pedersen, I.N. and Scheiby, B.B. (1983) 'Vi zoomer os ind på musikterapi.' *Modspil 23* (temanummer om musikterapi). Publimus. Aarhus.

Pedersen, I.N. and Scheiby, B.B. (1999) 'Inter Music Therapy in the Training of Music Therapy Students.' *Nordisk Tidsskrift for musikkterapi 8,* 1, 59–72.

Persoons, J. and De Backer, J. (1997) 'Vibroacoustic Therapy with Handicapped and Autistic Clients.' In T. Wigram and C. Dileo (eds) *Music, Vibration and Health.* Pennsylvania: Jeffrey Books.

Pine, F. (1990) *Drive, Ego, Object and Self. A Synthesis for Clinical Work.* N.Y.: Basic Books.

Plahl, C. (2000) *Entwicklung fördern durch Musik. Evaluation Musiktherapeutischer Behandlung.* Münster: Waxmann.

Pollack, N.J. and Namazi, N.H. (1992) 'The Effect of Music Participation on the Social Behavior of Alzheimer's Disease Patients.' *Journal of Music Therapy 29,* 1, 54–67.

Pontvik, A (1996) *Der tönende Mensch. Gesemmelte Musikterapeutische Schriften. Heidelberger Schriften zur Musikterapie. Band 9.* Stuttgart: Gustav Fischer Verlag.

Pratt, R.R. and Grocke, D. (1999) *MusicMedicine 2 & 3: MusicMedicine and Music Therapy: Expanding Horizons.* Melbourne: Faculty of Music, University of Melbourne.

Pratt, R.R. and Hesser, B. (eds) (1989) *Music Therapy and Music in Special Education: The International State of the Art.* St. Louis: MMB.

Pratt, R. and Jones, R.W. (1988) 'Music and Medicine: A Partnership in History.' *International Journal of Arts Medicine, 6,* 377–389.

Pratt, R.R. and Spintge, R. (eds) (1996) *MusicMedicine II.* Saint Louis: MMB Music.

Prickett, C.A. (1995) 'Principles of Quantitative Research.' In B. Wheeler (ed) *Music Therapy Research. Quantitative and Qualitative Perspectives.* Phoenixville: Barcelona Publishers.

Prickett, C.A. and Moore, R.S. (1991) 'The Use of Music to Aid Memory of Alzheimer's Patients.' *Journal of Music Therapy 28,* 2, 101–110.

Priestley, M. (1975) *Music Therapy in Action.* London: Constable.

Priestley, M. (1994) *Essays on Analytical Music Therapy.* Phoenixville: Barcelona Publishers.

Priestley, M. (1995) 'Linking Sound and Symbol.' In T. Wigram, B. Saperston and R. West (eds) *The Art and Science of Music Therapy: A Handbook.* London: Harwood Academic Publishers.

Proctor, S. (1999) 'The Therapeutic Musical Relationship: A Two-Sided Affair? A Consideration of the Significance of the Therapist's Musical Input in Co-improvisation.' *British Journal of Music Therapy 13,* 1, 28–37.

Radocy, R.E. and Boyle, J.D. (1988) *Psychological Foundations of Musical Behaviour.* Springfield, Illinois: Charles C. Thomas.

Raffman, D. (1993) *Language, Music, and Mind.* London: A Bradford Book.

Ragneskog, H., Kihlgren, M., Karlsson, I., and Norberg, A. (1996) 'Dinner Music for Demented Patients. Analysis of Video-recorded Observations.' *Clinical Nursing Research 5,* 3, 262–282.

Raijmaekers, J. (1993) 'Music Therapy's Role in the Diagnosis of Psycho-Geriatric Patients in The Hague.' In M. Heal and T. Wigram (eds) *Music Therapy in Health and Education.* London: Jessica Kingsley Publishers.

Raudsik, R. (1997) 'Vibroacoustic Therapy in General Medicine.' In T. Wigram and C. Dileo (eds) *Music, Vibration and Health.* Pennsylvania: Jeffrey Books.

Reyner, E. (1992) 'Matching, Attunement and the Psychoanalytic Dialogue.' *International Journal of Psychoanalysis 73,* 127–148.

Ricoeur, P. (1978) *The Rule of Metaphor. Multi-disciplinary Studies of the Creation of Meaning in Language.* London: Routledge.

Ridder, H.M.O. (2001a) *Musik & Demens. Musikaktiviteter og musikterapi med demensramte.* Denmark: FormidlingsCenter Nord. www.fcnord.dk.

Ridder, H.M.O. (2001b) 'Musikterapi med ældre.' In L. Bonde, I. Pedersen and T. Wigram (eds) *Musikterapi: når ord ikke slår til.* Århus: KLIM.

Rider, M. (1997) *The Rhythmic Language of Health and Disease.* Saint Louis: MMB Music.

Rider, M. (1999) 'Homeodynamic Mechanisms of Improvisational Music Therapy.' In C. Dileo (ed) *Music Therapy and Medicine: Theoretical and Clinical Applications.* Silver Spring, MD: American Music Therapy Association.

Riegler, J. (1980) 'Comparison of a Reality Orientation Program for Geriatric Patients With and Without Music.' *Journal of Music Therapy 17,* 1, 26–33.

Robarts, J. (1998) 'Music Therapy for Children with Autism.' In C. Trevarthen, K. Aitkin, D. Papoudi and J. Robarts (eds) *Children with Autism. Diagnosis and Interventions to Meet Their Needs.* London and Philadelphia: Jessica Kingsley Publishers.

Robarts, J.Z. (2000) 'Music Therapy and Adolescents with Anorexia Nervosa.' *Nordic Journal of Music Therapy 9,* 1, 3–12.

Robb, S. (1996) 'Techniques in Song Writing. Restoring Emotional and Physical Well-Being in Adolescents who have been Traumatically Injured.' *Music Therapy Perspectives 14,* 1, 30–37.

Robbins, C. and Robbins, C. (1980) *Music for the Hearing Impaired: A Resource Manual and Curriculum Guide.* Saint Louis: MMB Music.

Robbins, C. and Robbins, C. (eds) (1998) *Healing Heritage: Paul Nordoff Exploring the Tonal Language of Music*. Gilsum, NH: Barcelona.

Robertson, J. (2000) 'An Educational Model for Music Therapy: The Case for a Continuum.' *British Journal of Music Therapy 14*, 1, 41–46.

Rogers, C.R. (1951) *Client-centered Therapy*. Houghton Mifflin: Boston.

Rogers, P. (1993) 'Research in Music Therapy with Sexually Abused Clients.' In H. Payne (ed) *Handbook of Enquiry in the Arts Therapies*. London: Jessica Kingsley Publishers.

Rugenstein, L. (1996) 'Wilber's Spectrum Model of Transpersonal Psychology and its Application to Music Therapy.' *Music Therapy 14*, 1, 9–28.

Ruud, E. (1990) *Musikk som kommunikasjon og samhandling. Teoretiske perspektiv på musikkterapien*. Oslo: Solum Forlag.

Ruud, E. (1996) *Musikk og verdier. Musikkpedagogiske essays*. Oslo: Universitetsforlaget.

Ruud, E. (1997) *Musikk og identitet*. Oslo, Universitetsforlaget.

Ruud, E. (1998a) *Music Therapy: Improvisation, Communication and Culture*. Gilsum, NH: Barcelona Publishers.

Ruud, E. (1998b) 'Music and Identity.' In E. Ruud *Music Therapy: Improvisation, Communication and Culture*. Gilsum, NH: Barcelona Publishers.

Ruud, E. (2000) '"New Musicology", Music Education and Music Therapy.' Keynote ved 13th Nordic Musicological Congress, Århus August 18 – 2000. Også tilgængelig på *Nordic Journal of Music Therapy's* hjemmeside.

Ruud, E. (2000b) 'Music Therapy – History and Cultural Context. Two Major New Texts on Music Therapy.' *Nordic Journal of Music Therapy 9*, 2, 67–76.

Ruud, E. and Mahns, W. (1991) *Meta-Musiktherapie. Wege zur einer Theorie der Musiktherapie*. Oslo: Norsk Musikforlag.

Sacks, O. (1998) 'Music and the Brain.' In C.M. Tomaino (ed) *Clinical Applications of Music in Neurological Rehabilitation*. St. Louis: MMB Music.

Sambandham, M. and Schirm, V. (1995) 'Music as a Nursing Intervention for Residents with Alzheimer's Disease in Long-term Care.' *Geriatric Nursing 16*, 2, 79–83.

Sameroff, A.J. and Emde, R.N. (1989) *Relationship Disturbances in Early Childhood*. New York: Basic Books.

Saperston, B. (1989) 'Music Based Individualised Relaxation Training (MBIRT): A Stress Reduction Approach for the Behaviourally Disturbed Mentally Retarded.' *Music Therapy Perspectives, 6*, 26–33.

Saperston, B. (1995) 'The Effect of Consistent Tempi and Physiologically Interactive Tempi on Heart Rate and EMG Responses.' In T. Wigram, B. Saperston and R. West (eds) *The Art and Science of Music Therapy: A Handbook*. London, Toronto: Harwood Academic Publications.

Scartelli, J. (1989) *Music and Self-Management Methods: A Physiological Model*. St. Louis: MMB.

Scheiby, B.B. (1998) 'The Role of Musical Countertransference in Analytical Music Therapy.' In K.E. Bruscia (ed) *The Dynamics of Music Psychotherapy*. Gilsum, NH: Barcelona Publishers.

Schogler, B. (1998) 'Music as a Tool in Communications Research.' *Nordic Journal of Music Therapy 7*, 1, 40–49.

Schumacher, K. (1999) *Musiktherapie und Säuglingsforschung*. Frankfurt am Main: Peter Lang.

Schumacher, K. and Calvert-Kruppa, C. (1999) 'The "AQR" – an Analysis System to Evaluate the Quality of Relationship during Music Therapy.' *Nordic Journal of Music Therapy 8*, 2, 188–191.

Schwabe, C. (1985) *Rezeptive Musiktherapie. Musikpsychologie*. München: Urban & Schwarzenberg.

Schwabe, C. (1987) *Regulative Musiktherapie. 2., überarbeitete Aufl*. Leipzig: Thieme / Stuttgart: Fischer.

Sears, W. (1968/1996) 'Processes in Music Therapy.' *Nordic Journal of Music Therapy 5*, 1, 33–42.

Selman, J. (1988) 'Music Therapy with Parkinson's Disease.' *Journal of British Music Therapy 2*, 1, 5–9.

Shoemark, H. (1999) 'Indications for the Inclusion of Music Therapy in the Care of Infants with Bronchopulmonary Dysplasia.' In T. Wigram and J. De Backer (eds) *Clinical Applications of Music Therapy in Developmental Disability, Paediatrics and Neurology*. London and Philadelphia: Jessica Kingsley Publishers.

Siegal, L.S., Cartwright, J.S. and Katz, E. (1986) 'Where's the Research?' *Journal of Music Therapy 23*, 1, 38–45.

Siegelman, E. (1990) *Metaphor and Meaning in Psychotherapy*. New York: The Guildford Press.

Sikström, M. and Skille, O. (1995) 'The Skille Musical Function Test as a Tool in the Assessment of Psychological Function and Individual Potential.' In T. Wigram, B. Saperston and R. West (eds) *The Art and Science of Music Therapy: A Handbook*. London, Toronto: Harwood Academic Publications.

Silber, F. (1999) 'The Influence of Background Music on the Performance of the Mini Mental State Examination with Patients Diagnosed with Alzheimer's Disease.' *Journal of Music Therapy 36*, 3, 196–206.

Silber, F. and Hes, J.P. (1995) 'The Use of Songwriting with Patients Diagnosed with Alzheimer's Disease.' *Music Therapy Perspectives 13*, 1, 31–34.

Simpson, F. (2000) 'Creative Music Therapy: A Last Resort?' In D. Aldridge (ed) *Music Therapy in Dementia Care*. London: Jessica Kingsley Publishers.

Skille, O. (1982a) 'Musikkbadet – Anvendt for de Svakeste.' *Nordisk Tidsskrift for Speciale Pedagogikk 4*, 275–84.

Skille, O. (1982b) 'Musikkbadet – en musikkterapeutisk metode.' *Musikkterapi 6*, 24–27.

Skille, O. (1989a) 'Vibroacoustic research'. In R. Spintge and R. Droh (eds) *Music Medicine*. St. Louis: Magna Music Baton.

Skille, O. (1989b) 'Vibroacoustic therapy.' *Music Therapy 8*, 61–77. New York: AAMT.

Skille, O. (1992) 'Vibroacoustic research 1980–1991.' In R. Spintge and R. Droh (eds) *Music and Medicine*, (pp.249–266) St. Louis: Magna Music Baton.

Skille, O. and Wigram, T. (1995) 'The effects of music, vocalisation and vibration on brain and muscle tissue: studies in vibroacoustic therapy.' In T. Wigram, B. Saperston and R. West (eds) *The Art and Science of Music Therapy: a Handbook*, (pp.23–57) London: Harwood Academic Publications.

Skille, O., Wigram, T. and Weekes, L. (1989) 'Vibroacoustic therapy: The therapeutic effect of low frequency sound on specific physical disorders and disabilities.' *Journal of British Music Therapy 3*, 2, 6–10.

Skinner, B.F. (1953) *Science and Human behaviour*. New York: Macmillan.

Sloboda, J.H. (1991) Empirical Studies of Emotional Response to Music. In M. Riess-Jones (ed) *Cognitive Bases of Musical Communication*. Washington D.C.: American Psychological Association.

Sloboda, J.A. (1985) *The Musical Mind: The Cognitive Psychology of Music*. Oxford: Clarendon Press.

Sloboda, J.A. (1987) 'Music as a Language.' In F. Wilson and F. Rochmann (eds) *Music and Child Development: Proceedings of the 1987 Biology of Music Making Conference*. St Louis: Magna Music Baton.

Sloboda, J.A. (ed) (1988) *Generative Processes in Music. The Psychology of Performance, Improvisation and Composition*. Oxford: Clarendon Press.

Sloboda, J.A. (1995) *The Cognitive Psychology of Music*. Oxford: Oxford Science Publications.

Small, C. (1998) *Musicking*. Hannover NH: Wesleyan University Press.

Smeijsters, H. (1994) *Musiktherapie als Psychotherapie*. Stuttgart: G. Fischer.

Smeijsters, H. (1997a) *Multiple Perspectives. A Guide to Qualitative Research in Music Therapy.* Gilsum, NH: Barcelona Publishers.

Smeijsters, H. (1997b) *Musiktherapie bei Altzheimerpatienten. Eine Meta-Analyse von Forschungsergebuissen. Musikterapeutische Umschau 4,* 268–283.

Smeijsters, H. (1998) 'Developing Concepts for a General Theory of Music Therapy. Music as Representation, Replica, Semi-representation, Symbol, Metaphor, Semi-symbol, Iso-morphé, and Analogy.' 4th European Music Therapy Conference, Leuwen, Belgium. In D. Aldridge (ed) *Music Therapy Info CD-ROM II.* Witten/Herdecke: Universität Witten/Herdecke.

Smeijsters, H. (1999) *Grundlagen der Musiktherapie. Theorie und Praxis der Behandlung psychischer Störungen und Behinderungen.* Göttingen: Hogrefe.

Smeijsters, H. and van den Hurk, J. (1999) 'Music Therapy Helping to Work Through Grief and Finding a Personal Identity. Qualitative Single Case Research.' *Journal of Music Therapy 16,* 3, 222–252.

Smith-Marchese, K. (1994) 'The Effects of Participatory Music on the Reality Orientation and Sociability of Alzheimer's Residents in a Long-term Care Setting.' *Activities, Adaptation, & Aging 18,* 2, 41–55.

Spintge, R. (1982) 'Psychophysiological Surgery Preparation With and Without Anxiolytic Music.' In R. Droh and R. Spintge (eds) *Angst, Schmerz, Muzik in der Anasthesie.* Basel: Editiones Roche.

Spintge, R. (1988) 'Music as a Physiotherapeutic and Emotional Means in Medicine.' *International Journal of Music, Dance and Art Therapy 8,* 75–81.

Spintge, R. (1993) 'Music and Surgery and Pain Therapy.' Paper to the NAMT/AAMT/CAMT Conference on Music Therapy: 'Crossing Borders, Joining Forces'. Toronto 1993. Unpublished.

Spintge, R. and Droh, R. (1982) 'The Pre-operative Condition of 191 Patients Exposed to Anxiolytic Music and Rohypnol (Flurazepam) Before Receiving an Epidural Anaesthetic.' In R. Droh and R. Spintge (eds) *Angst, Schmerz, Muzik in der Anästhesie.* Basel: Editiones Roche.

Spintge, R. and Droh, R. (1992) *MusicMedicine.* St. Louis: MMB.

Standley, J.M. (1991a) 'The Effect of Vibrotactile and Auditory Stimuli on Perception of Comfort, Heartrate, and Peripheral Finger Temperature.' *Journal of Music Therapy 28,* 3, 120–134.

Standley, J.M. (1991b) 'The Role of Music in Pacification/Stimulation of Premature Infants with Low Birth Weights.' *Music Therapy Perspectives 9,* 19–25.

Standley, J.M. (1995) 'Music as a Therapeutic Intervention in Medical and Dental Treatment: Research and Clinical Applications.' In T. Wigram, B. Saperston and R. West.(eds) *The Art and Science of Music Therapy: A Handbook.* London: Harwood Academic.

Standley, J.M. (1998) 'The Effect of Contingent Music to Increase Non-nutrive Sucking of Premature Infants.' ISMM Congress, Melbourne University, 1998. Communication.

Standley, J.M. and Hanser, S.B. (1995) 'Music Therapy Research and Applications in Paediatric Oncology Treatment.' *Journal of Paediatric Oncology Nursing 12,* 1, 3–8.

Standley, J.M. and Moore, R. (1995) 'Therapeutic Effects of Music and Mother's Voice on Premature Infants.' *Paediatric Nursing 1,* 2, 90–95.

Standley, J. and Prickett, C. (eds) (1994) *Research in Music Therapy: A Tradition of Excellence. Outstanding Reprints from the Journal of Music Therapy 1964–1993.* Silver Spring, MD: NAMT.

Staum, M.J. and Brotons, M. (2000) 'The Effect of Music Volume on the Relaxation Response.' *Journal of Music Therapy 37,* 1, 22–39.

Steen-Møller, A. (1996) 'Music as Means of Contact and Communication with the Physically and Mentally Handicapped.' In I.N. Pedersen and L.O. Bonde (eds) *Music Therapy within Multi-Disciplinary Teams.* Aalborg Universitetsforlag.

Steiner, R. (1983) *The Inner Nature of Music and the Experience of Tone: Selected Lectures from the Work of Rudolf Steiner.* Spring Valley, NY: Anthroposophic Press.

Stern, D. (1985) *The Interpersonal World of the Infant: A View from Psychoanalysis and Developmental Psychology.* New York: Basic Books.

Stern, D. (1995) *The Motherhood Constellation.* New York: Basic Books.

Stern, D.N. (1989) 'The Representation of Relational Patterns: Developmental Considerations.' In A.J. Sameroff and R.N. Emde (eds) *Relationship Disturbances in Early Childhood.* New York: Basic Books.

Stern, D., Sander, L.W., Nehum, J.P., Harrison, A.M., Lyons-Ruyh, K., Morgan, A.C., Brunschweiler-Stern, N. and Tronic, E.Z. (1998) 'Non-Interpretive Mechanisms in Psychoanalytic Therapy.' *International Journal of Psychoanalysis 79*, 903–921.

Stewart, D. (2000) 'The State of the UK Music Therapy Profession. Personal Qualities, Working Models, Support Networks and Job Satisfaction.' *British Journal of Music Therapy 14*, 1, 13–31.

Stige, B. (1993) 'Changes in the Music Therapy "Space" – With Cultural Engagement in the Local Community as an Example.' *Nordisk tidsskrift for musikkterapi 2*, 2, 11–22.

Stige, B. (1995) 'Om Improvisational Assessment Profiles (IAP) Del I: Grunnlagsproblemer.' *Nordisk Tidsskrift for Musikkterapi 4*, 2, 55–66.

Stige, B. (1996) 'Om Improvisational Assessment Profiles (IAP) Del II: Klinisk og forskningsmessig relevans.' *Nordisk Tidsskrift for Musikkterapi 5*, 1, 3–12.

Stige, B. (1997) 'Music and infant interaction. Colwyn Trevarthen interviewed by Brynjulf Stige.' *Nordic Journal of Music Therapy 6*, 1, 61–65.

Stige, B. (1998a) 'Perspectives on Meaning in Music Therapy.' *British Journal of Music Therapy 12*, 1, 20–28.

Stige, B. (1998b) 'Aesthetic Practices in Music Therapy.' *Nordic Journal of Music Therapy 7*, 2, 121–134.

Stige, B. (1999) 'The Meaning of Music – From the Client's Perspective.' In T. Wigram and J. De. Backer (eds) *Clinical Applications of Music Therapy in Psychiatry.* London: Jessica Kingsley Publishers.

Stige, B. (2000) 'The Nature of Meaning in Music Therapy. Ken Bruscia interviewed by Brynjulf Stige.' *Nordic Journal of Music Therapy 9*, 2, 84–96.

Strange, J. (1999) 'Client-Centred Music Therapy for Emotionally Disturbed Teenagers with Moderate Learning Disability.' In T. Wigram and J. De Backer (eds) *Clinical Applications of Music Therapy in Developmental Disability, Paediatric and Neurology.* London: Jessica Kingsley Publishers.

Strauss, A. and Corbin, J. (1990) *Basics of Qualitative Research: Grounded Theory, Procedures and Techniques.* Newbury Park, CA: Sage.

Streeter, E. (1999a) 'Definition and Use of the Musical Transference Relationship.' In T. Wigram and J. De Backer (eds) *Clinical Applications of Music Therapy in Psychiatry.* London: Jessica Kingsley Publishers.

Streeter, E. (1999b) 'Finding a Balance Between Psychological Thinking and Musical Awareness in Music Therapy Theory – A Psychoanalytic Perspective.' *British Journal of Music Therapy 13*, 1, 5–20.

Summer, L. (1996) *Music: The New Age Elixir.* Amherst NY: Prometheus Books.

Sundin, K. (2001) *Sense of "Understanding and Being Understood" in the Care of Patients With Communication Difficulties.* Unpublished dissertation, Umeå Universitet, Sweden.

Sutton, J. (1993) 'The Guitar Doesn't Know This Song: An Investigation of Parallel Development in Speech and Language and Music Therapy.' In M. Heal and T. Wigram (eds) *Music Therapy in Health and Education.* London: Jessica Kingsley Publishers.

Swanwick, K. (1994) *Musical Knowledge, Intuition, Analysis and Music Education.* London: Routledge.

Tabloski, P., McKinnon-Howe, L. and Remington, R. (1995) 'Effects of Calming Music on the Level of Agitation in Cognitively Impaired Nursing Home Residents.' *The American Journal of Alzheimer's Care and Related Disorders & Research,* Jan./Feb., 10–15.

Tame, D. (1984) *The Secret Power of Music.* Wellington: Turnstone Press.

Taylor, D. (1997) *Biomedical Foundations of Music as Therapy.* St. Louis: Magna Music Baton.

Thaut, M.H. (1985) 'The Use of Auditory Rhythm and Rhythmic Speech to Aid Temporal Muscular Control in Children with Gross Motor Dysfunction.' *Journal of Music Therapy 22,* 3, 129–145.

Thaut, M.H. (1990) *Physiological Responses to Music Stimuli. Music Therapy in the Treatment of Adults with Mental Disorders.* New York: Schirmer Books.

Thaut, M.H., McIntosh, G.C., Prassas, S.G. and Rice, R.R. (1993) 'Effect of Rhythmic Cuing on Temporal Stride Parameters and EMG Patterns in Hemiparetic Gait of Stroke Patients.' *Journal of Neurologic Rehabilitation, 6,* 185–190.

Thaut, M.H., McIntosh, G.C., Rice, R.R., Miller, R.A., Rathbun, J. and Brault, J.M. (1996) 'Rhythmic Auditory Stimulation in Gait Training for Parkinson's Disease Patients.' *Movement Disorders 11,* 1–11.

Theilgaard (1994) *Metaforer I terapiens tjeneste.* Psyke and Logos 16: 164–173.

Thomas, D., Heitman, R. and Alexander, T. (1997) 'The Effects of Music on Bathing Co-operation for Residents with Dementia.' *Journal of Music Therapy 34,* 4, 246–259.

Tilly, M. (1948) 'Music Therapy.' *Notes for Californian Music Libraries 1,* 9, 1–9.

Tomaino, C. (1998) *Clinical Applications of Music in Neurological Rehabilitation.* St. Louis: Magna Music Baton.

Tomaino, C.M. (2000) 'Working with Images and Recollection with Elderly Patients.' In D. Aldridge (ed) *Music Therapy in Dementia Care.* London: Jessica Kingsley Publishers.

Trehub, S. E., Trainor, L.J. and Unyk, A.M. (1993) 'Music and Speech Processing in the First Year of Life.' *Advances in Child Development and Behavior 24,* 1–35.

Trevarthen, C. (1999) 'Musicality and the intrinsic motive pulse: Evidence from human psychobiology and infant communication.' *Musicæ Scientiæ* (Special issue 1999–2000), 155–215.

Trevarthen, C. and Malloch, S.N. (2000) 'The Dance of Wellbeing: Defining the Musical Therapeutic Effect.' *Nordic Journal of Music Therapy 9,* 2, 3–17.

Trolldalen, G. (1997) 'Music Therapy and Interplay. A Music Therapy Project with Mothers and Children Elucidated through the Concept of "Appreciative Recognition".' *Nordic Journal of Music Therapy 6,* 1, 14–27.

Turry, A (1999) 'A Song of Life: Improvised Music with Children with Cancer and Serious Blood Disorders.' In T. Wigram and J. De Backer (eds) *Clinical Applications of Music Therapy in Developmental Disability, Paediatrics and Neurology.* (pp.47–68) London and Philadelphia: Jessica Kingsley Publishers.

Tüpker, R. (1988) *Ich singe, was ich nicht sagen kann. Zu einer morphologischen Grundlegung der Musiktherapie.* Regensburg: Bosse.

Tyler, H.M. (1998) 'Behind the Mask. An Exploration of the True and False Self as revealed in music therapy.' *British Journal of Music Therapy 12,* 2, 60–66.

Tyson, F. (1981) *Psychiatric Music Therapy. Origins and Developments.* St. Louis: MMB.

Tønsberg, G.E.H. and Hauge, T.S. (1998) 'A response to "Music as a Tool in Communication Research".' *Nordic Journal of Music Therapy 7,* 2, 50–54.

Unkefer, R. (ed) (1990) *Music Therapy in the Treatment of Mental Disorders.* New York: Schirmer Books.

Voigt, M. (1999) 'Orff Music Therapy with Multi-Handicapped Children.' In T. Wigram and J. De Backer (eds) *Clinical Applications of Music Therapy in Developmental Disability, Paediatric and Neurology.* London: Jessica Kingsley.

Waldon, E.G. (2001) 'The effects of Group Music Therapy on Mood States and Cohesiveness in Adult Oncology Patients.' *Journal of Music Therapy 38,* 3, 212–238.

Wallerstein, R.S. (1988) 'One Psychoanalysis or many?' *International Journal of Psychoanalysis 69,* 5–21.

Wallin, N., Merker, B. and Brown. S. (eds) (2000) *The Origins of Music.* Cambridge MA: MIT Press.

Warwick, A (1995) 'Music Therapy in the Education Service: Research with autistic children and their mothers'. In T. Wigram, B. Saperston and R. West *The Art and Science of Music Therapy.* Harwood Academic: Toronto, London.

West, T.M. (1994) 'Psychological issues in hospice music therapy. Special Issue: Psychiatric music therapy.' *Music Therapy Perspectives 12,* 2, 117–124.

Wheeler, B. (1988) 'An Analysis of Literature from selected music therapy journals.' *Music Therapy Perspectives 5,* 94–101.

Wheeler, B. (1995) *Music Therapy Research: Quantitative and Qualitative Perspectives.* Phoenixville: Barcelona Publishers.

Wheeler, B. (1999) 'Experiencing Pleasure in Working with Severely Disabled Children.' *Journal of Music Therapy 36,* 1, 56–80.

Wigram, A. (1988) 'Music Therapy Developments in Mental Handicap.' *The Bulletin of the Society for Research in Psychology of Music and Music Education 16,* 1, 42–52.

Wigram, T. (1991a) 'Music Therapy for a Girl with Rett's Syndrome: Balancing Structure and Freedom.' In K. Bruscia (ed) *Case Studies in Music Therapy.* Phoenixville: Barcelona Publishers.

Wigram, A. (1991b) 'Die Wirkung von Tiefen Tonen und Musik auf den Muskel-Tonus und die Blutxirkulation.' ÖBM. *Zeitschrift des Österreichischen Berufsverbandes der Musiktherapeuten (2–91),* 3–12.

Wigram, T. (1991c) 'Die Bedeutung musikalischen Verhaltens und Empfanglichkeit im Verlauf der Differentialdiagnose von Autismus und anderen Retardierungen.' ÖBM. *Zeitschrift Des Österreichischen Berufsverbandes der Musiktherapeuten (1–91),* 4–18.

Wigram, A. (1992a) 'Aspects of Music Therapy Relating to Physical Disability.' Keynote paper to the 1991 Annual Congress of AMTA, Sydney, Australia. *Australian Journal of Music Therapy 3,* 3–15.

Wigram, A. (1992b) 'Differential Diagnosis of Autism and Other Types of Disability.' Keynote paper to the 1991 Annual Congress of AMTA, Sydney, Australia. *Australian Journal of Music Therapy 3,* 16–26.

Wigram, T. (1993a) 'Music Therapy Research to Meet the Demands of Health and Education Services: Research and Literature Analysis.' In M. Heal and T. Wigram (eds) *Music Therapy in Health and Education.* London: Jessica Kingsley Publishers.

Wigram, T. (1993b) 'Observational Techniques in the Analysis of Both Active and Receptive Music Therapy with Disturbed and Self-Injurious Clients.' In M. Heal and T. Wigram (eds) *Music Therapy in Health and Education.* London: Jessica Kingsley Publishers.

Wigram, T. (1994) 'Improvvisazione tematica: Transfert e controtransfert positivo e negativo.' In G. Di Franco and R. de Michele (eds) *Musicoterapia in Italia: Scuola Handicap Salute Mentale.* (Thematic Improvisation: Positive and Negative Transference and Countertransference in the Music Therapy Process. Paper to the Italian National Congress of Music Therapy. June 1994. Napol). Napoli: Idelsen.

Wigram, T. (1995a) 'A Model of Assessment and Differential Diagnosis of Handicap in Children Through the Medium of Music Therapy.' In T. Wigram, B. Saperston and R. West (eds) *The Art and Science of Music Therapy: A Handbook*. London: Harwood Academic.

Wigram, T. (1995b) 'Musicoterapia: Estructura y Flexibilidad en el proceso de Musicoterapia.' In P. del Campo (ed) *La Musica como proceso humano*. (Music Therapy: Structure and Flexibility in the Music Therapy Process. In P. Del Campo (ed) *Music and the Human Process*. Vitoria, Spain.) Amaru Ediciones, Salamanca, Spain.

Wigram, T. (1996a) '"Becoming Clients": Role playing clients as a Technique in the Training of Advanced Level Music Therapy Students.' In I.N. Pedersen and L.O. Bonde (eds) *Music Therapy in Multi-Disciplinary Teams*. Aalborg Universitetsforlag.

Wigram T. (1996b) *The Effect of Vibroacoustic Therapy on Clinical and Non-Clinical Populations*. PhD. Psychology research thesis. St George's Medical School. University of London. CD-ROM *Music Therapy Info II*. Witten-Herdecke Universität.

Wigram, T. (1997a) 'The Effect of VA Therapy on Multiply Handicapped Adults with High Muscle Tone and Spasticity.' In T. Wigram and C. Dileo (eds) *Music, Vibration and Health*. New Jersey: Jeffrey Books.

Wigram, T. (1997b) 'Foundations of Vibroacoustic Therapy.' In T. Wigram and C. Dileo (eds) *Music, Vibration and Health*. New Jersey: Jeffrey Books.

Wigram, T. (1997c) 'The Effect of Vibroacoustic Therapy Compared with Music and Movement Based Physiotherapy on Multiply Handicapped Patients with High Muscle Tone and Spasticity.' In T. Wigram and C. Dileo (eds) *Music, Vibration and Health*. New Jersey: Jeffrey Books.

Wigram, T. (1997d) 'The Measurement of Mood and Physiological Responses to Vibroacoustic Therapy in Non-Clinical Subjects.' In T. Wigram and C. Dileo (eds) *Music, Vibration and Health*. New Jersey: Jeffrey Books.

Wigram, T. (1997e) 'The Effect of Amplitude Modulation of the Pulsed Sinusoidal Low Frequency Tone as a Stimulus in Vibroacoustic Therapy.' In T. Wigram and C. Dileo (eds) *Music, Vibration and Health*. New Jersey: Jeffrey Books.

Wigram, T. (1997f) 'The Effect of Vibroacoustic Therapy in the Treatment of Rett Syndrome.' In T. Wigram and C. Dileo (eds) *Music, Vibration and Health*. New Jersey: Jeffrey Books.

Wigram, T. (1997g) 'Equipment for Vibroacoustic Therapy.' In T. Wigram and C. Dileo (eds) *Music, Vibration and Health*. New Jersey: Jeffrey Books.

Wigram, T. (1997h) 'Sound Sensations: The Physical Effect of Sound in the Treatment of Hyperarousal and Motor Disorders.' III Congress Nazionale de Musicoterapia: Metodologie, Ricerche Cliniche ed Interventi. Turin: Italy (awaiting publication).

Wigram, T. (1999a) 'Contact in Music: The Analysis of Musical Behaviour in Children with Communication Disorder and Pervasive Developmental Disability for Differential Diagnosis.' In T. Wigram and J. De Backer (eds) *Clinical Applications of Music Therapy in Developmental Disability, Paediatrics and Neurology*. London: Jessica Kingsley Publishers.

Wigram, T. (1999b) 'Music Therapy in Diagnostic Assessment: Analysis of Musical Material Using the IAP's for Assessing and Diagnosing Communication Disorder and Autism.' In D. Aldridge (ed) *Kairos V Beiträge zur Musiktherapie in Der Medizin*. Bern: Verlag Hans Huber.

Wigram, T. (1999c) 'Assessment Methods in Music Therapy: A Humanistic or Natural Science Framework?' *Nordic Journal of Music Therapy 8*, 1, 6–24.

Wigram, T. (1999d) 'Muziektherapie en Improvisatie: Therapeutisch improviseren op de piano.' (Clinically related piano improvisation.) *ADEM Driemaandelijks Tijdschrift voor muziekcultuur*. 99/4, 200–203.

Wigram, T. (1999e) 'Variability and Autonomy in Music Therapy Interaction: Evidence for Diagnosis and Therapeutic Intervention for Children with Autism and Asperger Syndrome.' In

R. Pratt and D. Erdonmez Grocke (eds) *MusicMedicine 3: MusicMedicine and Music Therapy: Expanding Horizons.* Melbourne: Faculty of Music, University of Melbourne.

Wigram, T. (1999f) 'La Scienza, l'arte e le aplicazioni cliniche della musicoterapia.' (The Art, Ccience and Clinical Application of Music Therapy.) *Journal of the Italian Confederation of Music Therapy (CONFIAM).* Musicoterapia: News: 2–4.

Wigram, T. (1999g) *Moments of Change: Structured and Free Improvisation in Group Music Therapy. Techniques, Frameworks and Transitions – Clinical Improvisation Skills.* World Congress of Music Therapy. Washington DC, 1999 (unpublished).

Wigram, T. (2000a) 'A Method of Music Therapy Assessment for the Diagnosis of Autistic and Communication Disordered Children.' *Music Therapy Perspectives 18,* 1, 13–22.

Wigram, T. (2000b) *Assessment and Evaluation in the Arts Therapies: Art Therapy, Music Therapy and Dramatherapy.* Radlett: Harper House Publications.

Wigram, T. (2000c) 'Music Therapy Education in Scandinavia.' *World Federation of Music Therapy Symposium on Training and Education in Music Therapy.* Washington DC: WFMT Publications.

Wigram, T. (2000d) 'Minimum Requirements for Qualifications of Heads of Training and Lecturers on Music Therapy Training Courses.' *World Federation of Music Therapy Symposium on Training and Education in Music Therapy.* Washington DC: WFMT Publications.

Wigram, T. (2000e) *Theory of Music Therapy: Lectures to Undergraduate and Post-graduate Students, University of Aalborg* (unpublished communication).

Wigram, T. (2001a) *Potentialer i Musikterapi med børn indenfor det Autistiske Spektrum.* Keynote Presentation to the 1st Danish Kongress of Musikterapi. Brandbjerg Højskle. Musikterapeuternes Landsklub: Storvede. Og Dansk Forbund for Musikterapi: Grindsted.

Wigram, T. (2001b) 'The Evidence from Clinical Practice: Music Therapy's Inspiration for the 21st Century.' In D. Aldridge, G. di Franco, E. Ruud and T. Wigram (eds) *Music Therapy in Europe.* Rome: Ismez.

Wigram, T. and Cass, H. (1995) 'Music Therapy Within the Assessment Process of a Therapy Clinic for People with Rett Syndrome.' 1995 BSMT Conference. London: BSMT Publications. In press.

Wigram, T. and De Backer, J. (eds) (1999a) *Clinical Applications of Music Therapy in Developmental Disability, Paediatrics and Neurology.* London: Jessica Kingsley Publishers.

Wigram, T. and De Backer, J. (1999b) *Clinical Applications of Music Therapy in Psychiatry.* London: Jessica Kingsley Publishers.

Wigram, T., De Backer, J. and Van Camp, J. (1999) 'Music Therapy Training: A Process to Develop the Musical and Therapeutic Identity of the Music Therapist.' In T. Wigram and J. De Backer (eds) *Clinical Applications of Music Therapy in Developmental Disability, Paediatrics and Neurology.* London: Jessica Kingsley Publishers.

Wigram, T. and Dileo, C. (1997) 'Clinical and Ethical Considerations.' In T. Wigram and C. Dileo (eds) *Music, Vibration and Health.* Pennsylvania: Jeffrey Books.

Wigram, T. and Dileo, C. (1997) *Music, Vibration and Health.* New Jersey: Jeffrey Books.

Wigram, T., McNaught, J. and Cain, J. (1997) 'Vibroacoustic Therapy with Adult Patients with Profound Learning Disability.' In T. Wigram and C. Dileo (eds) *Music, Vibration and Health.* New Jersey: Jeffrey Books.

Wigram, T., Saperston, B. and West, R. (1995) *The Art and Science of Music Therapy: A Handbook.* London, Toronto: Harwood Academic Publications.

Wigram, T., Saperston, B. and West, R. (2000) *Manuele di Arte e Scienza della Musicoterapia.* Roma: Ismez.

Wigram, T. and Weekes, L. (1985) 'A Specific Approach to Overcoming Motor Dysfunction in Children and Adolescents with Severe Physical and Mental Handicaps using Music and Movement.' *British Journal of Music Therapy 16*, 1, 2–12.

Wilber, K. (1986) *Transformations of Consciousness.* Boston, MA: Shambhala.

Wilber, K. (1998) *The Marriage of Sense and Soul.* Boston, MA: Shambhala.

Wilber, K. (2000a) *Integral Psychology.* Boston, MA: Shambhala.

Wilber, K. (2000b) *Collected Works Vol. III.* Boston, MA: Shambhala.

Wilber, K. (2000c) *Collected Works Vol. IV.* Boston, MA: Shambhala.

Wilber, K. (2000d) *Sex, Ecology, Spirituality. The Spirit of Evolution 2nd Edition.* Boston, MA: Shambhala.

Wilson, B.L. and Smith, D.S. (2000) 'Music Therapy Assessment in School Settings: A Preliminary Investigation.' *Journal of Music Therapy 37*, 2, 95–117.

Wilson, G.T. (1989) 'Behaviour Therapy.' In J.C. Corsini and D. Wedding (eds) *Current Psychotherapies.* Illinois: Peacock Publishers.

Wilson, M.D. *et al.* (eds) (1990) *Music and Child Development: The Biology of Music Making.* 1987 Conference Proceedings. Saint Louis: MMB Music.

Winn, T., Crowe, B. and Moreno, J. (1989) Shamanism and Music Therapy: Ancient Healing Techniques in Modern practice.' *Music Therapy Perspectives 3*, 2, 67–71.

Winnicott, D.W. (1971) *Playing and Reality.* New York: Basic Books.

Woodward, S. (2000) 'A Response to James Robertson's "An Educational Model for Music Therapy: the Case for a Continuum".' *British Journal of Music Therapy 14*, 2, 94–98.

World Federation of Music Therapy (1996) 'Definition of Music Therapy.' *www.musictherapyworld.de.*

World Health Organization (1992) *International Statistical Classification of Diseases and Related Health Problems* (tenth edition.)Geneva.

Wrangsjö, B. (1994) 'När själven möts uppstår musik – Daniel Sterns självteori.' *Nordic Journal of Music Therapy 3*, 2, 79–83.

Wrangsjö, B. and Körlin, D. (1995) 'Guided Imagery and Music (GIM) as a Psychotherapeutic Method in Psychiatry.' *Journal of the Association for Music & Imagery 4*, 79–92.

Wulff, H.A., Petersen, S.A. and Rosenberg, R. (1990) *Medicinsk filosofi.* Kbh.: Munksgaard.

Wylie, M. and Blom, R. (1986) 'Guided Imagery and Music with Hospice Patients.' *Music Therapy Perspectives 3*, 25–28.

Zelazny, C.M. (2001) 'Therapeutic Instrumental Music Playing in Hand Rehabilitation for Older Adults with Osteoarthritis: Four Case Studies.' *Journal of Music Therapy 38*, 2, 97–113.

Contents of accompanying CD
(all durations are approximate)

18 (1:25) Case: Joel, ex. 12, see page 256

19 (0:50) Case: Joel, ex. 13, see page 256

Ex. 20-21 Music therapy in social work (music therapist: Ole Agger)

20 Ludwig (Text/Music: Steffen Lyckegaard, 4:13) From the CD Sange fra hjertet

21 Jeg vil ud (Text/Music: Nete Leth Rasmussen & Lars Sletten Thomsen, 4:52)

From the CD Sange fra hjertet (Songs from the heart), see pages 203–4

22-25 Selected classical music for Guided Imagery and Music

22 J. Pachelbel: Canon in D (5:04) Performed by Orchestre de Chamber, conducted by Jean-Francois Paillard – from RCA Victor 09026 654682. see page 106

23 J.S. Bach/L. Stokowskij: Passacaglia and Fugue in C minor (14:57) Performed by Leopold Stokowski – From RCA Victor LRM 7033, see page 107

24 J.S. Bach: Air (from Orchestral Suite No. 3) (6:00), Performed by Orchestre de Chamber, conducted by Jean-Francois Paillard – from RCA Victor 09026 654682. see page 108

25 Intuitive music (3:21) Con Fuoco: Vand (Water) (concert excerpt), see page 273

Copyright:

1-10: Inge Nygaard Pedersen.

11-19: Tony Wigram

20-21: The authors and composers mentioned above. The CD (UCCD 1001) is released by Ungdomscentret I

22 Orchestre de Chambre Jean-Fancois Paillard/Paillard (RCA Victor: 09026654682)

23 Orchestra/Leopold Stokowski (RCA Victor: LRM-7033)

24 BBC Chorus/New Philharmonia Orchestra/Otto Klemperer (EMI: 7633642)

24 Orchestre de Chambre Jean-Fancois Paillard/Paillard (RCA Victor: 09026654682)

25 Con Fuoco (six music therapy students from AAU, live recording 1.4.2000)

Mini Biographies of the Authors

Professor Tony Wigram PhD, LGSM (MT), SRAsT(M), RMT

Professor of Music Therapy and Head of PhD Studies in Music Therapy in the Institute for Music and Music Therapy, Department of Humanities, University of Aalborg, Denmark. He is Head Music Therapist at the Harper House Children's Service, Hertfordshire, England, and Research Advisor to the Horizon NHS Trust. He is Past President of the European Music Therapy Committee and Past President of the World Federation of Music Therapy.

He read Music at Bristol University, undertook post-graduate study in Music Therapy at the Guildhall School of Music under Juliette Alvin, and took a qualifying degree in Psychology at Royal Holloway and Bedford New College, London University. He took his Doctorate in Psychology at St. George's Medical School, London University.

He is a Visiting Lecturer in Music Therapy, Child Assessment, Learning Disability and Vibroacoustic Therapy in universities and music therapy programs in England, Australia and Belgium, and an Adjunct Professor in Music Therapy at CRM, Naples, Italy, and the Escuela de Musicoterapia, University of the Basque Country, Vitoria-Gasteiz, Spain. He is a Research Fellow in the Faculty of Music, Melbourne University.

He is a former Chairman of the Association of Professional Music Therapists, and of the British Society for music therapy, and a Churchill Fellow of 1985. He has edited seven books on Music Therapy, and authored many articles. His research interests include the physiological effect of sound and music, assessment and diagnosis of autism and communication disorder, Rett syndrome, methods of training and advanced level training in music therapy, and thematic improvisation.

Main Publications: 1991–2001

Wigram, T. (1991) 'Music Therapy for a Girl with Rett's Syndrome: Balancing Structure and Freedom.' In K. Bruscia (ed) *Case Studies in Music Therapy*. Phoenixville: Barcelona Publishers.

Heal, M. and Wigram, T. (1993) *Music Therapy in Health and Education*. London: Jessica Kingsley Publishers.

Wigram, T., Saperston, B. and West, R. (1995) *The Art and Science of Music Therapy: A Handbook*. London, Toronto: Harwood Academic Publications.

Wigram, T. (1995) 'Psychological and Physiological Effects of Low Frequency Sound and Music.' *Music Therapy Perspectives – International Edition*. USA: NAMT Publications.

Wigram, T. (1995) 'Musicoterapia: Estructura y Flexibilidad en el proceso de Musicoterapia.' In P. Del Campo (ed) *La Musica como proceso humano*. Salamanca, Spain: Amaru Ediciones. (Music Therapy: Structure and Flexibility in the Music Therapy Process. In P. Del Campo (ed) *Music and The Human Process*. Salamanca: Amarú Ediciones.

Wigram, T. (1996) '"Becoming Clients": Role Playing Clients as a Technique in the Training of Advanced Level Music Therapy Students.' Paper to the 3rd European Music Therapy Conference, Aalborg, Denmark. In L.O. Bonde and I.N. Pedersen. *Music Therapy Within Multi-Disciplinary Teams*. Aalborg: Aalborg University Press.

Wigram, T. (1996) *The Effect of Vibroacoustic Therapy on Clinical and Non-Clinical Populations*. PhD. Psychology research thesis. St George's Medical School. University of London.

Wigram, T. and Dileo, C. (1997) *Music, Vibration and Health*. Pipersville, Pennsylvania: Jeffrey Books.

Wigram, T. and De Backer, J. (1999) *Clinical Applications of Music Therapy in Developmental Disability, Paediatrics and Neurology*. London: Jessica Kingsley Publishers.

Wigram, T. and De Backer, J. (1999) *Clinical Applications of Music Therapy in Psychiatry*. London: Jessica Kingsley Publishers.

Wigram, T. (1999) 'Assessment Methods in Music Therapy: A Humanistic or Natural Science Framework?' *Nordisk Tidsskrift for Musikterapi*, 8, 1, 6–24.

Wigram, T. (2000) 'A Method of Music Therapy Assessment for the Diagnosis of Autistic and Communication Disordered Children.' *Music Therapy Perspectives 18*, 1.

Wigram, T. (ed) (2000) *Assessment and Evaluation in the Arts Therapies: Art Therapy, Music Therapy and Dramatherapy*. Radlett: Harper House Publications.

Bonde, L., Nygaard Pedersen, I. and Wigram, T. (2001) Musikterapi: *Når Ord ikke Slår Til: En handbøg i Musikterapiens teori og praksis i Danmark*. (Music Therapy: When Words are Not Enough. A Handbook of Music Therapy Theory and Practice in Denmark.) KLIM: Århus.

Aldridge, D., Di Franco, G., Ruud, E. and Wigram, T. (2001) *Music Therapy in Europe*. Rome: Ismez.

Associate Professor Inge Nygaard Pedersen

Inge Nygaard Pedersen was employed at Aalborg University in 1981 for the task of building up an MA program in music therapy. She became Associate Professor in 1986. With only few interruptions she functioned as the head of the program from 1982 to 1995. Since 1995 she has functioned as Head of the Music Therapy Clinic – a centre of treatment and research which is a joint institution between the University of Aalborg and Aalborg Psychiatric Hospital. From 1993 to 1996 she was a co-ordinator of the Nordic Research Network (NorFA) and since 1997 she has been active in the Research Unit for Psychiatric Research in the county of North Jutland. She is a regular visiting teacher in Germany, Sweden and Norway and, since 1988, a permanent visiting teacher on the Institute of Art and Psychology (Art therapy) in Denmark. She has a MA degree in Music Science from Copenhagen University (1981) and became a Diplomad Music Therapist from the 'Mentor Education', Herdecke, Germany, in the same year. Additionally she is an examined relaxation teacher (1976) and a GIM therapist (2002). She has edited and been co-editor of five books and has written a number of articles in national and international journals on issues such as: music therapy education, music therapy in Denmark, autism, music therapy in psychiatry, the therapist's way of being present, listening attitudes, and teaching methodology in music therapy training programs at an advanced level.

Selected publications

Pedersen, I.N. and Scheiby, B.B. (1981) *Musikterapeut-Musik-Klient.* Aalborg Universitetsforlag. (med Lydbånd).

Pedersen, I.N. (1987) *Musikterapi-en uddannelse under udvikling. Et nyt skud på stammen af universitetspædagogiske traditioner.* Upubl rapport. Inst. for Musik og Musikterapi. Aalborg Universitet.

Pedersen, I.N. (1991) 'Væren, bevægelse og samværsidentitet i fritonal improvisation.' I konferencerapport: *Levanda musik,* Nordisk Musikkterapikonference 1991. Høgskuleutdanninga på Sandane.

Pedersen, I.N. (1992) 'Musikterapi med autistiske klientmålgrupper.' *Nordisk Tidsskrift for Musikkterapi 1,* 1.

Pedersen, I.N. and Mahns, W. (1996) *Nordic Network in Music Therapy Research 1993–1996.* Aalborg University.

Pedersen, I.N. (1997) 'The Music Therapist's Listening Perspectives as Source of Information in Improvised Musical Duets with Grown-up, Psychiatric Patients, Suffering from Schizophrenia.' *Nordic Journal of Music Therapy 6,* 2, 98–111.

Pedersen, I.N. (ed) (1998) *Indføring i musikterapi som en selvstændig behandlingsform. Musikterapi i psykiatrien. Årsskrift 1998.* Aalborg Psykiatriske Sygehus – Aalborg Universitet.

Pedersen, I.N., Frederiksen, B. and Lindvang, C. (1998) 'Musikterapiens indplacering i Danmark. I: *Musikterapi i psykiatrien. Årsskrift 1998.* (s. 21–45).

Pedersen, I.N. (1999) 'Music Therapy as Holding and Re-organising Work with Schizophrenic and Psychotic Patients.' In T. Wigram and J. De Backer (eds) *Clinical Applications of Music Therapy in Psychiatry.* London: Jessica Kingsley Publishers.

Pedersen, I.N. (2000) 'Inde-fra eller ude-fra – orientering i terapeutens tilstedeværelse og nærvær.' In *Musikterapi i psykiatrien. Årsskrift 2000.* Aalborg Psykiatriske Sygehus. Aalborg Universitet. (s. 81–103).

Pedersen, I.N. (2002) 'Analytical Music Therapy (AMT) with Adults in Mental Health and Counselling Work.' In M.J. Eschen (ed) *Analytical Music Therapy.* London: Jessica Kingsley Publishers.

Pedersen, I.N. (1996, 2002) 'Psychodynamic Movement – A Basic Training Methodology for Music Therapists.' *Analytical Music Therapy.* Eschen, J. (ed) London: Jessica Kingsley Publishers.

Pedersen, I.N. (1993, 2002) 'Self Experience for Music Therapy Students. Experiential Training in Music Therapy as a Methodology – A Compulsory Part of the Music Therapy Programme at Aalborg University.' *Analytical Music Therapy.* Eschen, J. (ed) London: Jessica Kingsley Publishers.

Associate Professor Lars Ole Bonde

Lars Ole Bonde is Associate Professor at the Music Therapy Program, Aalborg University. MA in Musicology and Nordic Literature, AU 1979. Music therapist (GIM, FAMI) 1999. Upper-secondary school teacher 1979–1981. Associate Professor in Musicology, Aalborg University 1981–1987. Music producer in the Danish Broadcasting Corporation 1987–1993. Concert producer and artistic opera director 1993–1995. Associate Professor in Music Therapy from 1995. Head of PhD Studies 1995–1997, Head of Studies since 1997. Teaching areas: music education, music psychology, music history, theory of science, music therapy theory. PhD supervision and courses in advanced literature searching. GIM courses and workshops in Denmark, Norway and Finland. Papers at national and international conferences. Danish editor of *Nordic Journal of Music Therapy*. Member of the arr. Committee, 3rd European Music Therapy Conference, Aalborg 1995, and 4th European GIM Conference, Elba 2000. Member of ESCOM. Board member, The Danish GIM Society. Chairman of the Board, Aarhus Summer Opera and GAIA Vocal Ensemble. Has published a number of books and articles within music history, opera, music education and music therapy.

Selected publications (within music education and music therapy)

Jespersen, H.T. *et al.* (1987) *Man skal høre meget. Musikaliteten i fokus. En bog om lærere og undervisning.* Kbh.: Chr. Ejlers Forlag.

Bonde, L.O. (1992) 'Sol- og måneskinshistorier – musikterapi i 90-årenes Europa.' *Nordisk tidsskrift for musikkterapi 2,*1, 33–37.

Bonde, L.O. (1993) *Musikterapilitteratur. Lille bibliografi og Vejledning i litteratursøgning.* AUC Institut 10.

Bonde, L.O. (1994) 'Oplysning – Oplevelse – Oplivelse. Fællesoppgaver i undervisning og terapi.' *Nordisk Tidsskrift for Musikk og Musikkterapi 4,* 1, 13–18.

Bonde, L.O. (1996) 'Sound and Psyche. Impressions from the 8th World Congress of Music Therapy in Hamburg, July 14th–20th 1996.' *Nordic Journal of Music Therapy 5,* 2, 122–127.

Bonde, L.O. and Pedersen, I.N. (eds) (1996) *Music Therapy Within Multi-Disciplinary Teams.* Proceedings of the 3rd European Music Therapy Conference, Aalborg, June 1995. Aalborg University Press.

Bonde, L.O. (1997) 'Music Analysis and Image Potentials in Classical Music.' *Nordic Journal of Music Therapy 6,* 2. Also available from www.hisf.no/njmt.

Bonde, L.O. (1998) 'Musikterapiforskning ved Aalborg Universitet.' *Dansk Årbog for Musikforskning XXIV,* 79–80.

Bonde, L.O. (1999) 'Metaphor and Metaphoric Imagery in Music Therapy Theory: A Discussion of a Basic Theoretical Problem – With Clinical Material from GIM Sessions.' 9th World Congress of Music Therapy, Washington DC, November 17–22, 1999. D. Aldridge (ed) CD-ROM *Music Therapy Info Vol. III.*

Bonde, L.O. (1999) 'Music Therapy, The Internet and Other Electronic Resources – An Update.' *Nordic Journal of Music Therapy 8,* 1, 100–104.

Bonde, L.O. (ed) (1999) *Nordic Journal of Music Therapy*. 8(1) Special Issue: Music Therapy in Aalborg University. Nordic Journal of Music Therapy. Sandane.

Bonde, L.O. (2000) 'Metaphor and Narrative in Guided Imagery and Music.' *Journal of the Association for Music and Imagery 7*, 59–76.

Bonde, L.O. (2000) 'Mozart-Effekten – et notat.' *Musik & Terapi 27*, 1, 25–29.

Bonde, L.O. (2001) 'Steps Towards a Meta-Theory of Music Therapy? An Introduction to Ken Wilber's Integral Psychology and a Discussion of its Relevance to Music Therapy.' *Nordic Journal of Music Therapy 10*, 2, 176–187.

Subject index

Author index